CONTACT LENSES:
Procedures and Techniques

Gerald E. Lowther, O.D., Ph.D.
Professor, Ferris State College
College of Optometry
Big Rapids, Michigan

BUTTERWORTHS
Boston • London
Sydney • Wellington • Durban • Toronto

*Every effort has been made to ensure that the drug dosage
schedules within this text are accurate and conform to standards accepted at time of publication. However, as treatment
recommendations vary in light of continuing research and clinical experience, the reader is advised to verify drug dosage
schedules herein with information found on product information sheets. This is especially true in cases of new or infrequently
used drugs.*

Library of Congress Cataloging in Publication Data

Lowther, Gerald Eugene.
  Contact lenses.

  Includes index.
    1. Contact lenses. 2. Optometric assistants.
  I. Title. [DNLM: 1. Contact lenses. 2. Physicians' assis-
  tants. WW 355 L922c]
  RE977.C6L68 617.7'523 81–18101
  ISBN 0–409–95012–2   AACR2

Butterworth Publishers Inc.
80 Montvale Avenue
Stoneham, MA 02180

10 9 8 7 6 5 4 3 2

Printed in the United States of America

CONTENTS

LIST OF TABLES

PREFACE

The assistant or technician in the contact lens practice can be invaluable in providing good, efficient, professional service. The more education obtained, the better the service that can be provided and the more enjoyable and challenging the tasks become. This book is intended to provide the basic background in the field of contact lenses to enable an individual to become a clinically proficient assistant or technician in a contact lens practice.

Basic concepts from the most elementary terms and procedures to the more complex ones are covered. For experienced technicians, some chapters may be read quickly, or only chapters of particular interest need be consulted. The chapters have been written to cover definitive areas so that anyone desiring to study one given topic can go directly to the appropriate chapter. For an individual not familiar with contact lens terminology, Chapter 2 should be studied before other technical chapters are attempted.

Tradenames and specific company products are, for the most part, avoided throughout the text since there are so many companies around the world providing contact lenses and related products. Only those concepts that will remain constant and give a proper background to deal with companies and laboratory representatives are provided.

This book is not intended to teach all the theory and detail required to provide total patient care. If this is desired, one should consult *Contact Lens Correction* by Norman Bier and Gerald Lowther as this is the companion text for the licensed practitioner.

Without the encouragement and help of many people this book would not have been possible. I would like to thank Norman Bier for his encouragement and use of photographs and sections from *Contact Lens Correction*. Thanks also to Fred Nista, George Milkie, Clifford Brooks, and Rita Pierce for the many hours reading the manuscript and making suggestions and corrections. Also to Betty Dever for doing much of the typing of the manuscript. I am grateful to Dean Jack Bennett and the faculty, staff, and students of the Ferris State College, College of Optometry, for their encouragement. I am particularly indebted to my wife and family for their encouragement and for tolerating the many hours I was away from family endeavors.

Gerald E. Lowther, O.D., Ph.D.

1

HISTORICAL DEVELOPMENT OF CONTACT LENSES

EARLY DEVELOPMENT

Correcting refractive errors by placing a lens on the eye was described many years before a practical method to accomplish this feat was developed. As with any complex technology, many steps occurred in the development of materials, manufacturing, fitting techniques, and solutions. Hundreds of individuals have been involved in these developments. It is not possible to acknowledge all of these people and each step in the process. Only the major contributions will be covered to give an overall concept of the development and time periods involved. Other sources are available for more detailed histories (1, 2, 3). (See Table 1–1 for a summary of the historical development of contact lenses.)

The earliest reference to contact lenses was by Leonardo da Vinci in 1508. He described using glass contact lenses to neutralize (eliminate the refractive power) the cornea. da Vinci developed the concept that the front of the contact lens replaces the optical power of the cornea (4, 5).

For more than a hundred years there cannot be found any further reference to the development of contact lenses. Then, in 1636, René Descartes, the French mathematician and philosopher, described a tube of water placed on the eye neutralizing the human cornea and using the exposed end of the tube as the new optical surface (6, 7). The next development occurred in 1801 when Thomas Young used the principle de-

Table 1-1. Summary of historical development of contact lenses.

Year	Individual(s)	Development
1508	Leonardo da Vinci	Described glass contact lens
1636	René Descartes	Tube of water used to neutralize the cornea
1801	Thomas Young	Used Descartes principle to study the eye
1827	John Herschel	Described how a contact lens could be ground; concept of molding the eye
1887	F. E. Muller	Fitted a glass blown lens for a patient to protect the eye
1888	A. E. Fick	Described first glass lens to be worn to correct vision
1888	E. Kalt	Designed and fitted glass corneal lenses. Used ophthalmometer to fit lenses
1936	W. Feinbloom	Made lens with glass central optic and plastic surround (first plastic used in contact lens)
1938	Mullen and Obrig	First all-plastic (PMMA) contact lens
1947	N. Bier	Fenestrated minimum-clearance haptic lens
1947	K. Touhy	All-plastic corneal lens
1950	Butterfield	Designed corneal lens to parallel the cornea. Used peripheral curves
1960	Wichterle and Lim	Hydrogel polymers for contact lenses
1968		U.S. FDA became involved in regulating contact lenses
1971	Bausch and Lomb, Inc.	First hydrogel lens approved in United States
1970s	J. DeCarle	Extended wear with high water content hydrogel lenses
1970s	Rynco Scientific	Use of CAB polymer for contact lenses
1970s		First clinical marketing of soft silicone lenses
1978	Danker Laboratories	U.S. FDA approval of CAB lenses.
1979	Syntex Ophthalmics	U.S. FDA approval of a PMMA-silicone copolymer lens

scribed by Descartes to neutralize the cornea to study the principles of accommodation, astigmatism, and refraction.

In 1827, John Herschel, an English astronomer, described how a glass contact lens could be ground to match the shape of the cornea to neutralize its power (8). He also described how a transparent animal jelly could be placed between the cornea and the lens surface. In addition, Herschel suggested that a lens might be designed if a mold of the eye were made.

In 1887, F. E. Muller of Germany, a maker of artificial glass eyes, made a glass blown lens with a clear optical portion for a patient whose lids had been surgically removed. The lens protected the eye and kept it moist. This patient was reportedly able to wear the lens for the remaining 20 years of his life.

In 1888, two investigators working independently furthered the development of contact lenses. A. Eugen Fick (Switzerland), in his paper entitled "A Contact Spectacle," described the first glass contact lens to be worn to correct vision (9). He experimented with both small glass lenses that rested only on the cornea and larger lenses that covered the cornea but rested on the sclera (called haptic or scleral lenses). He found the larger scleral lenses to be better supported and more comfortable. The lenses, fabricated by Zeiss Optical Works of Germany, were at first blown; later they were ground and polished. Patients were required to use solutions to fill the space between the lens and the eye. Fick designed the lenses based on molds taken of animal and cadaver eyes.

E. Kalt (Germany), contemporaneously with Fick, designed and fitted glass corneal contact lenses. The fitting of these lenses was based on measurements of the corneal curvature using a ophthalmometer. The patient's tears were used as the fluid between the lens and the eye, not auxiliary solutions. The lenses in use at this time were not of the quality or comfort known today. They were primarily used on patients with keratoconus and other distorted corneal conditions where spectacles would not give adequate vision.

From the early 1890s until the 1930s only some minor advances were made in the design and fabrication of contact lenses, mainly by the scientists at Carl Zeiss Optical Works.

PLASTIC SCLERAL LENSES

In 1936, a United States optometric pioneer in the contact lens field, William Feinbloom, utilized a new synthetic plastic in the fabrication of contact lenses. Plastic offered greater latitude in fabrication and fitting, as it could be ground, polished, and molded easily. Feinbloom manufactured a scleral (haptic) lens. A scleral lens is relatively large and covers a portion of the sclera as well as the whole cornea. The central optical portion of this scleral lens was glass and the surrounding portion a white translucent acrylic plastic—thus, the beginning of the use of plastic lenses. At about this same time, a clear transparent polymethylmethacrylate

(PMMA) plastic was introduced by Rohm and Haas Co. (USA) for use in aircraft canopies. This plastic was also suited for contact lenses because of its light weight and ease of fabrication.

Muller and Obrig (U.S.A.), in 1938, constructed the first all-plastic scleral contact lenses (10). They used the method of taking eye impressions developed by Dallos first to make a cast of the individual's eye. Then, heated, softened plastic was molded over the cast to obtain a lens that would fit the eye. Scleral lenses were also formed by lathe cutting.

During the 1940s, plastic scleral contact lenses were fitted with a relatively large fluid-filled space between the lens and the cornea. These were commonly called vaulted or fluid scleral lenses. One of the significant problems with this type of lens was that corneal swelling (edema), which causes blurred vision and discomfort, occurred after a few hours' wear, thus limiting wearing time. Much experimentation took place utilizing different fluids under the lens to obtain increased wearing time, but with no success. It was later discovered the edema was the result of lack of oxygen supply to the cornea.

In 1947, Norman Bier (12) (England) revolutionized the fitting of scleral contact lenses with his discovery of the need to have a good fluid exchange under the lens. He accomplished this by using a design with very little tear fluid between the lens and the eye. This is referred to as a minimum-clearance corneal fit. Tears under the lens were exchanged on blinking to supply the eye with oxygen to prevent edema. To facilitate this, apertures or fenestrations (small holes drilled through the contact lens at the periphery of the corneal section) were used. This increased wearing time and comfort of the lenses.

CORNEAL LENSES

The next significant contribution to the contact lens field occurred in 1947. Kevin Touchy (USA) developed and manufactured the first all-plastic corneal contact lens. This lens was much smaller than the scleral lens and rested on the cornea. It closely resembled the contact lenses presently utilized; although numerous changes in design have occurred. Over the next several years considerable controversy developed over whether the fluidless scleral or the corneal lens should be used. In the long run, the corneal lens won out, but even so, today there are still indications for the use of scleral lenses.

Touhy developed a relatively large lens. It was fitted so the lens back radius was longer than the corneal radius, that is, fitted flatter than the cornea (see Chapter 6). Butterfield (USA), in 1950, designed a lens to be fitted to parallel the curvature of the cornea with longer radius peripheral curves on the back surface of the lens near the edge to give more edge clearance. This advancement, along with the design of much smaller lenses, such as the microcorneal contact lenses by Sohnges (Germany), increased the comfort and wearability of corneal lenses. Sohnges, Moss (USA), and Bier further refined fitting of the smaller corneal lens with the contour fitting technique. The idea was to fit a lens that conformed to the eye as closely as possible over the central corneal area with slight edge stand-off. This would allow tear exchange with blinking, preventing corneal edema and increasing wearing time.

Hundreds of practitioners, researchers, and manufacturers have contributed to the advancement of corneal contact lens development over the years. Some of these contributions include the use of fluorescein, the use of the biomicroscope, methods of inspecting lenses, manufacturing of thin lenses, aspheric lenses, toric lenses, bifocal lenses, fitting techniques, and physiological considerations.

HYDROGEL LENSES

During the 1950s and 1960s, these various refinements in lenses made of PMMA were occurring. The next major change in the contact lens field was the introduction of hydrogel contact lenses. In the late 1950s, Otto Wichterle of Czechoslovakia experimented with hydrogel polymers for various medical uses. These plastics differ considerably from the PMMA plastic in that the hydrogels absorb relatively large quantities of water (30 to 85 percent by weight) and become soft and flexible. PMMA lenses only absorb about 1.5 percent water and remain rigid. Hydrogel materials can dehydrate, becoming hard and brittle, but can then be rehydrated, returning to a soft and pliable form. In 1960, Wichterle and Lim (Czechoslovakia) published an article (13) on the hydrophilic gels. In the same year, these chemists, along with an ophthalmologist, Dreifus (Czechoslovakia), described the use of these materials for contact lenses (14). The plastics in these early lenses were not as refined as those of today. They were quite thick and not well designed, but a new era in contact lenses was initiated.

The first 6 to 8 years of the use of hydrogel lenses were disappointing. Even though they were usually quite comfortable, obtaining satisfactory vision was often a problem. Because of their soft nature, the lenses often lost their original shape and distorted vision. As with any new development, refinements followed. With better chemistry, manufacturing, and lens design, vision and wearability improved. Hydrogel lenses are usually made as large as the cornea or larger so they will be comfortable and stay centered on the eye. Thus, they are considerably larger than the standard rigid corneal contact lens but not as large as the scleral lens.

From 1961 to 1964, there was only limited use or experimentation with the hydrogel lenses. In 1964, the National Patient Development Corporation (USA) acquired the rights to the hydrogel material (15), as developed in Czechoslovakia, for use in the Western Hemisphere. The chemical name of the material is hydroxyethylmethacrylate, usually referred to as HEMA. The National Patent Development Corporation did some initial development of the HEMA lenses, but in 1966 granted exclusive sublicense to Bausch and Lomb, Inc., to manufacture and sell HEMA lenses in the United States.

Bausch and Lomb further developed the manufacturing of the soft lenses and worked with ophthalmic practitioners to determine their clinical effectiveness. In December 1968, another development occurred that would make a major change in the contact lens field in the United States. The U.S. Food and Drug Administration (FDA) declared that soft contact lenses were a drug. This required extensive testing of the lenses and FDA approval before being marketed. These procedures are to assure that a relatively safe and effective product is provided to the practitioner and patient. Unfortunately, the testing and approval process is very expensive and time-consuming. Prior to 1968, there was no significant federal regulation of the contact lens field.

Finally, in March 1971, the Soflens® HEMA lens developed by Bausch and Lomb was approved. In the meantime, considerable clinical experience was gained by companies and practitioners outside the United States, where there were no regulatory restraints on manufacturing and fitting. Therefore, many of the clinical advances in the field were occurring in other countries of the world. In 1974, another soft contact lens for correction of refractive errors was approved, and by 1976, numerous soft lens manufacturers were applying for approval by the FDA (16). The chemical composition of these lenses varies slightly as does the amount of water they absorb and their design.

As clinical experience grew with hydrogel lenses, several problems were encountered. These included physiological changes in the cornea, most notably corneal edema. Soft lenses did not always allow enough oxygen to reach the cornea. To increase oxygen transmission, some companies manufactured very thin hydrogel lenses, often referred to as ultrathin. They are 0.04 to 0.08 mm thick (standard thickness lenses are 0.10 mm and thicker). Another method to increase oxygen transmission is to increase the water content; consequently, high water content lenses came into use.

Another problem was the development of deposits on the lens surface. These deposits or coatings developed in a few months, causing some patients to experience decreased visual acuity, comfort, lens positioning, and physiological acceptance of the lens. Different cleaning methods, including surfactant and enzyme cleaners, were developed in the 1970s to decrease the problem of lens deposits. Other polymer types and polymer modifications have also been experimented with to eliminate the coating problem, yet it still persists.

Spherical hydrogel lenses will not correct asigmatism as rigid lenses usually will. Thus, for the first years of hydrogel lens use patients with significant astigmatism could not be corrected. The development of toric hydrogel lenses to correct astigmatism occurred during the 1970s, particularly in Europe and Australia. By the late 1970s, several toric hydrogel lenses were available in the United States. There are design and fitting problems with these lenses that limit their use. Bifocal hydrogel lenses are a recent development.

The extended wear of contact lenses, wearing the lenses for days, weeks or months at a time without removal, also received a great deal of attention and experimentation during the 1970s. John DeCarle of England was the leader in this field with his high water content Permalens®. The use of extended wear increased with the development of other high water content lenses and high oxygen permeable materials such as silicone. Physiological requirements for extended wear are very demanding since very little oxygen is available with the eye closed during sleep.

Waste products of metabolism can build up in the cornea and trauma from lens wear has no recovery opportunity. Thus, there can be numerous problems with extended wear that limit the number of individuals who can wear the lenses. Severe complications can arise if strict precautions are not followed. There has been some controversy within the ophthalmic professions and among scientists about the advisability of extended wear. For patients requiring contact lens correction but not having the dexterity for placement and removal of the lenses, extended wear can be a solution to their problem. Many thousands of people around the world are wearing lenses on an extended schedule. Further research and development are occurring in this field, and many advances are expected in the future.

NEWER RIGID LENS MATERIALS

Along with the development of hydrogel lenses, experimentation and development have continued on rigid lens plastics and flexible materials that do not absorb water. Even though hydrogel lenses were a great advancement, they did not solve all the clinical problems and did not present the best correction for all patients. Rigid lenses often give better vision and do not require as frequent replacement.

The main problem with the standard rigid PMMA lens was persistent corneal edema from insufficient oxygen supply to the cornea. The developers of new polymers had as their main goal the increase of oxygen supply through the lens material to the cornea. One of the first innovations was the use of cellulose acetate butyrate (CAB) polymer for contact lenses. Rynco Scientific Corporation (USA) began the initial development of this material in the early 1970s, as did other companies throughout the world. The first CAB lenses were approved by the FDA in the United States in 1978. They were manufactured by Danker Laboratories. Other companies later also had CAB lenses approved. This material allows a small amount of oxygen diffusion, which is helpful in preventing corneal edema. The plastic, however, is not as stable as PMMA; therefore, the lenses often flatten or warp slightly when soaked in solution or worn on the eye. To minimize this problem, CAB lenses are often made thicker than lenses of other materials. This increased thickness can introduce other fitting problems and discomfort.

Silicone, a polymer with extremely high oxygen permeability, has been utilized in combination with PMMA to increase the oxygen transmission. The first lens of this type was developed by Syntex Ophthalmics, Inc. (Polycon® lens). It was approved by the FDA in 1979. Other companies have developed similar combinations. The oxygen permeability of this material is in the same range as the CAB lenses but is a more stable material and can be made much thinner. This increases the comfort and oxygen transmission.

Another new rigid contact lens material is a pure silicone lens developed by Dow Corning, Inc. (USA). Because of its composition more oxygen is transmitted than with other rigid lenses. Since silicone is very hydrophobic (does not absorb or hold water on the surface), the surfaces of these lenses must be treated so the tear film can form over the lens to make it comfortable.

SOFT SILICONE LENSES

The soft silicone contact lens is a lens with the highest oxygen permeability of all the materials available. Work began in the early 1960s on lenses of this material, with patents granted in 1963 in England and 1966 in the United States. Silicone only became a viable clinical entity, however, in the late 1970s, with the marketing of silicone lenses in Germany and Japan. One of the main problems with soft silicone material is its hydrophobic (water-repelling) nature. Surface treating techniques had to be developed to overcome this problem. In addition, fabrication is more difficult than with other lens materials because the lenses must be formed in molds under heat and pressure. Fitting can be more difficult because of the material's high elasticity. Further development of this material is expected to result in greater clinical use for both daily and extended wear.

REFERENCES

1. Graham R. The evolution of corneal contact lenses. Am J Optom 1959; 36:55–72.
2. Silbert M. Optometric contributions to the development of contact lenses I–XVIII. Optical journal and review of optometry April 1, 1965 (Vol. 102, No. 7), through March 1, 1966 (Vol. 103, No. 5).
3. Mandell RB. Contact lens practice hard and flexible. 2nd ed. Springfield, Ill.: Thomas, 1974.
4. da Vinci L. Codex of the eye. Manuscript D (circa 1508).
5. Hofsetter HW. Graham R. Leonardo and contact lenses. Am. J. Optom. 1953; 30:41–44.
6. Descartes R. Methods of correcting vision in Discourse de la methode. 1636, Discourse 7, La dioptrique, p. 147.
7. Enoch JM. Descartes contact lens. Am J Optom 1956; 33:77–85.
8. Young T. On the mechanisms of the eye. Philos Trans R Soc Lond 1801; 91:23–88; reprinted in Surv Ophththalmol 1961; 6:383–91.
9. Fick AE. Eine contactbrille. Arch f Angenheilk 1888; 18:279–89; trans in Arch Ophththalmol 1888; 17:215–26.
10. Obrig T. Salvatoric P. Contact lenses. 3rd ed. New York: Obrig Laboratories, 1957.
11. Dallos J. Uber haftglaser u kontaktschalen. Klin Monatsbl Angenheilkd 1933; 91:640; English trans in Arch Ophththalmol 1936; 15:617–23.
12. Bier N. The tolerance factor and Sattler's veil as influenced by a new development of contact lens making. Am J Optom December 1947.
13. Wichterle O. Lim D. Hydrophilic gels for biological uses. Nature (Lond) 1960; 183:117.
14. Dreifus M. Wichterle O. Lim D. Intracasmeral lenses of hydrocolloid acrylates. Cesk Oftalmol 1960; 16:154–59.
15. Soft contact lens. Hearings before the Subcommittee on Government Regulation of the Select Committee on Small Business, United States Senate, Ninety-second Congress, July 6 and 7, 1972.
16. Bailey NJ. Contact lens update. Contact Lens Forum 1979; 4:25–32.

2
CONTACT LENS TERMINOLOGY AND TYPES

In order to communicate with contact lens practitioners, laboratories, and patients, it is necessary to have an understanding of contact lens terminology, which can be confusing since several different contact lens terms have been used to designate the same lens dimension or condition. To confuse the field further, some manufacturers have coined their own trade names for lens designs and parameters. Once lens design is understood and the common terms become familiar, however, it is easy to determine the meaning of unfamiliar terms used by different individuals and manufacturers.

Before discussing lens terminology, it is important that some basic ophthalmic concepts and terms be understood. When light from a distant object enters the eye, refraction (deflection or bending of the light) occurs. If the image of this light is refracted (bent) and focused directly on the retina, the condition is called emmetropia. An emmetrope, generally speaking, does not need glasses. If the light from a distant object does not fall on the retina, the condition is called ametropia. An ametrope, generally speaking, requires glasses or contact lenses. There are three types of refractive ametropia: myopia, hyperopia, and astigmatism.

Myopia is commonly called nearsightedness and is the most common visual problem for which contact lenses are prescribed. For the myopic patient, distant objects are blurred because the images of these objects are brought to focus in front of the retina (the sensitive nerve layer at the posterior part of the eye) instead of on it (Figure 2–1). If an object is brought close to the eye, then it may be clear since the image falls on the retina. How close the patient must hold the object depends on the amount of myopia. To compensate the myopic patient, a minus or negative lens is used. This particular lens causes light to diverge, resulting in image movement back to the retina. The center of such a lens is thinner than the edge.

Hyperopia or farsightedness implies the vision at far is often clear, but the near vision is poor. When the hyperopic patient looks at a distant object, the image will fall behind the retina (Figure 2–1) and be blurred. The patient may be able to clear the image of a distant object by changing the shape of the crystalline lens in the eye (see Chapter 4). The change is called accommodation. This takes effort and can cause eyestrain and discomfort. To focus on close objects even more accommodation is required. To compensate for hyperopia, a plus or positive lens is required. This type of lens causes light to converge, resulting in image movement forward to the retina. In this case the lens is thicker in the center than at the edges.

A third type of refractive error (need for glasses or contact lenses) is astigmatism. This is a condition where the light rays from an object are focused at different distances from the retina depending on the point

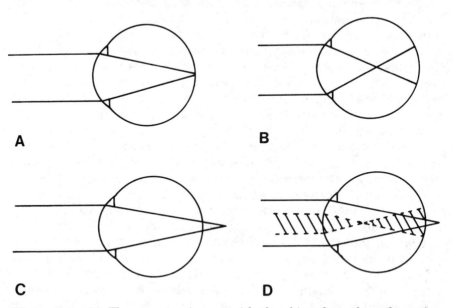

Figure 2–1. (a) The emmetropic eye, with the object focused on the retina; (b) The myopic eye, with the image focused in front of the retina; (c) The hyperopic eye, with the object focused behind the retina; (d) The astigmatic eye, with the light focused at different points

they enter the eye (Figure 2–1). For example, light rays entering the eye in the vertical plane may focus in front of light entering in the horizontal plane. The result is somewhat blurred vision at all distances. The most common cause of significant amounts of astigmatism is the cornea. This clear front layer of the eye (see Chapter 4) is not round or spherical, like a section of a basketball, but shaped like the side of a football. To correct this problem, a similarly designed spectacle lens or contact lens must be used. A patient can have astigmatism and myopia or astigmatism and hyperopia, but not both myopia and hyperopia in the same eye.

One of the changes experienced with age is the gradual loss of accommodation. This gradual loss progresses until it is difficult to focus (see clearly) at the normal reading distance by the age of 40 to 45 years. At this time, patients need an additional lens to focus close objects if they are to read fine print. This condition is called presbyopia. One method of compensation is with bifocal lenses. This loss of ability to accommodate happens to everyone.

A common problem occurs in older age when the crystalline lens becomes cloudy or opaque, obscuring vision. This is called a cataract. No lens placed in front of the eye can compensate or correct this condition. In order to restore vision, the cloudy lens must be surgically removed, resulting in the condition termed aphakia. In order to correct aphakia a high plus lens (one very thick in the center) is usually required. The condition can also occur in young individuals as a result of certain systemic diseases, injury, chemicals, or congenital problems. Aphakic spectacles generally cause visual distortion problems that are minimized by contact lenses or lenses implanted inside the eye (called intraocular lenses or IOLs).

Throughout the text many other ocular conditions and terminology will be introduced and defined.

There are certain standard terminology lists available for describing contact lenses such as those by the American National Standards Institute, Inc. (1), Standards Association of Australia (2), British Standards (3), and others. The following definitions and descriptions utilize the terms proposed by these standards as well as others in common usage. Table 2–1 summarizes many of these interchangeable terms.

CORNEAL LENSES

Corneal contact lenses are usually smaller than the diameter of the cornea. This section will cover the terminology for rigid lenses. Hydrogel lens terminology will be covered later, although many terms are interchangeable.

Table 2–1. Common contact lens terms and abbreviations.

   I. Maximum external dimension
      Overall size (OS)
      Diameter (D)
      Lens diameter (LD)
      Overall diameter (OAD)
  II. Posterior central optic portion of lens
      Posterior central curve (PCC)
      Optic zone (OZ)
      Back central optic portion (BCOP)
 III. Linear dimension of posterior central optic zone of lens
      Posterior optic zone diameter (POZD)
      Optic zone diameter (OZD)
      Optic zone width (OZW)
      Back central optic diameter (BCOD)
 IV. Radius of posterior central optic portion
      Posterior central curve radius (PCCR)
      Base curve radius (BCR)
      Base curve (BC)
      Back central optic radius (BCOR)
  V. Back peripheral curve portion of lens
      Posterior secondary curve (PSC)
      Posterior peripheral curve (PPC)
      Peripheral curve width (PCW)
      Back peripheral optic portion (BPOP)
 VI. Radius of peripheral curve portion of lens
      Posterior secondary curve radius (PSCR)
      Posterior peripheral curve radius (PPCR)
      Back peripheral optic radius (BPOR)
VII. Central anterior optic portion of lens
      Anterior central curve (ACC)
      Optic cap (OC)
      Reduced optic (RO)
      Anterior optic bowl
      Front central optic portion (FCOP)
VIII. Linear dimension of central anterior optic portion
      Anterior optic zone diameter (AOZD)
      Optic cap diameter
      Reduced optic diameter
      Front central optic diameter (FCOD)
 IX. Radius of central anterior optic portion
      Anterior central curve radius (ACCR)
      Optic cap radius
      Front central optic radius (FCOR)

Table 2–1. (continued).

   X.   Anterior peripheral portion of lens
         Anterior peripheral curve zone (APCZ)
         Front peripheral optic portion (FPOR)
 XI. Radius of anterior peripheral portion of lens
         Anterior peripheral curve radius (APCR)
         Carrier radius
         Front peripheral optic radius (FPOR)

Posterior Central Curve

A corneal contact lens is composed of curved surfaces that are either spherical or nonspherical. The back (concave) surface of a spherical contact lens can have one or more curves (Figure 2–2). The central most radius can be called the posterior central curve radius (PCCR), base curve (BC), base curve radius (BCR), back central optic radius (BCOR), or central posterior curve (CPC). This radius is best specified in millimeters

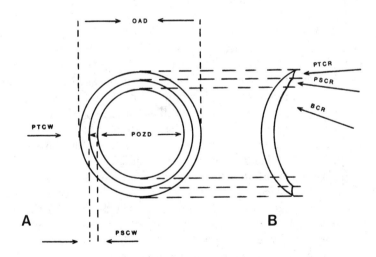

Figure 2–2. (a) Frontal view of a corneal contact lens showing the posterior optical zone diameter, peripheral curves, and overall diameter. (b) Cross-sectional view showing the radii of the different portions of the lens

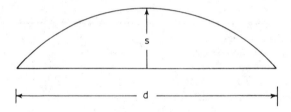

Figure 2–3. Sagittal depth(s) of a radius with a chord of d

(mm). Some practitioners designate it in diopters (D) corresponding to the dioptric power as read with a keratometer or ophthalmometer, an instrument used to measure the cornea. The use of this instrument and the conversion between diopters and millimeters are discussed in Chapter 5.

Another concept sometimes associated with the base curve radius and posterior optical zone is sagittal depth. This is the measurement of the distance from a line (called the chord) drawn between the outer edges of the optical zone up to the center of the back surface (Figure 2–3). The shorter (steeper) the base curve radius is, the greater the sagittal depth. Also, the larger the optical zone diameter, the greater is the sagittal depth. It is specified in millimeters.

For most contact lenses, the posterior central curve radius (base curve) is spherical. The surface is specified with one radius, meaning the surface is like a section of the inside of a round ball. It is possible to have a toric back central curve, indicating that the surface cannot be specified with one radius value; two must be used. In this case the surface is not the shape of a round ball, but like the surface of a football. In this situation the radius in the smallest dimension and radius in the largest dimension must be specified. Toric lenses may be used on the patients with large amounts of corneal toricity or astigmatism. If the back or front surface of the contact lens is toric, the lens is said to be back toric or front toric, respectively. If both sides are toric, the lens is bitoric.

Another shape that may be generated on the back surface of the lens is an aspheric surface. With this type of lens there is a gradual lengthening of the radius from the center toward the edge of the lens. In this case the radius value for the very center of the lens is given, along with a further description of how fast the radius changes as it moves away from the center. A more detailed description of such surfaces is given later.

Posterior Peripheral Curve Radii

Peripheral to the central curve there are usually one or more additional curves (Figure 2–2) called posterior peripheral curves. One way to specify these curves is to designate the first curve beyond the central base curve the posterior secondary curve radius (PSCR) (or peripheral curve radius), or the posterior peripheral bevel (or bevel). Another method is to call the curves back peripheral optic radii (BPOR) and number them starting with the first one beyond the back central optical radius—for example, BP_1OR, BP_2OR, and so on.

Normally the posterior peripheral curve radii are specified in millimeters (mm) of radius. Occasionally they will be specified in terms of millimeters flatter than the central base curve radius. Still another method is to specify them in terms of diopters flatter than the posterior central curve. Each diopter flatter is approximately 0.2 mm flatter. In all cases the peripheral curves have longer radii (are flatter curves) than the posterior central base curve and each peripheral curve progressing from the center outward is longer than the preceding one.

Posterior peripheral curves are used to give a better match between the shape of the back surface of the lens and the cornea. They also give edge clearance of the lens from the cornea to allow proper tear exchange under the lens.

Blends

Where two posterior surface radii meet, such as between the base curve radius and the secondary curve radius, there may be a distinct junction. When there is a significant difference in radii between the two curves this junction may be sharp and must be smoothed out or blended. Blends are narrow zones where a curve with a radius between the two adjacent curves is polished on the lens. Blends are usually specified in one of three ways: light, medium, or heavy; one, two, or three; or A, B, or C. Light, A, or number-one blend designates only a very slight smoothing of the curves. The heavy, C, or number-three blend specifies the transition between the curves as indistinguishable.

Aspheric or Continuous Curve Lenses

To obtain about the same effect as using spherical base curve radii and peripheral curve radii, it is possible to fabricate an aspherical surface. If the whole back surface of the lens is aspheric, there is a gradual lengthening (flattening) of the surface from the center toward the edge (Figure 2–4), with no transition zones. The rate of flattening can be varied, depending on the characteristics of different eyes.

Most aspheric surfaces approximate sections of a cone called conic sections (Figures 2–5 and 2–6). Conic sections are either elliptical, parabolic, or hyperbolic surfaces. These terms are often used to describe the

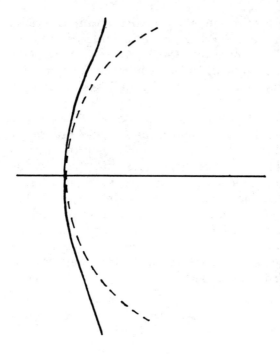

Figure 2–4. An aspheric curve (solid line) compared to a spherical curve (dotted line)

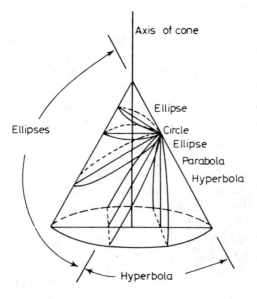

Figure 2–5. Conic sections formed by cutting a right perpendicular cone with planes

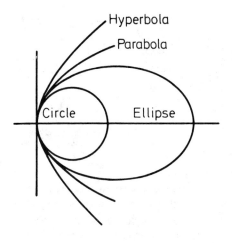

Hyperbola

Parabola

Circle   Ellipse

Figure 2–6.   Relative shapes of conic sections

surfaces. A method of specifying an aspherical curve is to give the apical radius (a millimeter value for the spherical curve that matches the curve at the center of the lens) along with what is called an e-value. The larger the e-value, the greater the rate of flattening from center to edge. An e-value of zero specifies a spherical surface, e-values between zero and 1.0 are elliptical surfaces, an e-value of 1.0 is a parabolic surface, and greater than 1.0 is a hyperbolic surface. The aspheric surfaces used clinically usually have e-values between 0.5 and 1.5. An example of specifying the back surface of an aspheric lens could be a 7.50 mm apical radius and e = 0.70. Many laboratories supplying aspheric lenses may provide only one or a few e-values and may use their own trade names or terms on those provided.

It is also possible to have regular spherical posterior central curve radii with an aspheric peripheral curve. The aspheric peripheral curve can be specified in the same fashion as the full back surface aspheric.

Overall Size

The linear measurement of the greatest distance across a lens from outside edge to outside edge (Figure 2–2) is the diameter (D), lens diameter (LD), overall size (OS), or overall diameter (OAD). This dimension is specified in millimeters (mm).

If the outside dimension of the lens is oval instead of round, then the widest and narrowest dimensions must be specified. In some cases one portion of the lens is removed (Figure 2–7), to give a flat side. This is called truncation. Two sides may also be removed, giving what is called a double truncated lens.

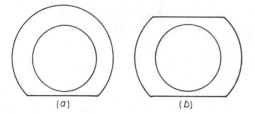

Figure 2-7. (a) Single truncated lens. (b) Double truncated lens

(a)   (b)

Posterior Optical Zone Diameter

The linear dimension of the lens that contains the posterior central curve radius (base curve radius) can be called the posterior optical zone diameter (POZD), optical zone diameter (OZD), back central optical diameter (BCOD), optical zone width (OZW), or simply optical zone (OZ). This dimension is specified in millimeters.

The optical zone is usually circular (round) and centered with respect to the outside circumference of the lens. In some cases the optical zone may be oval in shape. In this case both the longest and shortest dimensions are specified. This means that some of the curves (radii) on the back surface are toric. If the optical zone is not centered in relation to the outside circumference, then the amount of decentration as well as the optical zone diameter must be specified.

If there is only one curve on the back surface of the lens (there is only the posterior central curve and the posterior optical zone diameter equals the overall diameter) the lens is said to be a monocurve lens.

Peripheral Curve Widths

The width of each peripheral curve can be specified. These are labelled in the same order as the radii, that is, the posterior secondary curve width (PSCW) or just secondary curve width (SCW), posterior teritary curve width (PTCW), posterior peripheral curve width (PPCW), or back peripheral optical portion (PB_1OP, BP_2OP, etc.). This dimension is specified in millimeters.

If the lens has only one peripheral curve, then the sum of the optical zone diameter plus twice the peripheral curve width equals the overall diameter (Figure 2-8). Where there are several peripheral curves, twice the width of each must be added to the optical zone to equal the overall diameter.

When there is only one peripheral curve, the lens is called a bicurve lens; with two peripheral curves its a tricurve lens.

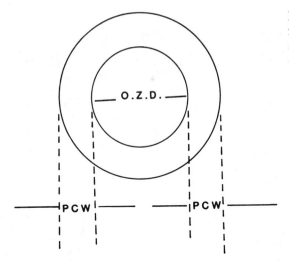

Figure 2-8. Twice the peripheral curve width must be added to the optical zone to obtain the lens diameter

Anterior Lens Surface

Many rigid corneal contact lenses have only one radius on the front surface; however, others may have two or more radii. The anterior central curve radius (ACCR) is usually not specified by the practitioner because if the base curve radius, center thickness (ct), and lens power (D) are specified, then there is only one possible anterior central curve radius that the laboratory can use. If the front surface radius is specified, it is given in millimeters of radius. The front surface can be toric, in which case two anterior central curve radii must be given, one for each major meridian. Another term for the anterior central curve radius is the front central optic radius (FCOR).

When the front surface is divided into two zones (Figure 2–9), the lens is a lenticular design. The central zone contains the optical portion that corrects the patient's refractive error. This region is called the anterior optical zone, front central optic portion (FCOP), front optic zone, reduced optic, optic bowl, or optic cap.

The front peripheral zone is often called the carrier with plus powered lenses. The main reason for using a lenticular lens with plus prescriptions is to reduce the thickness and weight of the lens. The radius of the peripheral zone of the lens can be varied to give different thickness and contour variations. For example, the front peripheral radius may approximate the radius of the back surface of the lens in this region, resulting in a regular lenticular lens (Figure 2–9). Another common form is to fabricate the lens with the front peripheral radius longer than the back surface of the lens in this region, giving a thicker edge (Figure 2–9).

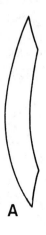

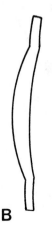

Figure 2–9. Lenticular lens designs: (a) single cut lens; (b) regular carrier lenticular; (c) minus carrier lenticular; (d) minus lens design

A

B

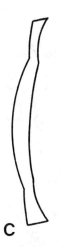

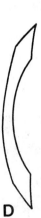

C

D

This is a minus carrier lenticular lens. This design aids in centering the lens on the cornea since the upper eyelid will hold the lens better.

With high minus prescription lenses, the lens edges can be very thick unless an anterior peripheral curve radius is used to decrease the edge thickness (Figure 2–9). This results in a minus lenticular design. The anterior peripheral curve radius in this case is shorter (steeper) than the central anterior radius. With minus lenses where the anterior peripheral curve is very narrow, such a curve is often called a bevel, anterior bevel, or CN bevel.

All of the dimensions of the front surface of the lens are given in millimeters. This includes the radii of the anterior central optical zone and anterior peripheral curve width. Normally a practitioner will specify the diameter of the anterior central optic and the type of lenticular design but leave the other front surface specifications for the laboratory to determine. The anterior optical zone diameter is usually made a few tenths of a millimeter larger than the posterior optical zone diameter.

Thickness

The thickness of a contact lens can be very important in determining lens centration and comfort. If a lens is thicker than necessary, it will be heavy and tend not to stay centered on the cornea. If the edge is too thick, it will likely be uncomfortable and may cause corneal damage.

The center thickness (ct) is determined mainly by the dioptric power and diameter. The center will be thicker with plus lenses and thinner with minus lenses (Figure 2–10). If the lens diameter of a plus lens is increased, the center thickness must be increased to maintain an acceptable edge thickness. The center thickness of a minus lens need not be changed if a larger-diameter lens is made, but the edge will become thicker. The center thickness for standard mid-range minus powered corneal lenses (– 2.50 D and greater) is 0.10 to 0.12 mm. Ultrathin lenses are usually 0.06 to 0.08 mm thick. Lenses of high plus prescriptions for aphakic patients (+ 10.00 to + 15.00) may be 0.30 to 0.60 mm thick.

The edge on plus lenses is usually 0.10 to 0.12 mm thick before being rounded. Thinner edges may be uncomfortable and tend to chip easily. The edge thickness increases as the minus prescription increases. At edge thickness between 0.20 to 0.30 mm anterior bevels or minus lenticular designs are used to thin the edge.

The optical zone diameter, peripheral curve widths, and radii affect center and edge thickness. If the posterior peripheral curve of a lens is widened, the edge thickness is decreased. This may not create any prob-

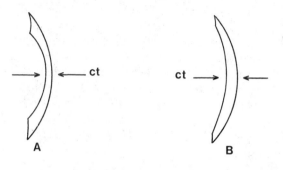

Figure 2–10. (a) Minus lens design. (b) Plus lens design

lems with a minus lens if there was sufficient edge stock initially. If the edge is initially thin, however, as with a plus lens, the edge may become too thin. The lens must be redesigned with a thicker center to maintain the minimum edge thickness. Likewise, if the posterior peripheral curve is made longer (flatter), the edge will be thinned.

The junction thickness, the thickness where the anterior central and peripheral curves meet, is important with plus lenticular designs. Common junction thicknesses are 0.12 to 0.15 mm. If the junction is thinner, the lens will tend to break at this point. If junction thickness is increased, however, then effectively a layer of additional plastic is added over the whole lens surface. Thus, a small increase in junction thickness greatly increases the lens weight.

The center, edge, and junction thicknesses can be calculated. The methods of making these determinations are described in other texts, and tables are available (4, 5).

Refractive Power

The dioptric power of a contact lens is important in terms of correcting a patient's refractive error. If the power is incorrect, the patient will usually be aware of the problem immediately, for vision will be blurred. The diopter is the standard unit for specifying the focusing power of a lens. Dioptric power of a lens is determined by dividing the focal length of the lens specified in meters into 1.0. Thus, if a lens focuses a distant object at one meter from the lens, it is a 1.00 diopter lens (note: dioptric power is written to two decimal places). If the distant object is focused at 0.5 meters from the lens, it is a 2.00 diopter lens. The shorter the focal length, the higher the dioptric value. Plus lenses focus the image behind the lens. They are used to compensate the hyperopic and aphakic patient. Minus lenses form a virtual image in front of the lens and compensate for myopia.

The focal length of a lens can be clinically measured from either the front surface of the lens of the back surface. Normally the back lens surface is used as the reference point, and the term back vertex power (BVP) is used. In actual practice, a lensometer or vertexometer (see Chapter 7) is utilized to measure lens power. To determine the BVP, the back surface of the lens is placed against the lens stop of the instrument. Some laboratories, in their manufacturing process, will measure front vertex power (FVP) by placing the front surface of the lens against the stop of the lensometer. With low prescriptions, 4.00 diopters or less, there is essentially no difference between FVP and BVP. With high prescriptions, however—for example, aphakic lenses (+12.00 to +20.00 D)—there may be over 1.00 D difference between front and back vertex powers. Thus, any high prescription, plus or minus, should be specified as to FVP or BVP.

In addition to spherical powers, cylindrical powers can be fabricated in contact lenses. A cylindrical power results from a toric lens surface and compensates for astigmatism. In this case, two dioptric powers must be specified for the lens, a power for the major and minor meridians of the lens cylinder. Remember, a surface with a cylindrical power is shaped like the side of a football, one direction having a long radius and the direction (meridian) 90 degress away having a short radius. The power in each of two major meridians must be specified.

One method of specifying the cylindrical power is to give the power in each meridian, for example, $-2.00/-3.00$. This is usually used when a toric base curve lens is fitted. Another method is to give the power and axis, which is common when the base curve radius is spherical, the front surface is toric, and prism is used as a ballast to prevent the lens from rotating. In this case the lens power may be written as -2.00 -1.00 $\times$ 090, for example. This is the same as the $-2.00/-3.00$ notation, but is more specific about the meridian (axis) of the cylinder (90 degrees in this example). Of course, the powers and axis will vary depending on the lens and patient's prescription. The axis can be anywhere from 1 to 180 degrees. The zero axis is in the horizontal meridian of the eye to the right as you face the patient (Figure 2–11) and progresses counterclockwise to the 180° meridian. Zero meridian is the same as the 180-degree meridian; therefore, zero is not used.

A further complication of cylindrical corrections is that they can be written in either a minus cylinder form or a plus cylinder form. To convert from minus cylinder to plus cylinder form the cylinder power (-1.00 in the above example) is added to the spherical power (-2.00 above) to give the new spherical power, -3.00 D. The sign of the cylinder is changed to plus, but the amount remains the same, in this example it is now $+1.00$. The cylinder axis is then changed 90 degrees to 180 degrees. Thus, the minus cylinder notation, -2.00 -1.00 $\times$ 090 becomes -3.00 $+1.00$

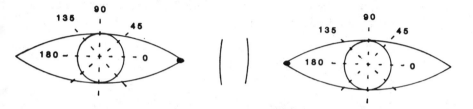

Figure 2–11. Convention for specifying axis of cylindrical corrections

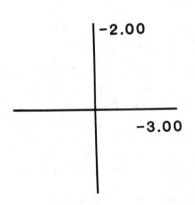

Figure 2–12. Optical cross designation of the cylindrical power given in the examples in the text

× 180 when written in the plus cylinder form. The powers can be placed on an optical cross (Figure 2–12) so that a graphical representation can be seen.

In addition to spherical and cylindrical power, it is possible to incorporate prismatic power into the lens. With contact lenses, prism is most often used to prevent lens rotation so that a cylindrical or bifocal correction can be held in the proper position on the eye. It can also be used to correct a vertical phoria. This is a condition where one eye tends to turn up slightly in relation to the other. A lens with prism has a gradual increase in thickness from the apex of the prism to the base. Prism power is specified as prism diopters (one prism diopter will displace an object 1 cm when the object is 1 m from the lens). Prism power can be read directly from the lensometer (see Chapter 7). When on the eye, the base of the prism will usually ride at or near the bottom of the cornea in the 90 degree meridian.

Fenestrations (Apertures)

Occasionally holes (called fenestrations or apertures) are drilled or placed through a lens with a laser or sparks. These holes are used to increase tear flow under the lens so that oxygen from the air reaches the cornea. It also changes the fluid forces involved.

Tints

Many rigid contact lenses are prescribed with tints. There are several colors available (blue, green, gray, brown, and pink). Normally, there are three shades of each color designated as number one or light, number two or medium, and number three or dark. Some laboratories also make available half shades. The pigment (coloring) is within the plastic and is not a surface coating. Thus, two lenses may be made from the same shade of plastic, but if one is thicker than the other, it will be darker. This can be a problem with high prescriptions, where even the lightest tint may be too dark. These standard tints normally do not change eye color, but make it easier to find lost lenses. Many lenses made of new plastics have no tint at all.

Special colorations may be used. For example, there is a deep red lens (trade name X-Chrom®) that is used to aid some color-deficient (color-"blind") patients in distinguishing objects of different colors. There are also cosmetic lenses that are fitted to cover a scarred or disfigured eye and painted to match the good eye. Contact lenses are also used to change eye color and appearance. Cosmetic lenses are frequently used in the movies and television to create special effects.

BIFOCAL LENSES

To compensate for presbyopia, the loss of the ability to focus at near, two different lens powers are required, one prescription for distance and a second one for near. With spectacles this is accomplished by placing a zone of more plus power (near segment or add) in the lower part of the lens for near vision. These are known as bifocals or multifocals. The same procedure is used with contact lenses. Just as with spectacle lenses, the size and shape of the bifocal segment can be varied (Figure 2–13).

With bifocal contact lenses, the dimensions of the lenses are smaller

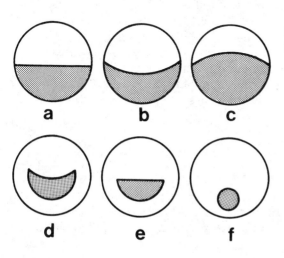

Figure 2–13. Different bifocal segment designs

than those of spectacles; therefore, the manufacturing process is very critical. The segment may be fused into the main body of the lens. The near portion is of a different kind of plastic than the distance portion. Another method of manufacturing bifocal contact lenses is to have two different radii on the front surface resulting in different powers. These are often called cut bifocals as opposed to fused bifocals.

These bifocals must be fitted so the near segment stays down toward the lower lid and does not rotate. To accomplish this, prism is used. To function properly when the patient looks down, the lens must be pushed up by the lower eyelid so the near segment moves in front of the pupil. A refinement of these bifocals is called "no-jump", or monocentric design. This is an optical principle of lens design. It prevents the apparent jump or movement of viewed objects when the line dividing the distance and near portion moves across the patient's pupil. The design and fitting of these bifocal designs are exacting.

Another bifocal design is called a concentric bifocal. In this case the near portion is a zone around the entire central area of the lens. This lens can rotate, and prism is not needed. The lens must move up on down gaze so the near portion covers the pupil. The types of bifocals described are sometimes called alternating because the lens must move between the distance and near portions.

Another design is the simultaneous or bivision bifocal. Both the distance and near portion of the lens are in front of the pupil at all times. In this situation, when the patient looks at a distant object, light rays passing through the distance portion of the lens will be in focus while the rays passing through the near portion will be out of focus. When viewing near objects, the opposite is true. The patient must learn to utilize the in-focus image and ignore the out-of-focus image. Some patients are able to do this, but others cannot. Concentric designs with small central optics or highly aspheric lenses are usually used as simultaneous bifocals.

Another method used to compensate for presbyopia is called the monovision technique. Here one eye is corrected for distance vision and the other eye for near. This interrupts binocular vision (functioning of the two eyes together). Some patients are able to adapt to this procedure while others are not.

HYDROGEL LENSES

Hydrogel (also called hydrophilic or soft) contact lenses are made of polymers (plastics) that absorb water. These lenses may absorb up to 90 percent water. This makes the lenses relatively soft and flexible, so they must be handled and fitted somewhat differently than are rigid lenses.

Hydrogel lenses are usually larger than rigid lenses, normally cover all the cornea, and often extend out onto the sclera, the white part of the eye. Hydrogel lenses smaller than the diameter of the cornea (less than about 12.0 mm) are termed corneal hydrogel lenses. These are seldom used because it is difficult to keep them centered on the cornea. Many of the hydrogel lenses are 12.5 to 13.5 mm in overall diameter and may be called limbal lenses since the edge of the lens is approximately at the limbus (the junction between the cornea and sclera). Larger lenses (13.5 to 16 mm) are called paralimbal or semiscleral.

The terminology of hydrogel lens specifications is essentially the same as for rigid corneal lenses with some dimension variations.

HAPTIC (SCLERAL) LENSES

The haptic or scleral lens is a large-diameter lens, about 25 mm (1 inch). It rests on the sclera. This was the first type of contact lens to be routinely fitted. Today this design is mainly used for patients with certain types of ocular diseases or injuries, for some athletes, for cosmetic reasons and other special reasons.

Haptic lenses can be fitted by using a diagnostic set of lenses to determine which lens best fits the patient's eye. Lenses fitted in this fashion are called preformed lenses. The other method of fitting the haptic lens is to make a mold or impression of the eye. In this case, a compound, which when put into the eye has a thick, creamy consistency, will form a soft, rubbery mold of the eye. From this a lens can be formed after several additional steps are executed. A lens fitted with this method is called a molded or impression haptic lens.

Haptic lens terminology is essentially the same as for other lens types. The section of the lens covering the sclera is called the haptic. The region between the back central optic portion (base curve) and the haptic is called the transition zone. Most haptic lenses have at least one relatively large (about 1 mm diameter) fenestration.

LENS MATERIALS

Contact lenses are made of polymers (also called plastics, acrylics, or resins). Chemically, these are very long molecules made up of small units that are repeated over and over in long chains. These small repeating units are called monomers. There can be just one monomer or small chemical structure used to make the polymer, or there may be two or more different ones utilized. The chemical nature of the monomer or monomers and the ways they are connected determine the properties of the plastic and lens. These long molecules may have a branching pattern or adjacent molecules may be connected by cross-linking molecules, giving the polymer different properties.

There are many important properties of these polymers that must be considered when used in the manufacturing of contact lenses. The various contact lenses on the market today are made of different polymers. Some polymers, for example, have different refractive indices (usually symbolized by n), which affects the ability of the material to bend light rays. Others have different surface wetting ability. This is important for comfort and vision. Tears may not develop a uniform film over the lens surface but instead bead up, allowing the lens surface to dry. This will make the lens uncomfortable. Debris from the tear film may dry on the lens surface, and the patient will complain of blurred vision. The ability of a lens surface to wet is described by its wetting or contact angle. This is measured by placing a drop of water or solution on the surface and measuring the angle between the lens and drop at the edge of the drop of solution (Figure 2–14). If this angle is less than about 70 degrees, then the tears will usually form a thin film over the lens. If the angle is greater (the water beads up like drops of water in a skillet), the lens surface will not be wetted properly. When a film will not form, clinicians will say the surface is hydorphobic ("water hating"); if the tears spread evenly, the lens surface is said to be hydrophilic.

Another property of a lens material is its ability to absorb water. Some polymers absorb little or no water, such as the standard rigid lens. This material (PMMA) will take up about 1.5 percent water by weight. Some materials will absorb as much as 80 to 90 percent water by weight. There is a whole spectrum of materials with water absorptions between these extremes. The polymers that absorb significant amounts of water are called hydrogels. Usually the more water a lens absorbs, the softer it becomes. Likewise it may become more fragile.

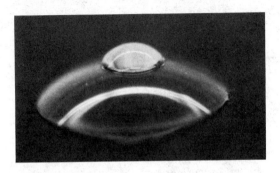

Figure 2–14. A drop of water on a lens surface showing how the water does not completely wet the surface. The angle between the surface and the drop is the contact angle

A property which has received much attention in recent years is the oxygen permeability of lens materials. In order for the cornea to remain in its normal state it must receive oxygen from the air. With a lens on the eye, oxygen can reach the cornea via tears flowing under the edge of the lens or by going through the lens. If the lens is impermeable to oxygen, then all the oxygen must reach the cornea by pumping action of the lens on blinking, causing a flow of tears. If enough tear exchange does not occur, corneal swelling (called edema) develops. The eyes become uncomfortable and permanent corneal damage can occur.

Many of the new lens materials have been developed to allow some oxygen to go through the lens. The ability of oxygen to move through a material is termed permeability. This is a property of the material, and is often called the DK value, where D is the diffusion coefficient and K is the solubility of oxygen in the material. Another term is oxygen transmissibility, which is a specification of how much oxygen goes through a lens. It is the DK value divided by the lens thickness. Both of these values are given by some companies for their lenses. The higher the values, particularly the transmissibility, the better the oxygen transfer to the cornea. Another method of specifying the oxygen available to the cornea under a lens is by equivalent oxygen percent (EOP). Air is about 21 percent oxygen, which is available to the cornea when there is no lens on the eye. With a lens on the eye this may be only 2 percent; thus, the EOP is said to be 2 percent.

There are many other lens properties that may be important, such as lens elasticity, strength, heat (thermal) conductivity, scratch resistance, permeability to molecules in the tear film, and density. In addition, the safety of the material is quite important. Some polymers may be toxic; they may damage tissues with which they are in contact. If any lens material dissolves out into the tear film (often termed leaching) it may cause a tissue reaction. Likewise, if solutions or medications, which are commonly used with the lens, react with the polymer, problems may develop. Therefore, the lens material and solutions must be extensively tested in the chemistry laboratory and with animals to assure its safety on humans.

Rigid Materials

Lenses that are fairly stiff and do not tend to take the shape of the eye were essentially the only type used prior to the late 1960s. Such lenses generally result in good optics with no distortion. They are easy for the patient to handle, do not absorb significant amounts of fluids or other substances, and can be easily manufactured and modified. Thus, rigid lenses have served many patients well for many years. With new, better polymers being developed, rigid lenses should continue to serve as a good mode of correction for a large number of future patients.

Polymethymethacrylate (PMMA) is the main polymer that has been used in the manufacture of contact lenses over the years. It is a very transparent polymer with a refractive index of 1.49. The polymer is non-toxic, stable, and resistant to most solutions and chemicals with the exception of organic solvents such as acetone. It has a contact angle of 60 to 70 degrees, which allows the tear film to wet the surface. Different tints can be polymerized into the material. The main disadvantage of PMMA as a contact lens material is its lack of permeability to oxygen. There is, for clinical purposes, no oxygen transmission through the lenses. In many cases this results in corneal edema. For this reason, the use of PMMA has been decreasing in favor of the rigid oxygen permeable lens.

Cellulose acetate butyrate (CAB) is a transparent polymer that has some oxygen transmission and has found considerable use as a contact lens material in recent years. It is made up of three monomers (cellulose, acetate, and butyrate) and forms a very tough polymer. CAB lenses are quite strong, but still scratch as easy or easier than PMMA. CAB has greater thermal conductivity than PMMA. CAB lenses are not generally as stable as PMMA, and this can result in flattening of the base curve radius or distortion when the lens is hydrated and worn. In order to make the lens more stable, a thicker lens may be used. This can add weight and increase edge thickness, with accompanying fitting and comfort problems. The contact angle of CAB is less than with PMMA. Material from the tear film tends to collect on the lens surface, causing blurred vision in some cases. Even though some of the properties of CAB are not as good as those of PMMA, the increased oxygen transmission outweighs the disadvantages for many patients.

PMMA-silicone copolymers are also clear materials that can be used for contact lenses. Silicone and its derivatives have extremely high oxygen permeability. As a result of the combination of PMMA and silicone, the oxygen transmission is increased due to the silicone while the properties of PMMA such as stability, wettability, optical properties, machining, and ability to be modified have been maintained. These lenses are generally made thinner than CAB lenses and have greater stability.

Rigid silicone resin lenses are also being manufactured. The main advantage of using this material is the relatively high oxygen transmission, higher than that of the CAB and PMMA-silicone combination lenses, but not as high as that of soft silicone lenses. A problem with silicone is the highly hydrophobic nature of the lens surface. In order to obtain wettability of the lens surface, the surface chemistry of the lens must be changed. Such treatments make the lens very wettable and clinically valuable. This does prevent major modifications of the lens, however, because if this superficial layer is polished off, the lens will no longer wet. In other aspects this material is very stable, transparent, and lightweight and appears to have a place in the clincial practice.

Other oxygen-permeable polymers and different mixtures of the above polymers are being used. Advances in technology including additional materials continue.

Hydrogel Lens Materials

Hydroxyethylmethacrylate (HEMA) was the first hydrogel lens polymer used for contact lenses. This polymer, or copolymers of HEMA, is still the major hydrogel material used. Its introduction opened up a whole new area in the contact lens field. For the first time there was a soft contact lens that would conform to the shape of the eye. This meant that fitting techniques had to change from those used with rigid lenses.

It is best to refer to these lenses as hydrogel lenses rather than soft or flexible lenses as there are soft and flexible lenses that do not absorb significant amounts of water. Members of the general public, as well as many professionals, refer to these lenses simply as soft lenses. This terminology will probably continue. Hydrophilic is another term in common use but again is not as correct as hydrogel.

Since hydrogel lenses absorb water as well as other chemicals, the care of the lenses is different from that for rigid lenses. To disinfect (kill all the microorganisms that might cause eye infections) the lenses, they must be heated or placed in solutions with preservatives (chemicals preventing the growth of organisms). Since solutions are absorbed by the polymer, the use of chemicals can cause eye irritation as they slowly leach out of the lens while the patient wears it. Regular sodium fluorescein dye used to evaluate the fit of rigid lenses cannot be used with hydrogel lenses because it will be absorbed by the lens. Only a special large-molecule fluorescein can be used. Hydrogel lenses must be kept in a solution with the proper salt concentration (called tonicity). This prevents the lens from sticking to the eye or causing discomfort when first placed on the cornea.

A hydrogel lens will lose water and dehydrate if not kept in solution. If the lens is allowed to dehydrate, it will become very distorted and brittle (Figure 2–15). It can be rehydrated and made soft and usable by placing it in saline solution. Most hydrogel lenses are manufactured in the hard, dehydrated state and then hydrated prior to being sent to the practitioner.

Different hydrogel polymers absorb different amounts of water.

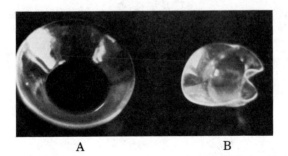

Figure 2-15. (a) A normally hydrated hydrogel lens. (b) A hydrogel lens that has been allowed to dry

A   B

Presently on the market are lenses with water contents of 20 to 90 percent. Usually the more water the lens contains, the softer and more fragile the lens. Oxygen permeability increases with increased water uptake. For this reason, high water content contact lenses are often used for extended wear. The patient wears the lenses continuously for days, weeks, or months without removal. Extended or prolonged wear are terms preferred over permanent wear since no lenses are actually worn permanently.

Some hydrogel lenses are also made very thin (0.04 to 0.08 mm) to increase oxygen transmission. These are commonly called ultrathin lenses.

There are many different hydrogel lenses with different chemical compositions and water contents. Additional variations continue to be developed and different designs manufactured. Lenses to correct astigmatism, cosmetic hydrogel lenses and bifocal hydrogel lenses are all being utilized.

Silicone Elastomer Lenses

Silicone lenses are made from inorganic polymers. The other contact lens polymers are called organic. The long molecular chain of organic polymers is made up of carbon atoms. The long silicone polymers are made up of silicone and oxygen atoms. The great advantage of silicone as a contact lens material is the extremely high oxygen permeability. Even a very thick silicone elastomer lens will transmit more than enough oxygen to the cornea.

Silicone elastomer lenses are flexible. Silicone resin lenses can be rigid, as previously discussed. The soft silicone lenses will conform to the shape of the cornea and have a greater elasticity than other contact lenses. Silicone is a rubber material. It can be stretched like a rubber band and will then return to the original shape. This is an advantage as the lens is very tough and difficult to tear or damage. This property may also demand more accurate fitting than is required for a hydrogel lens.

Silicone is a very hydrophobic material that does not absorb water. The surface, therefore, does not wet well without being treated, although a properly treated surface is hydrophilic and quite functional. The lens cannot be manufactured by lathe cutting, similar to most rigid and hydrogel lenses. This lens is formed in a closed mold under heat and pressure.

Since the lens does not absorb solutions, it can be treated very much like the rigid lenses. Ordinary fluorescein dye can be used to evaluate the fit, as for rigid lenses.

Silicone elastomer lenses are good candidates for extended wear because of their high oxygen permeability and lack of absorption of solutions or other materials from the tear film.

REFERENCES

1. Prescription Requirements for First Quality Contact Lenses. Z80.2–1972, American National Standards Institute, Inc., 1430 Broadway, New York, NY 10018

2. Australian Standard Specification for Contact Lenses, Standards Assoc. of Australia, P.O. Box 458, North Sydney, 2060 Australia

3. British Standards 3521:Section 14, 1962

4. Bier N. Lowther, GE. Contact lens correction. London Butterworth, 1977.

5. Creighton CP. Contact lens fabrication tables. 2nd ed., Alden Optical Laboratories, Alden, N.Y., 1976.

3

OPTICAL PRINCIPLES OF CONTACT LENSES

The overwhelming majority of patients are fitted with contact lenses to compensate for their refractive errors. This chapter concentrates on the optical principles involved.

OPTICS OF THE EYE

The eye is designed to focus images of objects in space on the retina. Nerve signals generated in this light-sensitive layer are then transmitted, via a complex nervous system, to the brain. In order for a useful image to be coded and transmitted, a good optical image must be present.

The most important surface of the eye in focusing light rays from a distant object is the cornea (see Chapter 4). This clear, anterior window, being exposed to air, provides the greatest bending of the light rays. The ability of a surface or lens to bend light or focus it is called refractive power. The refractive power of a surface is dependent upon the curvature of the surface and the refractive index of the media on both sides of the surface. The refractive index of a material is a specification indicating its ability to slow and bend light waves. The higher the refractive index, the greater the slowing and bending of the light waves. For example, the refractive index of air is 1.0, water 1.33, and PMMA contact lenses 1.49. The greater the difference in refractive index on the two sides of a surface, the greater the bending of the light. Also, the steeper (shorter the radius) the surface, the greater the bending of the light. The refractive power of a surface is determined by the following formula: $F = \frac{n' - n}{r}$, where F is the refractive power in diopters, n' the refractive index of the second media, n the refractive index of the first media, and r the radius of curvature of the surface in meters. The radius of the cornea varies in different patients, but the average radius is 7.8 mm or .0078 m. The refractive index of the cornea can be assumed to be 1.3375 and air is 1.0, therefore $F = \frac{1.3375 - 1.0}{0.0078}$, or $F = 43.27$ diopters. This amount represents over two-thirds of the refractive power of the eye.

The back of the cornea is not as strong a refractive surface as the front surface. This is because the differences in refractive indices between the posterior cornea and aqueous humor, which bathes the back of the cornea, are small.

The crystalline lens, a biconvex lens that lies just behind the iris, contributes a total of about 19.00 diopters of refractive power to the eye. This is the structure that can become cloudy and opaque (called a cataract). It then must be removed. To compensate for the loss of its refractive power, strong spectacle lenses, contact lenses or intraocular lenses must be used.

The combination of the refractive powers of different surfaces of the eye and its length determine if distance objects will be focused on the retina. For a given refractive power, if the eye is too long, the image is focused in front of the retina resulting in myopia (see Chapter 2). When the eye's refractive power is too strong, a negative-powered lens must be placed in front of the eye to compensate. For hyperopia (farsightedness) the opposite is true, and a plus lens must be used.

LENS POWER

A contact lens has a certain specified refractive power dependent upon the refractive index of the material, front and back surface radii, and the lens thickness. If the lens front radius is shorter than the back surface radius, it will have plus refractive power (Figure 3–1). If the front surface radius is longer than the back surface radius, the lens has minus refractive power (Figure 3–1). The refractive power of a lens can be calculated by knowing the dimensions, but, clinically, the dioptric power is determined directly by using the lensometer, a lens power measuring device, (see Chapter 7). This instrument gives the power of the contact lens in air.

RIGID CONTACT LENSES ON THE EYE

It is possible to fit a contact lens so that the back central radius (base curve) is either longer (flatter) than the corneal curvature, the same as the cornea (called "on K" fit), or shorter (steeper) than the cornea (Figure

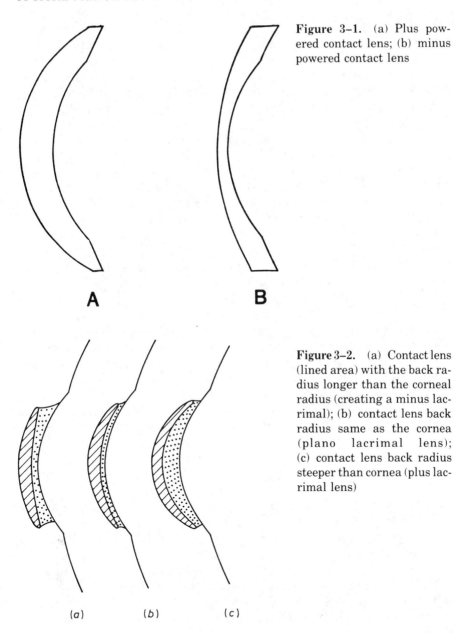

Figure 3–1. (a) Plus powered contact lens; (b) minus powered contact lens

A B

Figure 3–2. (a) Contact lens (lined area) with the back radius longer than the corneal radius (creating a minus lacrimal); (b) contact lens back radius same as the cornea (plano lacrimal lens); (c) contact lens back radius steeper than cornea (plus lacrimal lens)

(a) (b) (c)

3–2). The term K refers to the corneal radius as determined by using the keratometer (see Chapter 5). In the case of a toric cornea, the K value is the longest radius of the cornea.

The curve of the contact lens in relation to the curvature of the cornea affects the total power of the contact lens-eye system. If the contact lens back surface is flatter than the radius of the cornea, tears that pool between the contact lens and cornea (called tear or lacrimal lens) form a minus lens. For example, a patient might need a -1.00 D spectacle lens. The contact lens fitted may be flatter than the cornea; thus, the lacrimal lens adds minus power to the system. When the contact lens is fitted so the lacrimal lens has a -1.00 D power, then the eye would need no power in the contact lens to neutralize the refractive error. A lens with no or zero power is termed a plano lens.

To determine how much refractive power is contributed by the lacrimal lens, a comparison of the back curvature of the contact lens to the front of the cornea must be made. The easiest way to do this, clinically, is to determine the dioptric power of the cornea with the keratometer. The dioptric power of the contact lens back surface can be determined from its base curve radius. The refractive index that the keratometer is commonly based on is 1.3375. Thus, if the back radius of the contact lens is 7.50 mm, the dioptric power of this surface is $F = \frac{1.3375 - 1.00}{0.0075m}$. The power is 45.00 diopters. By convention, the lens is said to have a 45.00 D base curve. If the cornea has a dioptric power of 46.00 D (7.34mm radius), the contact lens is said to be 1.00 D flatter than the cornea. This results in a lacrimal lens power of -1.00 D. As with the above example, if the patient required a -1.00 D correction with the 45.00 D base curve lens on the eye, the contact lens would have to be plano.

To more conveniently convert the back central radius of the contact lens to diopters, a table can be used (see Appendix I). It must be remembered that this is not the actual dioptric power of the back surface of the contact lens because the index of 1.3375 is used. The actual contact lens index is higher depending on the material used (1.49 for PMMA, for example).

For example, when the contact lens base curve radius is the same as the corneal radius (the cornea is 46.00 D and the lens back surface is 46.00 D), the lacrimal lens power is zero. Therefore, to obtain a correction of -1.00 D the contact lens must have a -1.00 D power as measured with the lensometer.

The third situation would be to fit this patient (a 1.00 D myope) with a contact lens that has a 47.00 D (7.18 mm) base curve. The lens would be 1.00 D steeper than the cornea (47.00 vs. 46.00 D). The lacrimal lens will have a $+1.00$ D power; therefore, to fit this patient properly, the contact lens must have a -2.00 D power, -1.00 to compensate for the $+1.00$ D lacrimal lens plus another -1.00 for the patient's myopia.

It can be readily seen that the power of a contact lens may not be the same as the patient's spectacle prescription. By knowing the patient's spectacle prescription, the patient's K-reading, and the way the contact lens is fitted (base curve radius), the power that must be ordered in the contact lens can be determined.

Another clinical situation involves the need for additional power added to a diagnostic lens used in fitting or a lens the patient has been wearing. For example, the patient is wearing a − 3.00 D contact lens and, on evaluation of the patient's vision with the lens in place, it is found that an additional − 0.50 D (the overrefraction) is required to give the patient the best visual acuity. In this case, if the same base curve radius lens is to be used, a − 3.50 D lens would be ordered for the patient.

What happens in the above case if the base curve radius is changed in order to improve the lens fit? For example, the original lens on the patient's eye has a 7.85 mm radius (43.00 D). It is decided to order the new lens with a 7.67 mm radius (44.00 D). The new lens will be 1.00 D steeper than the first lens, giving a lacrimal lens change of + 1.00 D (the difference between the 43.00 and 44.00 D). Now, in addition to the − 3.00 D in the original lens and the − 0.50 D overrefraction, an additional − 1.00 D is required for maximum visual acuity. Therefore, a − 4.50 D lens with a 44.00 D (7.67 mm) base curve must be ordered for the patient. This can be summarized as

original lens:	− 3.00 D
over-refraction:	− 0.50 D
lacrimal lens compensation:	− 1.00 D
New lens power:	− 4.50 D

The opposite effect applies if the base curve radius is flattened. For example, if the patient has a 7.85 mm radius (43.00 D), − 3.00 D lens on the eye with − 0.50 D overrefraction and it is decided to fit 8.04 mm radius (42.00 D) lens, an appropriate power compensation must be made. In this situation, the second lens will be 1.00 D flatter than the original.

The change in lacrimal lens power would be − 1.00 D; therefore, the power required for the 42.00 D base curve lens is − 2.50 D. This can be summarized as

original lens:	− 3.00 D
over-refraction:	− 0.50 D
lacrimal lens compensation:	+ 1.00 D
New lens power:	− 2.50 D

From the above examples it can be seen that the lens power required can be determined by placing a contact lens on the eye and refracting over it (called over refraction). With this procedure, the curvature of the cornea does not need to be known and is not used in the calculations. The spectacle correction is likewise not used.

There are two methods of determining the lens power to be ordered—spectacle prescription–corneal curvature–lens base curve method and the diagnostic lens–overrefraction procedure. Both should agree very closely. If both ways are evaluated during a contact lens fitting but do not agree, an error was probably made in one of the tests. By using both techniques, mistakes can be detected before an improper lens is ordered.

SPHERICAL RIGID LENS ON A TORIC CORNEA

As many as 85 percent of patients will have some degree of corneal toricity and astigmatism. This slightly complicates the optical situation when a rigid, spherical contact lens is placed on the cornea. The power of the lacrimal lens will be a cylindrical power. This is easily handled by considering each major meridian separately.

For example where the patient's K-reading is 43.00 D in the 180-degree (horizontal) meridian and 44.00 D in the 90-degree (vertical) meridian. This is commonly called with-the-rule corneal toricity (the horizontal meridian is flatter than the vertical). If this patient needs a spectacle correction of $-2.00 -1.00 \times 180$ and a 43.00 D (7.85 mm) base curve lens is to be fitted, what contact lens power will be required? The same procedure, as previously outlined, can be followed, but must be calculated separately for each major meridian. In the horizontal 180° meridian, the patient needs -2.00 D. The lens base curve (43.00 D) is the same as the corneal curvature in the horizontal meridian; thus, the lacrimal lens power is zero. Therefore, the power needed in the horizontal meridian of the contact lens is -2.00 D. In the vertical (90-degree) meridian, the patient requires -3.00 D (the power of a cylinder prescription is 90 degrees away from its axis). Thus, the power in the meridian 90 degrees from the cylinder axis is the sum of the prescriptions, the spherical and cylinder components, -2.00 D sphere in this example plus the cylinder power, -1.00 D. The power along the prescription axis (180° meridian in this example) is only the spherical component, a -2.00 D sphere. In the vertical meridian the contact lens base curve (43.00 D) is one diopter flatter than the cornea (44.00 D), so the lacrimal lens in this meridian is -1.00 D (remember, a $+1.00$ D must be used to neutralize this power). Since a total power of -3.00 D is needed in this meridian, the contact lens power must be -2.00 D. Therefore, the contact lens power required fully to correct both meridians is the same. This is commonly true because significant amounts of astigmatism are usually due to corneal toricity. Corneal toricity is neutralized by the lacrimal lens created with a rigid spherical base curve. To make power determinations of toric corneas and cylindrical corrections easier, it helps to draw optical crosses and label them appropriately (Figure 3–3). This may be summarized as

	180	90
spectacle prescription:	−2.00	−3.00
lacrimal lens compensation:	0	+1.00
contact lens power:	−2.00	−2.00

Often, a contact lens is fitted so the base curve differs from the corneal curve. In the previous example the 43.00 by 44.00 D cornea can be fitted with a 43.50 D (7.76 mm) base curve lens. In this case the lens is 0.50 D steeper than the cornea in the horizontal meridian, resulting in a +0.50 D lacrimal lens (Figure 3–4). Since a spectacle lens power of −2.00 D is required, the contact lens must be −2.50 D (an additional −0.50 D to compensate for the +0.50 D lacrimal lens plus the −2.00 D spectacle correction). In the vertical meridian, the base curve is 0.50 D flatter than the cornea, giving a −0.50 D lacrimal lens power. The spectacle prescription in this meridian is −3.00 D, so −2.50 D is required in

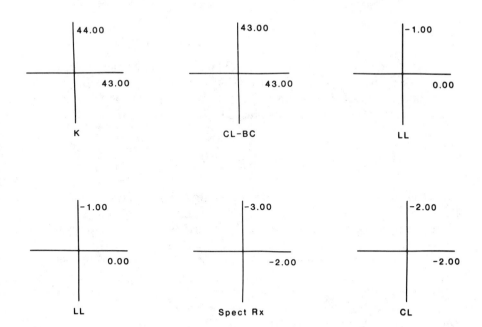

Figure 3–3. Optical crosses used to calculate the required contact lens power (see text). K: keratometer reading; CL–BC: contact lens base curve; LL: lacrimal lens power; CL: contact lens power; spect Rx: spectacle lens power

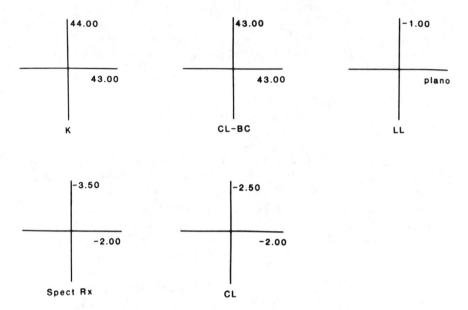

Figure 3–4. Optical crosses used to calculate the required contact lens power (see text)

the contact lens (-0.50 D is obtained from the lacrimal lens). Again, it can be seen that a spherical contact lens will fully correct the patient even though it is steeper than the flattest corneal meridian. A flatter lens would do the same, except less spherical power would be required.

RESIDUAL ASTIGMATISM

In the previous two examples the spectacle cylinder correction equaled the corneal toricity; therefore, a spherical, rigid contact lens alleviated all the astigmatism. In many cases there is at least a small discrepancy between the corneal toricity and the spectacle astigmatism. An example would be where the corneal curvature is 43.00 @ (along the) 180 and 44.00 @ 090. The spectacle correction is $-2.00 - 1.50 \times 180$. If a spherical 43.00 D (7.85 mm) base curve lens is placed on the cornea, there would be no lacrimal lens power in the horizontal meridian. The contact lens power in this meridian should be -2.00 D. In the vertical meridian the lacrimal lens power would be -1.00 D (43.00 D lens on a 44.00 D cornea). The power required in this meridian is -3.50 D (spectacle correction @ 90). The contact lens power required in this meridian is -2.50 D

(Figure 3–5). Now, a − 2.00 D is needed in the horizontal meridian and − 2.50 D in the vertical meridian of the contact lens. In such a situation, a cylindrical contact lens is usually not a practical solution. Instead, a spherical contact is used with a 0.50 DC (diopters of cylinder) remaining uncorrected. For example, a − 2.00 D contact lens may be ordered. If an overrefraction is performed, a − 0.50 DC × 180 will be found. This is called residual astigmatism. A − 2.25 D contact lens could be ordered, resulting in a spherical equivalent prescription (the spherical equivalent is the spherical power resulting from adding one-half the cylinder power to the sphere). It must be remembered that even when the spherical equivalent power is used, the cylindrical error is still present. If the − 2.25 D lens were used, an examination with the lens in place would indicate a + 0.25 − 0.50 × 180 refractive finding. Note the − 0.50 D.C. × 180 is still present.

It is also helpful to be able to predict the expected amount of residual astigmatism. This helps counsel the patient as to potential success with contact lenses. It also helps in the decision as to which type of lens to place on the patient first. A spherical, rigid contact lens placed on a toric cornea will correct an astigmatic error (spectacle astigmatism) equal to the amount of corneal cylinder. For example, the cornea may have one

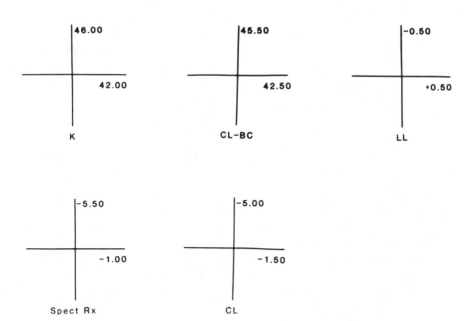

Figure 3–5.   Optical crosses used to calculate the required contact lens power (see text)

diopter of toricity, 45.00 D @ 180 and 46.00 D @ 090, and a spectacle correction of plano -1.00×180. In this case, there is one diopter corneal cylinder and the same amount spectacle cylinder at the same axis; therefore, no residual astigmatism. A 45.00 D spherical cornea with a plano -1.00×180 spectacle correction gives a different result, however. With no corneal toricity none of the required spectacle cylinder will be compensated, so there will be -1.00×180 of residual astigmatism. This is the calculated or predicted residual astigmatism. In some cases, it can be slightly different from the measured residual astigmatism.

The calculated residual astigmatism can be determined by using the above reasoning or it can be determined by formula. The formula is: residual astigmatism (RA) equals the spectacle cylinder (SC) minus the corneal cylinder (CC) or RA = SC − CC. For example, if the cornea is 45.00 @ 180 and 46.00 @ 090 with a spectacle correction of plano -1.00×180, then RA = $(-1.00 \times 180) - (-1.00 \times 180) = (-1.00 \times 180) + (+1.00 \times 180) = 0.0$

Another example would be a corneal toricity (K-readings) of 44.00 @ 180 and 44.75 @ 090 with a spectacle cylinder of -1.25×180. Then, RA = $(-1.25 \times 180) - (-0.75 \times 180) = (-1.25 \times 180) + (+0.75 \times 180) = -0.50 \times 180$.

SEMI-FLEXIBLE LENSES

The above calculations hold true for lenses that do not flex or bend on the cornea. If the lens does bend, this must be taken into account. Very thin lenses of PMMA or other normally rigid lenses will flex partially to take the shape of the toric cornea. When this happens, both the front and back surface of the lens bends, but since there is air in front of the contact lens and tears behind, a cylindrical correction is created. The amount of cylinder introduced can be determined by using the keratometer to measure the bending of the front surface of the lens while it is on the eye.

A cornea is 42.00 D @ 180 and 44.00 D @ 090 and the spectacle correction is plano -2.00×180. With a lens that does not flex on the eye, there would be no residual astigmatism. If, however, it does flex, say 0.50 D, which would be in the same direction as the corneal toricity, the result would be -0.50×180. A 0.50 D residual astigmatism would be created. In this case, the flexing of the lens is detrimental to a good optical correction. In some cases it can be an advantage, however. For example, in the above case, if the spectacle correction were a -1.50 D.C. $\times$ 180 (instead of -2.00 D.C. $\times$ 180), the residual astigmatism, with a nonflexing lens, would be -0.50×90 (or $+0.50 \times 180$, which is the same but in plus cylinder form. When the lens flexes, however, the -0.50 D $\times$ 180 compensates for the $+0.50 \times 180$ present without flexing, thus fully correcting the patient. As can be seen, lens flexing can be an advantage or disadvantage depending on the optical situation.

HYDROGEL AND OTHER VERY FLEXIBLE LENSES

When a very soft and flexible lens, such as the hydrogel lens, is placed on a cornea, it will usually conform to the shape of the cornea. There is only a very thin tear layer under the lens that has no power. In this case, there is no lacrimal lens power. Thus, a -3.00 D soft lens can be placed on an eye with a corneal curvature of 42.00 @ 180 and 43.00 @ 90 and a spectacle correction of $-3.00-1.00 \times 180$. The expected residual astigmatism would be -1.00×180 since none of the cylinder is corrected because no lacrimal lens exists.

Spherical hydrogel lenses are best used on patients with little or no spectacle cylinder. Most patients have no difficulty if a half- (0.50) diopter of residual astigmatism is present. Many find no problem with as much as three-quarters diopter. If there is 1 diopter or more, however, many patients will complain of blurred vision and/or eyestrain and headaches while reading.

An example of a situation where a spherical hydrogel lens results in better optical correction than a spherical rigid lens is where there is corneal toricity and a spherical spectacle correction. If the cornea is 42.00 @ 180 and 43.00 @ 90 with a spectacle correction of -3.00 D sphere, there would be 1.00 diopter of residual astigmatism with a rigid lens but none with the soft lens.

CYLINDRICAL CORRECTION

In order to compensate residual astigmatism, a cylindrical contact lens may be used. If a spherical base curve is used (as is usually done with less than 2.00 diopters of corneal toricity when rigid lenses are fitted) prism is added to prevent lens rotation. Then the cylinder correction is ground on the front surface of the lens. When a cylinder is put on the lens front surface, it is a plus cylinder. Some laboratories prefer that when such a lens is ordered the prescription be written in plus cylinder notation. This is accomplished by adding the cylinder power to the sphere, changing the sign of the cylinder and then changing the axis of the cylinder by 90 degrees. This process is called transposing. For example, $-1.00 -2.00 \times 180$ becomes $-3.00 +2.00 \times 90$.

With soft lenses, prism ballast-cylindrical lenses may be made with either front or back surface torics. Optically, it does not make much difference because the lenses flex on the eye.

TORIC BASE CURVE LENSES

In some cases, where there is considerable corneal toricity (at least 2.00 D or more), a toric base curve rigid lens is fitted. In this case, the lens power must be determined in each meridian. For example, if the corneal curvature is 44.00 @ 180 and 47.00 @ 090 with a spectacle correction of −1.25 −3.00 × 180 and a contact lens with base curve radii of 7.66 mm (44.00 D) and 7.18 mm (47.00 D), the lens power must be calculated. For the horizontal meridian, the spectacle lens power is −1.25 D and the lacrimal lens power is plano (44.00 D lens base curve). The flat meridian of the lens will align with the flat meridian of cornea, as will the steep lens meridian with the steep corneal meridian. This is like putting a saddle on a horse: it will not position sideways. Thus, in the above example a −1.25 D power is required in the 44.00 D meridian. In the vertical meridian, both the lens and cornea have curvatures of 47.00 D giving a plano lacrimal lens. The contact lens thus requires a −4.25 D power in this meridian. In order for the laboratory to fabricate the 44.00/47.00 base curve and the −1.25/−4.25 lens a toric front surface is required— that is, a bitoric lens.

Another example would be a corneal curvature of 42.00 @ 180 and 46.00 @ 90 and a spectacle correction of −1.00 −4.50 × 180. If the eye was fitted with a 42.50/45.50 base curve lens the lacrimal lens power in the horizontal meridian is +0.50 D (42.00 D cornea and 42.50 D lens base curve). Since the spectacle correction is −1.00 D, a −1.50 D power will be required in the horizontal meridian of the lens. In the vertical meridian the lens, 45.50 D base curve, is 0.50 D flatter than the cornea (46.00 D); thus, the lacrimal lens is −0.50 D. Since the spectacle power in this meridian is −5.50 D, the contact lens power must be −5.00 D to give maximum vision. It makes it much easier and avoids confusion with powers and radii if the optical cross is used.

Another method of determining lens power is to place a diagnostic contact lens on the eye, either spherical or toric, and overrefracting. Then, by adding the lens power, overrefraction power, and any change in lacrimal lens power, the required prescription for the final lens can be determined. This is the same procedure as for spherical lenses on spherical corneas, except that it is calculated for each major meridian. The important thing to remember with toric lenses is that they are no more complicated than spherical lenses. Treat each meridian as a separate lens.

VERTEX DISTANCE

When a patient wears spectacles to alleviate ametropia, the lenses are usually 9 to 15 mm in front of the corneal apex. This separation is called the vertex distance. A contact lens is positioned at the corneal apex. The effective power of the prescription required changes with the position of the lens in front of the eye. With lenses below ±4.00 D, the change in power between spectacle and corneal plane is clinically insignificant. Compensation in power is needed, however, if greater than 4.00 D in the spectacle plane (see Appendix II).

This clinically important optical principle is easily understood through the relationship of the secondary focal point of the correcting lens with respect to the far point of the eye. This is a point in space for which the eye is correctly focused when accommodation is completely relaxed (Figure 3–6). The secondary focal point of the correcting lens must therefore fall at the far point of the patient's eye to correct a re-

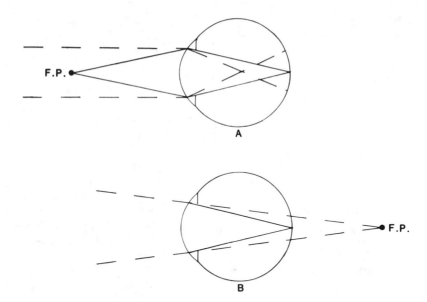

Figure 3–6. (a) Far point (FP) of a myopic eye is in front of the eye. Light rays emitting from this point (solid lines) will be in focus on the retina. Light rays from a distant object (dotted lines) focus in front of the retina, giving a blurred image on the retina. This is true when no correcting lens is used. (b) Far point of a hyperopic eye is behind the eye. Light rays directed toward this point (solid lines) are bent by the eye and focus on the retina. Light rays from a distant object focus toward this point and give a blurred retinal image when no correcting lens is used

fractive error. In this case of the hyperope this is behind the eye, at infinity for the emmetrope, and in front of the eye for the myope.

For example, if a patient requires a +15.00 D spectacle correction positioned 12 mm in front of the croneal apex, what power is needed at the cornea? From Figure 3–7, it can be seen that the secondary focal point of the spectacle lens falls 6.667 cm behind the corneal apex (f = 1/F, where f is in meters and F in diopters) or at the far point of the eye. Since a contact lens will be positioned at the corneal apex, its secondary focal length will have to be shorter than when the lens is in the spectacle plane (by 12 mm in this case) if the secondary focal point of the lens is to remain at the far point of the eye. Thus, the secondary focal length of the contact lens must be 5.467 cm, which when converted to diopters $\frac{1.0}{0.05467}$ is +18.29 D. With a difference of 3.29 D in this case, it can be seen that the vertex distance can be very significant. Figure 3–7 shows that if the spectacle lens is moved back to the cornea without a change in power, the secondary focal point will no longer fall at the far point of the eye.

In the case of the myopic patient, the far point of the eye falls in front of the cornea (Figure 3–8). For example, if a patient requires a −10.00 D spectacle lens at a vertex distance of 12 mm, the far point of the eye is 11.2 cm in front of the corneal apex. If the lens is moved back to the cornea, the secondary focal length must be 11.2 cm, or the power −8.93 D instead of −10.00 D.

With high plus corrections the contact lens must have a higher

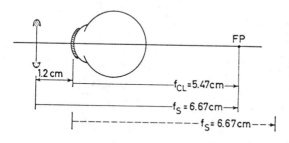

Figure 3–7. A +15.00 DS spectacle lens at a vertex distance of 1.2 cm and then on the cornea. FP: far point of the eye; f_s: focal length of the spectacle lens; f_{cl}: focal length of the contact lens

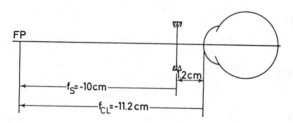

Figure 3–8. A −10.00 D spectacle lens at a vertex distance of 1.2 cm and then on the cornea

dioptric power than the spectacle lens, whereas minus corrections will have a lower dioptric value.

In high astigmatic corrections the effect of vertex distance must be taken into account for each meridian. This means that the same cylinder correction will not be required at the cornea as in the spectacle plane. Assume a lens of $+14.00 -5.00 \times 180$ in the spectacle plane and a vertex distance 12 mm. With this example, the $+14.00$ D in the 180 meridian moved to the cornea results in a power of $+16.83$ D. In the other meridian the $+9.00$ D at the spectacle plane calls for a $+10.09$ D at the cornea. Thus, the cylinder needed at the cornea is 6.74 D and not 5.00 D as in the spectacle plane.

The effect of vertex distance changes can be calculated using the following formula:

$$F_c = \frac{F_s}{1 - dF_s}$$

where:

F_c = power at cornea in diopters
F_s = power of spectacle correction in diopters
d = vertex distance in meters.

Confusion may be prevented if the principle is understood, rather than relying on the formula.

ACCOMMODATION

When a young individual focuses from a distant object to one up close, the ciliary muscle in the eye contracts, changing the shape of the crystalline lens to give a clear image of the near object. This is called accommodation. With increasing age, the ability to accommodate is gradually lost until objects at the reading distance cannot be focused easily (called presbyopia). This usually occurs around the age of 40 to 45 years. Because of the optics involved, a myope does not have to accommodate as much to focus a near object as a patient who does not need a spectacle correction or a hyperope. Therefore, the spectacle-corrected myope can usually delay the need for a bifocal for near tasks longer than the spectacle-wearing hyperope. The opposite is true of these individuals corrected with contact lenses. A myope will need more accommodation to focus a near object when wearing contact lenses than when wearing spectacles. The higher the correction, the greater the difference in accommodation.

The changes in accommodative requirements become particularly important when a patient is first fitted with contact lenses at about the age of 40. A relatively high myope may have no problems reading with spectacles. As soon as contact lenses are fitted, however, difficulty with close work may occur. On the other hand, a relatively high hyperopic patient may be able to delay the need for a bifocal correction with contact lenses longer than with a spectacle correction.

OTHER OPTICAL PROPERTIES

There are several differences in optical characteristics between spectacles and contact lenses. One difference is in the magnification of objects. A minus prescription makes objects in the field of view appear smaller. This is called minification. The change in the minification is less with contact lenses than with spectacle lenses because the contact lens is on the eye. For the hyperope, objects will appear larger with spectacles than with contact lenses (magnification). The effect is greater with higher prescriptions. The magnification effect is quite important with the aphakic patient because high plus prescription spectacle lenses greatly magnify. This makes it difficult for patients to move about in their environment without considerable adaptation. With contact lenses, however, the objects are not greatly magnified. Thus, there is a great advantage for the aphakic patient to have contact lenses.

The field of view is quite different for spectacles and contact lenses. With spectacles the frames and edge of the lenses limit the field of vision. In addition, magnification effects and decrease in quality of the spectacle lens optics in the periphery decrease the field of view. With contact lenses, the patient is using at all times the central part of the lens because the lens moves with the eye. Thus, the edge of the lens does not limit the field and peripheral lens aberrations do not affect vision as greatly as with spectacles.

SAMPLE PROBLEMS

1. The radius of the cornea is 7.50 mm. What is the dioptric power?
2. The K-reading of a cornea is 44.50 D. What is the radius of curvature?
3. A 44.00 D base curve rigid contact lens is placed on a cornea with a 43.50 D curvature. If the patient's spectacle correction is −1.25 D, what power should be ordered in the contact lens?
4. A patient's spectacle correction is +2.50 D and a 45.75 D base curve rigid lens is fitted on the patient's 45.25 D. cornea. What power is required in the contact lens?

5. A patient's spectacle correction is $+1.00$ D and K-reading is 46.25 D. If a rigid contact lens with a base curve of 46.00 D is fitted, what power is needed in the contact lens?

6. A -3.00 D. rigid contact lens with a 44.00 D base curve is placed on a patient's cornea. A refraction over the lens is -0.75 D. The contact lens to be ordered for the patient will have a 44.50 D base curve. What power should be ordered in this lens?

7. A patient's K-readings are 45.00 @ 180, 45.75 @ 90, and spectacle prescription of $-1.50 = -0.75 \times 180$. If a 45.25 D base curve rigid lens is fitted, what power is required? What residual astigmatism is expected?

8. A patient's spectacle refraction is $+2.00 = -1.00 \times 15$ and K-readings of 43.00 @ 15, 44.25 @ 105. If a 43.50 D base curve rigid lens is fitted, what lens power is required? What residual astigmatism is expected?

9. A 42.50 D base curve, -1.75 D rigid contact lens is on a patient's cornea. The overrefraction is $-0.50 = -0.25 \times 90$. If a 42.00 D rigid lens is to be ordered for this patient, what power should be ordered? What is the residual astigmatism?

10. A patient with a 44.50 D cornea with a -1.50 D spectacle correction is to be fitted with a 42.00 D base curve hydrophilic contact lens. What power would be required in the lens and what is the residual astigmatism?

11. A patient with a $+2.00 = -0.50 \times 135$ spectacle correction and a 43.00 @ 45, 43.75 @ 135 cornea is to be fitted with a 40.50 D base curve hydrophilic lens. What power is needed in the hydrophilic lens and what is the expected residual astigmatism?

12. A patient with a -3.50 spectacle correction and 46.00 @ 180, 47.00 @ 090 cornea is fitted with a 44.00 D base curve hydrophilic lens. What power is needed and what astigmatism is expected with the hydrophilic lens?

13. What if the patient in question 12 is fitted with a 46.25 D base curve rigid contact lens? What power would be needed and what residual astigmatism would be expected?

14. A patient has a 41.00 D base curve, -2.75 D. hydrophilic lens on and an overrefraction shows -0.50 D. $= -0.25 \times 180$. If a new hydrophilic lens with a base curve of 41.50 D is ordered for the patient, what power is needed and what residual astigmatism is expected?

15. A patient has K-readings of 41.00 @ 180; 44.00 @ 090, a spectacle correction of $+1.00 = -3.00 \times 180$, and is fitted with a rigid toric base curve lens of 8.13/7.67 (41.50/44.00). What power is required in the lens?

16. A patient has a spherical, rigid contact lens on the eye. The lens has a base curve of 7.58 mm (44.50 D) and has a power of −3.00 D. The overrefraction is +0.50 D = −1.00 × 90. If a 43.00/46.00 D base curve lens is to be fitted on this patient who has a highly with-the-rule toric cornea, what lens power is required?

17. A patient has a spectacle refraction of +12.50 D and the vertex distance is 13 mm. What power would this be at the corneal apex?

18. What is the prescription at the corneal plane if the spectacle correction is −10.00 = −5.00 × 180 and the vertex distance is 12 mm?

19. What is the following prescription written in plus cylinder form? −2.00 = −1.75 × 25.

Answers to Sample Problems

1. $F = \dfrac{1.3375 - 1.00}{0.0075} = 45.00$ D.

2. $r = \dfrac{1.3375 - 1.00}{44.50} = 0.00758$ m or 7.58 mm.

3. −1.75 D.
4. +2.00 D.
5. +0.75 D.
6. −4.25 D.
7. −1.75 D., no residual astigmatism.
8. +1.50 D., +0.25 × 15 or −0.25 × 105 residual astigmatism
9. −1.75 D., −0.25 × 90 residual astigmatism.
10. −1.50 D., no residual.
11. +2.00 D or +1.75 D if spherical equivalent is used. Residual astigmatism is −0.50 × 135.
12. −3.50 D., no residual astigmatism.
13. −3.75 D power or −4.25 D power if the spherical equivalent is used. The residual astigmatism is +1.00 × 180 or −1.00 × 90.
14. −3.25 power is needed (no lacrimal lens is present with the hydrophilic lens). The residual astigmatism is −0.25 × 180.
15. +0.50 D./−2.00 D.
16. −2.00/−4.00 D.
17. +15.00 D.
18. −9.00 = −3.75 × 180.
19. −3.75 = +1.75 × 115.

4

ANATOMY AND PHYSIOLOGY AS RELATED TO CONTACT LENS WEAR

A basic knowledge of the eye and its surrounding structures (adnexa) is required to understand the fitting, adaptation, and problems that occur with contact lens wear. To communicate with patients, it is important to understand the basic terminology and structural relationships as there are many misconceptions about the eye and vision. The assistant or technician has the unique opportunity to educate the patient about the eye.

The eye and surrounding structures are anatomically and physiologically complicated. In this chapter only some of the more common and important aspects will be covered. For more detailed ocular anatomy and physiology, books devoted to the topics can be consulted (1–4).

EYELIDS

The eyelids are important in protecting the eye. They act to keep foreign bodies out and the eye moist. The action of the lids causes tears to spread over the cornea, keeping it moist. If the cornea dries, discomfort results. Patients with lid injuries (lids are damaged and scarred) can lose vision from a secondary corneal scarring. Special contact lenses are often fitted just for protection of the eyes.

The eyelids are important in contact lens wear as they affect the wettability of the lens surface and also play a role in positioning the lens. Lid margins are quite sensitive and cause most of the discomfort when a contact lens is first placed on the eye. This is easily demonstrated by holding the lids open. The patient will usually not feel the lens. With repeated blinking over the lens edge, the lid sensitivity is decreased, with resultant comfort. This decrease in sensitivity usually occurs with several days of wear.

The outer layer of the lid consists of keratinized epithelial cells. This layer ends at the lid margin near the opening of the meibomian glands (Figure 4–1). This is the junction of the dry and moist portions of the lids. The eyelashes are two or three rows of hairs near the lid margins. The lashes are commonly darker than the hair on the head and normally do not turn gray like the hair with age. A lash will regrow in about 10 weeks

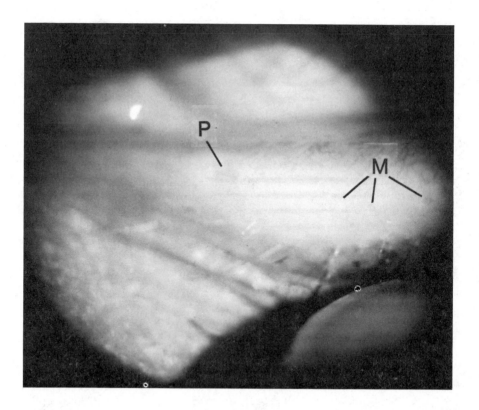

Figure 4–1. Lid margin showing the meibomian gland openings (M), puncta (P), and eyelashes

after removal. Its normal life is about 5 months. The skin at the root of the lashes has a rich nerve supply, and thus is very sensitive to any disturbance of the lashes.

Below the very thin layer of the lid's skin is a loose connective tissue layer. With injury this layer easily fills with blood (the "black eye") and fluid, which causes edema. Below this layer is a layer of muscle that causes closure of the eyelids. Behind the muscle is another layer of loose connective tissue. The next layer is a relatively stiff layer of fibrous tissue called the tarsal plates. These plates give the lid its stiffness. When the upper lid is everted to view the underside, the lid folds at the top of the tarsal plate (see Chapter 5). The meibomian glands are within the tarsal plates. There are about 25 meibomian glands in the upper tarsal plate and 20 in the lower. When the lid is everted, these glands can sometimes be seen as long, yellowish, vertical lines. They secrete a sebaceous material which is formed by the cells rupturing in the glands. This secretion is expelled through the glands on the lid margins. The openings of these glands can be seen as small spots along the margins (Figure 4–1). Sometimes a build-up of the sebaceous material can be seen at the opening of the glands (Figure 4–2). These glands can become plugged or infected, resulting in swelling. If the swelling occurs fairly rapidly (called acute) and is painful, this is an internal hordeolum. Irritation of the lids may initiate this. Warm compresses used for 10 to 15 minutes several times a day should clear the glands in a couple of days. If not, medical treatment may be necessary. If the gland gradually becomes swollen over a period of weeks without significant inflammation, it is called a chalazion. There

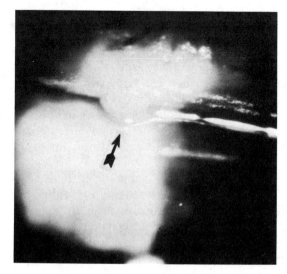

Figure 4–2. Build-up of se-beacous material at the opening of a meibomian gland

is not an effective treatment for this except surgical removal if it is large enough to be a cosmetic problem.

Occasionally, with contact lens wear these meibomian glands become engorged. Expression of the glands (squeezing material out of the glands) in such cases can improve the tolerance to contact lenses.

Another related lid problem is the external hordeolum or sty. This is an infection of the glands associated with the lashes. A sty, like the internal hordeolum, can be painful. The treatment is the same.

In addition to the openings of the glands along the lid margins, there is the punctum, a hole near the nasal side of each lid margin (Figure 4–1). Puncta, one each in the upper and lower lids, are where the tears flow from the eye through tubelike structures (lacrimal canals) into the nose.

The innermost layer of the lid, that surface against the eye, is called the palpebral conjunctiva. This is a thin, transparent tissue with a rich blood vessel supply. The blood supply gives the conjunctiva its reddish appearance. The palpebral conjunctiva folds over (point of fold is called the fornix) and is continuous with the bulbar conjunctiva, which covers the sclera. The fold from the lids to the eye forms what is called the cul-de-sac. The lower cul-de-sac is shallow and can be easily visualized by pulling the lower lid down (Figure 4–3). The upper cul-de-sac is deeper and not as easily seen. These folds keep any foreign bodies, including contact lenses, from getting behind the eye. Many new or prospective patients need to be reassured that a contact cannot be lost behind the eye.

TEAR FILM

The tear film is a thin, liquid layer that is essential in maintaining the cornea's optical quality as well as the health of the cornea and conjunctiva. If there is insufficient tear flow, the cornea can dry, resulting in its becoming rough and opaque (Figure 4–4). Milder areas of drying due to insufficient tearing or insufficient spreading of tears over the eye will result in epithelial damage. Epithelial cells of the cornea can rupture. When this occurs, the dye fluorescein can be absorbed into the tissue staining it.

Even though the tear film is very thin, it is composed of three basic layers (Figure 4–5). The outermost layer, exposed to the air, is called the oily or lipid layer, the middle layer is called the aqueous or lacrimal layer, and the innermost layer against the cornea is the mucoid layer. The outer lipid layer is formed by secretion of the meibomian glands. This lipid (fatty) material forms a very thin layer over the whole free surface of the

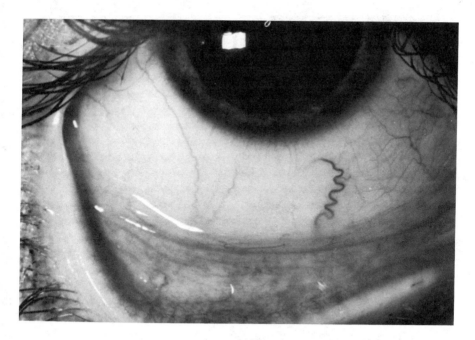

Figure 4–3.   View of the lower cul-de-sac

tear film. This material can sometimes be seen secreting from the gland openings and spreading over the tears.

The lipid layer slows evaporation of the tear film. Without it, rapid tear evaporation causes dry areas on the cornea and can result in discomfort and corneal damage. The lipid layer also helps prevent the tears from spilling onto the lids.

The central aqueous layer of the tear film makes up the majority of the thickness of the 7μm (0.0028 inch) thick layer. Under normal conditions, the major portion of this layer is produced by the accessory lacrimal glands (glands of Krause and Wolfring). They are in the palpebral conjunctiva. When there is excessive tearing, as with irritation of the eye, for example, or the placement of a contact lens or psychogenic crying, the aqueous portion of the tear layer is produced by the lacrimal gland in the upper, temporal portion of the upper cul-de-sac. In some individuals this gland can be seen on lid eversion as a soft, fleshy mass.

The aqueous layer of the tear film is mostly water (98.2 percent), but also has ions and other molecules. Sodium and potassium ions along with the protein concentration are important in controlling the osmolarity or tonicity of the tear film. If the concentration of these molecules is decreased, the tears become hypotonic and water flows into the cornea,

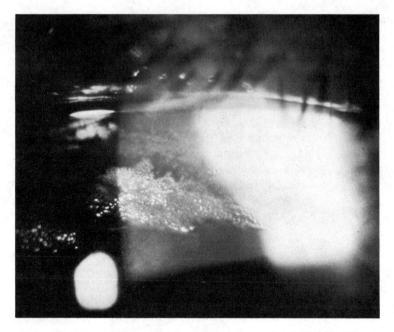

Figure 4–4.   A nonwetting, rough area of the cornea due to holding the eye open several minutes

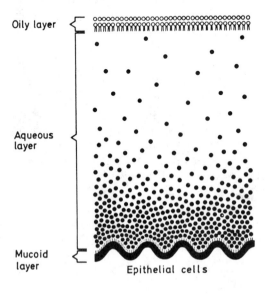

Oily layer

Aqueous layer

Mucoid layer

Epithelial cells

Figure 4–5.   Diagram of the tear film indicating the three basic layers

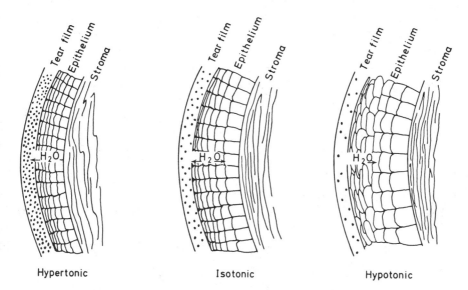

Figure 4-6. Effect of the tonicity of the tear film on water flow between the tears and corneal epithelium

causing the cornea to swell (Figure 4-6). This occurs, for example, with swimming when the individual opens the eyes under water. The water does not have many ions and is thus very hypotonic. Water then moves into the cornea, causing it to swell slightly, giving the person blurred or cloudy vision. The same thing happens to a lesser extent with excessive tearing. When tearing, normal evaporation does not occur and the tear film becomes hypotonic allowing slight swelling of the cornea. With normal tonicity of the cornea, called an isotonic tear film, an equal amount of water flows into and out of the cornea, keeping it at a normal thickness. An isotonic tear film has a tonicity equivalent of a 0.9 to 1.0 percent sodium chloride solution. A 0.9 percent solution is often called isotonic saline. A higher salt concentration solution (hypertonic), say 2 to 5 percent, placed on the cornea will draw water out causing a thinning of the tissue. This or other hypertonic solutions can be used on a swollen cornea to make it thin to a normal level.

Bicarbonate ions are also in the tears and act to keep the pH of the tears at the normal level (about 7.35). They keep the tears from becoming too acidic or too basic. This action is called a buffer and tends to neutralize chemicals, such as contact lens solutions, which may get into the eye.

The aqueous tear layer also contains proteins such as albumin, globulins, lysozyme, and enzymes, which are important for the functioning of the cornea. Other chemicals acting as nutrients, as well as waste products of metabolism, are also present. This layer acts as the main vehicle of exchange of materials across the corneal surface and in protection of the cornea.

The mucoid layer is immediately against the corneal and conjunctival epithelial cells. This layer is produced by goblet cells in the conjunctiva. The cells form and produce the mucoid material and then rupture onto the conjunctival surface. The lids spread the mucoid material over the conjunctiva and cornea. This material will attach to the lipid, hydrophobic surfaces of the epithelial cells and allow the aqueous layer to form. Without the mucoid layer, the tear film will break up very rapidly, resulting in drying and damage to the cornea. The time it takes from a blink until the tear film begins to break up (becomes discontinuous) is called the tear break-up time or BUT. A BUT of less than 5 to 10 seconds is abnormal. This can be measured clinically and will be discussed in the next chapter. Damage to the conjunctiva, as with chemical burns or vitamin deficiencies, will cause a short BUT. Lid deformities and incomplete blinking will result in a break-up of the tear film and corneal drying.

TEAR FLOW

The tears produced by the lacrimal and accessory lacrimal glands enter the eye in the superior cul-de-sac. The tears can be lost by evaporation into the air even with an adequate lipid layer and by absorption into the conjunctiva. A portion of the tears flow over the eye and around the cul-de-sac with the blinking action of the lids. The tears exit through the puncta into the nasolacrimal duct, which empties into the nasal cavity. The tears flow along the marginal tear strip, also called the tear prism, which forms along the point of contact between the lid margin and the eye (Figure 4–7). If the tear prism is viewed with magnification, small debris can be seen to move with a blink, but remain stationary between blinks. The same is true with the thin tear film over the cornea. The only time there is tear flow is with blinking, except when there is excessive reflex tearing. If the muscles that cause blinking are paralyzed, tears flow out over the lids (called epiphora) even when the puncta are open.

There is normally a flow of about 1 μl/minute (1 μl = one cubic mm) with about 7 μl of tears in the eye at one time. The cul-de-sac can hold about 24 μl maximum with excessive tearing. The turnover rate for the tears is about 5 to 6 minutes.

CORNEA

The cornea is a transparent tissue without blood vessels and forms the anterior refracting surface of the eye. It is of utmost importance to the

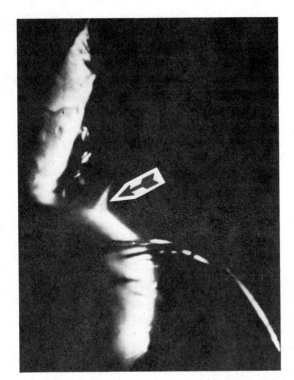

Figure 4–7. Tear prism formed along the lower lid margin

contact lens practitioner as the contact lens rests on this tissue. Ideally, a contact lens should not change the cornea's shape or metabolism since this could result in discomfort, damage, or decreased vision.

The cornea's shape (curvature or topography) is important since a contact lens must be fitted to this surface. Normally, it is not spherical from edge to edge. The radius of the cornea becomes longer (flatter) toward the periphery, giving an aspherical shape approximating an ellipse. There is considerable variation in shape between individuals and even between different meridians of the same eye (Figure 4–8). The central part of the cornea often approximates a sphere and is called the optic cap. The steepest point on the cornea is called the corneal apex. This may be in the center of the cornea or displaced from the center. A displaced apex can result in a poorly centered contact lens since a lens will usually center on the corneal apex.

The average central thickness of the cornea is 0.52 mm, increasing to about 0.65 mm at the limbus, the junction between the transparent cornea and the opaque sclera. There is considerable individual variation

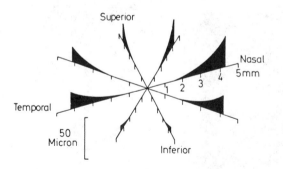

Figure 4–8. Mean corneal asphericities. The black curves indicate the variation from a spherical curve in each meridian (after Clark [5])

from these average values. Viewing the cornea from the front, it has an elliptical shape with an average horizontal diameter of 11.7 mm and 10.6 mm vertically. The normal range of horizontal diameters for corneas is 11.0 to 12.5 mm. When viewed from the back, the cornea is round and averages 11.7 mm. An extension of the scleral from the top and bottom of the cornea results in the smaller vertical dimension when viewed from the front. The clinically measured corneal dimension is often referred to as the visible iris diameter (VID) because the colored iris behind the cornea is used to gauge corneal diameter.

The cornea is composed of five basic layers. The epithelium is outermost, Bowman's layer next, then the stroma, Descemet's membrane, and the innermost layer, the endothelium (Figure 4–9).

CORNEAL EPITHELIUM

The epithelial layer is exposed to the tears. It is about five cell layers thick (0.05 mm or 50 μm) and makes up approximately 10 percent of the corneal thickness. The two surface cell layers are fairly large, thin cells called squamous cells (Figure 4–10). The cell surfaces have little projections called microvilli. These cells are continuously dying and sloughed off into the tear film. They are not as active metabolically as the deeper cells. The next two cell layers are called wing cells. They migrate up from the deepest layer and are metabolically active. The deepest layer is made up of columnar shaped cells called basal cells. These are the most active cells. In this layer, cells divide (called mitosis) and then migrate toward the surface. These cells also secrete a very thin membrane that lies between them and Bowman's layer. This basement membrane holds the epithelium tightly attached to Bowman's layer. If this membrane is damaged as when the eye is scratched, it will only be replaced slowly. The epithelium above the damaged area is easily pulled off by the action of

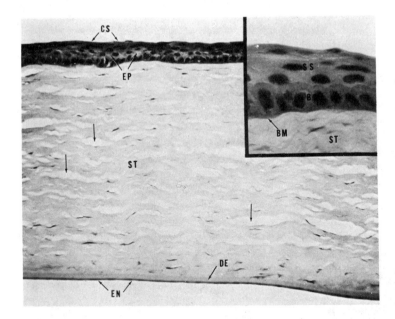

Figure 4-9. Cross-section of the cornea with the cornea surface (CS), epithelium (EP), stroma (ST), Descemet's membrane (DE), and endothelium (EN) indicated. The insert shows squamous cells (SS), basal cells (BC), and basement membrane (BM) of the corena (from Rengstorff, Sim, and Petrali by courtesy of the editor of Military Med 136:146, 1971)

the lid until the membrane is replaced. This is called a recurrent erosion. It is usually painful and commonly occurs in the morning on awakening. Sometimes solutions are used in the eye to keep the surface moist or soft contact lenses are fitted to protect the area from the lid action.

The epithelium does not allow water and other aqueous materials to pass easily. Cell membranes are a lipid material. They repel water and are very tightly attached to each other by small attachments called desmosomes. Cell membranes of adjacent cells are also interwoven. Thus, when an aqueous solution like the dye fluorescein is used to inspect the corneal surface for damage it stays in the tear film and does not penetrate healthy epithelium. When the dye enters the epithelium, it is called staining. If a particle has scratched the cornea or it has been scraped, there is an abrasion; thus, the epithelium will stain.

The epithelium has a remarkable ability to heal after being scratched. Usually within hours the scratched area is covered by surrounding epithelium cells, and within a day there is no sign of the abra-

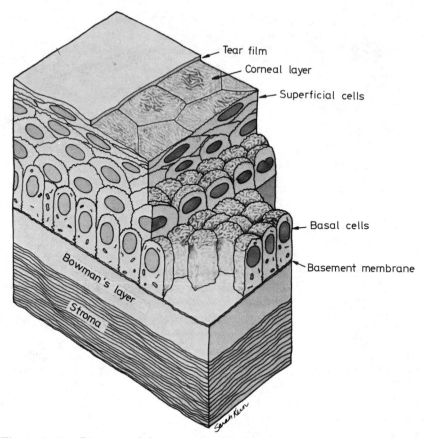

Figure 4-10. Diagram of the corneal epithelium

sion. The epithelium is thus quickly replaced and does not scar. In normally healthy epithelium the cells migrate from the basal layer and are sloughed off into the tear film in about 7 days.

BOWMAN'S LAYER

Bowman's layer is a modification of the underlying stroma and is only about 8 to 14 μm thick. It is made up of small collagen fibers and mucopolysaccride ground substance. If this layer is damaged as by a scratch or cut, it will not regenerate to its original form, thus scarring will occur.

STROMA

The stroma makes up the major portion of the corneal thickness, accounting for approximately 90 percent. It consists of 200 to 250 layers called lamellae, which lie parallel to the corneal surface. Each of the lamellae is made up of fibrils of the protein collagen surrounded by a viscous substance. There are a few cells, called fibroblasts, which produce the collagen. If the stroma is damaged by injury, scarring will occur and can make the cornea opaque. In addition to injury, long-term swelling or infection may cause blood vessels to invade the stroma. Blood vessels enter to supply oxygen and nutrients and can obscure vision. The growth of new blood vessels into the cornea is called neovascularization.

DESCEMET'S MEMBRANE

Descemet's membrane is the basement membrane of the endothelial cells and is 10 to 12 μm thick. This membrane is very resistant to damage and is elastic.

ENDOTHELIUM

The endothelium is made up of a single layer of relatively large cells. It rests on Descemet's membrane and is bathed in aqueous humor, the fluid in the chamber behind the cornea. This layer is very important in maintaining the normal water content of the stroma and is a very metabolically active layer. If endothelial cells are damaged and lost, surrounding cells spread out and cover the area. If extensive damage occurs, then corneal swelling and loss of corneal transparency results.

CORNEAL METABOLISM

For the cornea to retain its normal transparency and thickness the water content must be maintained at about 78 percent. If it increases from this relatively dehydrated state (often termed deturgescence) in comparison to other tissues, the cornea will become cloudy or opaque. To maintain this water content metabolic activity of the cellular layers, the epithelium and endothelium must be sustained. The endothelium is the most important layer in controlling corneal thickness. If it is damaged or not functioning, the cornea may swell two to three times its normal thickness.

With the endothelium functioning normally but without the activity of the epithelial cells, the cornea will swell only 20 to 30 percent.

Contact lenses tend to have the greatest effect on the epithelial cells. With contact lens wear the corneal thickness can increase 10 to 20 percent. Even though this is not a lot of swelling as compared to the case where the endothelium is damaged, it can cause cloudy vision, discomfort, epithelial abrasion, and general lens intolerance.

The cornea uses glucose as the main source of energy. The glucose reaches the epithelium by diffusion through the cornea from the aqueous humor. Very little glucose is utilized from the tears. The glucose is broken down in the epithelial cells by a complicated enzyme system. If the glucose must be broken down without oxygen present, the end product of the metabolism is lactic acid and 2 units of energy. This is a very inefficient system and the cells do not receive enough energy to do their work with corneal swelling resulting. If oxygen is supplied, the glucose is broken down into water and carbon dioxide, with 36 units of energy being produced. This makes the system more efficient and prevents swelling.

The oxygen that the epithelium utilizes is obtained from the atmosphere. The normal cornea uses about 5 milliliters of oxygen per square centimeter of corneal surface per hour ($ml/cm^2/hr$) and vents about 20 ml CO_2/cm^2 cornea/hr (Figure 4–11). A contact lens placed on the eye can prevent oxygen from reaching the epithelium. If the oxygen level is below the minimum required, the cornea will go into anaerobic metabolism (without oxygen). A gradual increase in corneal swelling will occur. If oxygen debt occurs from lens wear, the cornea will use oxygen at a much higher rate when the lens is removed. In the laboratory or clinical research setting this need for increased oxygen can be measured. If the need on removing a contact lens is the same as occurs, for example, with a 3 percent oxygen atmosphere in front of the cornea, the contact lens is said to supply an equivalent oxygen percentage (EOP) of 3 percent. If 3

Oxygen taken up and carbon dioxide expelled from the cornea

1 microlitre(μl) = 1 cubic millimetre of volume

Figure 4–11. Oxygen utilization and carbon dioxide efflux from the cornea

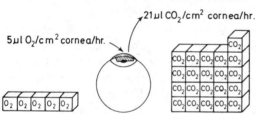

average corneal area = 1.3 cm^2

percent oxygen atmosphere is supplied to the cornea, clinical edema is usually not seen. This is much less oxygen presented to the cornea than the air usually supplies, which is about 21 percent oxygen. Thus, the cornea has a wide safety margin. During sleep, about 7 to 8 percent atmosphere is available to the cornea.

If no oxygen is supplied to the cornea, maximum swelling occurs in about 4 to 6 hours. It may take the cornea 12 to 24 hours to recover if the swelling is extensive.

THE LIMBUS

The limbus is the transition between the clear cornea and the translucent sclera (Figure 4–12). Anatomically, Bowman's layer and Descemet's membrane end at the limbus. There is not a sharp distinction between the cornea and sclera.

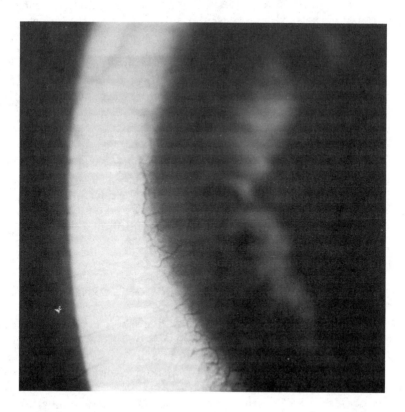

Figure 4–12. The limbus

The corneal epithelium begins to thicken at the limbus and becomes 10 to 12 cells thick over the conjunctiva. The stroma becomes more cloudy due to a loosening and intertwining of the collagen fibers, which causes more light scattering. The palisades of Vogt can be seen when examining the eye with magnification. They are spokelike patterns running perpendicular to the limbus and are formed by thickened portions of the epithelium. The palisades are about 0.5 mm wide and 1 to 2 mm long, being the easiest to see at the inferior limbus. They may be pigmented. Cornea nerves can also be seen entering the cornea at the limbus. They appear as small, white threads and are thicker at the limbus, becoming thinner as they extend into the cornea.

Blood vessels are prominent at the limbus. With ocular irritation such as allergies, infections, foreign bodies, contact lenses, and other problems, these vessels dilate. This is often called limbal engorgement. The same vessels in the conjunctiva also dilate, which is called conjunctival injection or just injection. If there is corneal disease or long-standing corneal edema, new blood vessels will start growing into the cornea from these limbal vessels. This neovascularization is, of course, undesirable.

CONJUNCTIVA

The conjunctiva is the rather soft, loose tissue covering the sclera and inside of the lids. The conjunctiva over the sclera is called the bulbar conjunctiva and is continuous with the palepral conjunctiva. There is a layer of epithelium over a connective tissue, which is rich in blood vessels. The conjunctiva can be moved slightly with digital pressure and the vessels can be seen to move. There are also deep blood vessels in the sclera. The scleral vessels are not as distinct due to the translucent sclera. These vessels will not move with finger pressure as do the surface vessels. Engorgement of the deep scleral vessels usually indicates more severe ocular disease or irritation.

OCULAR STRUCTURES BEHIND THE CORNEA

Contact lenses normally do not affect or disturb structures behind the cornea. Contact lens patients will often ask questions about other eye components, however, such as the pupil and crystalline lens. Therefore, it is important that the contact lens technician be knowledgeable of these and other ocular structures.

Immediately behind the cornea is the anterior chamber (Figure 4–13), which is filled with a clear liquid called the aqueous humor. The

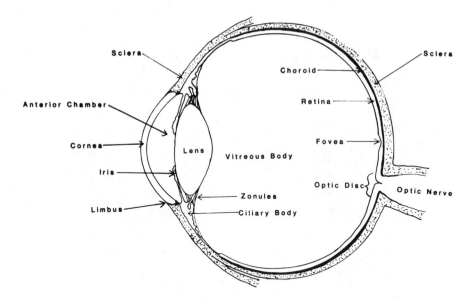

Figure 4-13. Cross-sectional view of the eye

aqueous humor is produced in the ciliary processes, which are behind the iris. The aqueous humor flows through the pupil and exists through the trabecular meshwork where the root of the iris meets the cornea at the anterior chamber angle. The fluid then flows into Schlemm's canal and ultimately to the venous blood vessels. If the aqueous is slow to flow through the meshwork or the iris closes off the angle, the pressure builds up in the eye. This increased pressure (glaucoma) can cause nerve damage in the retinal layer of the eye.

The normal aqueous humor is clear and nothing is seen in it. In addition to water, it has proteins, ions, oxygen, glucose and other molecules.

The iris is the tissue giving the eye color (Figure 4-14). It is a loose network of connective tissue, blood vessels, and muscles and controls the size of the pupil. It blocks extraneous light from entering the eye. Under low illumination situations the pupil becomes larger to allow more light to enter the eye, and under high illumination it constricts to decrease the light entering the eye. In some cases, as the result of heredity or trauma, the iris is missing. This is called aniridia. In such cases, cosmetic contact lenses with artificial pupils may be fitted. Sometimes with cataract surgery a section of the iris will be removed, creating a "keyhole" pupil (Figure 4-15). In other cases of cataract surgery or in surgery to alleviate glaucoma, a small triangular section of iris (called an iriodectomy) near

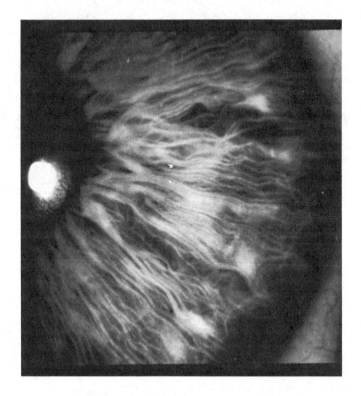

Figure 4–14. The iris

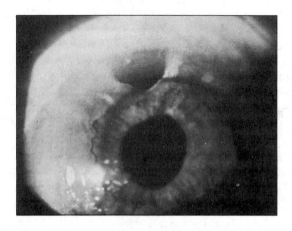

Figure 4–15. A superior keyhole pupil as the result of a sector iridectomy

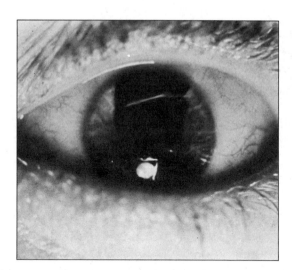

Figure 4–16. A peripheral iridectomy

the limbus will be removed to allow aqueous humor to flow from behind the iris to the front, preventing build-up of pressure (Figure 4–16).

Behind the iris is the crystalline lens. It is biconvex and made up of cell layers. The lens has no blood vessels and obtains nutrients from aqueous humor. It continues to grow and become more compact with age. This, as well as injury, systemic diseases, congenital problems, and chemicals, can cause the lens to become cloudy and opaque. This is a cataract, and in order to restore vision, it must be removed. After the lens is removed, the patient is said to be aphakic. As previously mentioned, contact lenses are often fitted after cataract surgery. Sometimes an artificial lens, called an intraocular implant, is surgically inserted in front of the iris to replace the natural lens.

As a result of ciliary muscle contraction, the normal crystalline lens becomes thicker in order to focus up close. The lens is attached to the ciliary muscle by suspensory ligaments. When the muscle contracts, the tension on the lens decreases and the lens becomes more convex due to its elastic properties. With age, the ability of the lens to change shape is reduced, requiring a plus power addition (bifocals) for near work.

Behind the lens is the vitreous body. It consists of a clear, gelatin material about the consistency of egg white.

The posterior portion of the eyeball which is visible when the eye is examined with the ophthalmoscope is the retina (Figure 4–17). This is the sensory nerve layer of the eye, which transposes the light image falling on it into the nerve impulses, which are transmitted to the brain. The retina is a sophisticated, multi-layered structure that is richly sup-

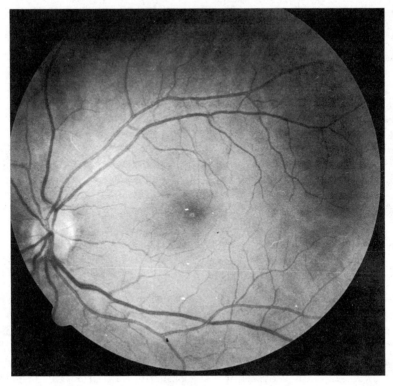

Figure 4-17. A view of the retina showing the blood vessels and optic nerve head

plied with blood vessels. These vessels are easily seen with the opthalmoscope and can be used in diagnosing systemic diseases such as diabetes and arteriosclerosis.

The nerve fibers of the retina go to the brain via the optic nerve. The head of the optic nerve can be seen as a white area (optic disc) on the retina. There is no retina over the disc; therefore, this is a blind spot in the visual field. The back of the eye is often referred to as the fundus. The small area of the retina used for critical seeing is called the macula or fovea. If the retina is damaged, vision is lost and will not be regained.

REFERENCES

1. Wolff E. (revised by Last RJ.). Anatomy of the eye and orbit. Philadelphia: Saunders, 1973.

2. Moses RA., ed. Adler's physiology of the eye. St. Louis: Mosby, 1975.
3. Davson H. The eye, vol. I vegetative physiology and biochemistry. 2nd ed. New York: Academic, 1969.
4. Fatt I. Physiology of the eye. Boston: Butterworth, 1978.
5. Clark BAJ. Topography of the normal human cornea. Ph.D. diss. University of Melbourne, 1971.

5

PRELIMINARY EXAMINATION AND CONSULTATION

The examination and recording of information prior to fitting a patient with contact lenses is extremely important. The information gained at this time helps determine if the patient is a good candidate for contact lens wear, gives an indication as to the type of contact lens that might be best for the patient, and indicates potential problems. Very importantly, the record gives the patient's baseline visual status, to which all later findings during adaptation and follow-up examinations can be compared. These data are necessary in order to determine the effect of a given lens type or design on the eye and visual system. This permits the practitioner to make the proper decisions concerning lens changes, wearing times, and other courses of action that may prove appropriate. This information can also be of legal importance. Therefore, records should be complete and in such a form as to be easily interpreted. The assistant or technician is invaluable in the contact lens practice in obtaining much of this information, recording data, and assuring that it is in proper order.

It is not the author's intention or within the scope of this book to cover all aspects of a vision examination. The particular aspects that deal directly with the fitting of contact lens will be discussed here. This does not mean that the general examination aspects of pathology, visual fields, intraocular pressure, binocular vision, refraction, and other aspects are not important. In fact, it must be remembered that a contact lens patient can have any of the ocular or systemic problems of any other patient plus any problems that might be associated with the wearing of contact lenses.

THE CASE HISTORY

Obtaining a complete history of the patient's general and ocular health is important in determining the patient's suitability for wearing contact lenses. The case history may help determine the type of lens to prescribe, the type of solutions to use, and the advice given to the patient concerning potential limitations and difficulties of lens wear. With some patients, one must be persistent in order to obtain the information and be a detective by questioning the patient in greater depth about facts that seem insignificant or unimportant to the patient. In some cases, the patient may feel more at ease and give more information to the assistant in the practice than to the doctor.

The general or systemic health of the patient must be known. The patient should be questioned about any allergies such as hay fever or allergies to medications, chemicals, or other substances. During periods of allergy attacks, the wearing of contact lenses may be uncomfortable or impossible. In addition, if the patient is allergic to medications or chemicals, there may also be a reaction to some of the solutions used with contact lenses. The patient should be questioned regarding previous sinus infections or related problems. The presence of systemic diseases must be known, especially hypertension and thyroid or metabolic disorders. With female patients the possibility of pregnancy must be considered. Normally, patients are not fitted during pregnancy due to possible ocular changes such as corneal edema that might adversely affect the lens fit and tolerance. Many patients who wear contact lenses and subsequently become pregnant have no difficulty wearing their lenses, but others have increased corneal edema, mucus build-up on the lenses, decreased comfort, and decreased lens tolerance.

The patient should be questioned regarding a history of convulsions or epilepsy, as identification should be carried on the individual indicating that he or she is wearing contact lenses. Any history of psychiatric treatment should also be known to discern the patient's apprehension and mental well-being, which may be affected during contact lens wear. This points out the importance of taking the history in a very professional manner. All communication and information gained about a patient must be kept in the utmost confidence. A patient's conditions, progress, or other information should not be discussed with anyone other than other professionals involved in the patient's care. Some patients can be upset over a discussion of what to you may seem to be a very normal condition or problem. Therefore, the rule must be no discussion of patients outside the office.

Patients must be asked about medications they may be taking. You must make it clear to the patient that this includes not only medications or drugs prescribed by a physician, but also over-the-counter drugs that may not have been prescribed. They should be asked about such medications as diuretics, thyroid medication, insulin, tranquilizers, allergy medications, antihistamines, cold remedies, and birth control pills. Many patients feel that antihistamines and birth control pills, for example, are not really medications and may not tell you they are taking them unless you specifically ask. These medications can affect the wearability of contact lenses by changing the tear film and cornea. Sometimes, by asking patients about medications you will find out about systemic problems of which they forgot to mention when asked about their general health.

The patient's ocular history should be evaluated with the same care as the general history. The patient should be asked about previous injuries to or around the eyes, ocular diseases such as styes, conjunctivitis ("pink eye"), glaucoma, detached retina, or other ocular problems. The patient should be questioned about dry or stinging eyes. You should also determine if the patient is using any ocular medication or "eye drops".

Patients should also be questioned about previous eye care. Have they ever worn or attempted to wear contact lenses? If so, with what results? Questions relating to type of lenses and length of wear should also be asked. Question them about spectacle wear: how long have they worn spectacles and how much of the time do they wear spectacles? A patient who does not wear spectacles all of the time may not need the correction badly enough to bother with contact lenses. It should be determined if a patient has had any special spectacle corrections, any binocular vision problems, or any visual training or other special visual care that could indicate possible problems when switched from spectacles to contact lenses.

The patients' present functioning with spectacles should be determined. Do they feel they have good vision with spectacles? Are they comfortable? Do they have eyestrain, headaches? Such information is important in determining the course of the vision examination and type of correction.

A patient's occupation, hobbies, and particular visual requirements may indicate possible problems or need for a specific type of lens. Both the practitioner and patient should be aware of this. For example, an accountant or secretary will perform different visual tasks than will a truck driver, construction worker, or professional athlete.

Motivation and reasons for desiring contact lenses are always relevant. If a patient merely seeks contact lenses because of encouragement by a member of the family or a friend, the motivation may be low and chances of success reduced. It is best when the patient has a real desire to wear lenses. If patients believe that contact lenses are less bothersome and less time-consuming than spectacles, they may quickly become disappointed and discontinue wear. The patient should understand that contact lenses are usually more time-consuming and bothersome than spectacles. If a patient discontinues wear because of an initial misunderstanding as to what is involved, it is unfortunate for both the patient and practitioner, as much time and money will be wasted. The patient should clearly be made aware of the procedures, care, and costs required to maintain lenses prior to fitting. There should always be a positive desire to wear contact lenses and no one should be talked or forced into wearing them. Most patients want contact lenses for cosmetic reasons or some special purposes such as sports. A few patients need them to rehabilitate sight or achieve adequate vision otherwise unobtainable. The reasons patients want lenses and their expectations from the lenses must be determined prior to fitting.

For most patients, contact lenses are a luxury. The patients should realize this and be willing to spend the time and money for proper care and upkeep of the lenses. If patients realize this prior to being fitted, they are less likely to be disillusioned later.

Table 5–1 summarizes the case history.

SPECIFIC EXAMINATION PROCEDURES

Visual Acuity

Visual acuity (VA) is the basic measurement of the functioning of the visual system. The visual acuity is usually one of the first and most repeated measurements taken since most procedures are to improve or maintain this function. The normal clinical measurement technique is to determine the smallest sized letters which the patient can read, usually specified as Snellen Visual Acuity. There are many aspects of visual acuity which are covered in detail in other texts.(1)

First of all, the visual acuity is usually given by the Snellen fraction, such as 20/20 in the English system or 6/6 in the metric system. The numerator (upper) portion of the Snellen fraction represents the distance at which the test is made (for example, 20 feet). The denominator (lower) portion represents the distance at which the smallest letter read subtends an angle of 5 seconds of arc. For example, if the chart is 20 feet from the patient and the patient can read a letter that is 0.35" (8.9 mm) high, the patient is said to have 20/20 visual acuity. This is considered the "normal" acuity, but in actuality, most people are able to read smaller letters. If a patient cannot read the 0.35" high letter, for example, but can only read a letter 3.5" high at 20 feet, then the patient is said to have 20/200 acuity because a 3.5" high letter subtends an arc of 5 seconds at 200 feet.

Table 5-1. Summary of case history.

A. General Health
  1. Allergies (hayfever, to medications, foods, other substances)
  2. Sinusitis
  3. Diabetes
  4. Thyroid imbalance
  5. Convulsions or epilepsy
  6. High or low blood pressure
  7. Psychiatric treatment
  8. Other:

B. Medications
  1. Insulin
  2. Thyroid
  3. Diuretics
  4. Birth control pills
  5. Antihistamines
  6. Cold medications
  7. Any ocular medications ("eye drops")
  8. Other:

C. Ocular health
  1. Any previous eye injuries
  2. Swollen or infected lids
  3. Conjunctivitis ("pink eye")
  4. Cataract
  5. Glaucoma (including family history)
  6. Dry eyes
  7. Any previous surgery to or around the eye
  8. Previous visual training or special corrections
  9. Other:

D. General
  1. Occupation (around chemicals, dust, special visual requirements)
  2. Hobbies
  3. Previous corrections (spectacles, contact lenses including types, success, and problems)

E. Reason for Wanting Contact Lenses
  1. Cosmetic
  2. Inconvenience of glasses
  3. Sports and recreation
  4. Occupation
  5. High Rx
  6. Aphakia
  7. Keratoconus

Table 5–1. Summary of case history (continued).

E. Reason for Wanting Contact Lenses (continued)
    8. Anisometropia
    9. Increased VA
    10. Myopia control
    11. Other:

Table 5–2. Snellen acuity notation, metric notion, and size of the letters at each acuity level when the chart is 20 feet (6 meters) from the patient.

Snellen acuity (feet)	Metric (meters)	Size of letter if chart is at 20 ft (6 m)	
		Inches	Millimeters
20/10	6/3	0.175	4.45
20/15	6/4.5	0.262	6.65
20/20	6/6	0.349	8.86
20/25	6/7.5	0.436	11.07
20/30	6/9	0.524	13.31
20/40	6/12	0.698	17.73
20/50	6/15	0.873	22.17
20/60	6/18	1.047	26.59
20/70	6/21	1.222	31.04
20/80	6/24	1.396	35.46
20/100	6/30	1.745	44.32
20/150	6/45	2.618	66.50
20/200	6/60	3.491	88.7
20/400	6/120	6.981	177.32

In other words, the "normal" patient should be able to read the 3.5" high letter if it is 200 feet away, but for this patient the 3.5" letter must be at 20 feet before it can be seen. The visual acuity chart is, of course, made up of lines and letters of different sizes giving visual acuities from about 20/10 to 20/400, with the 20/10 letters being the smallest and 20/400 being the largest. The metric system can also be used where the distances are indicated in meters where 20 feet equals 6 meters, so that 20/20 becomes 6/6. Table 5–2 gives the sizes the letters should be on a chart if the chart is 20 feet from the patient.

Often due to the size restrictions of the examination room, the visual acuity test is done at some distance other than 20 feet. In this case the size of the letters on the chart must be adjusted. For example, if a chart made for measuring acuity at 20 feet is used at 15 feet instead, the letters will be easier to read at the closer distance because they subtend a larger angle. To compensate for the closer viewing distance the letters must be made smaller. If a printed chart is used, a different chart is required for each distance or a computation must be made each time it is used. Most acuity charts used in professional practices are projection systems and the tubes on the projector can be adjusted to change the size of the letters. When an acuity chart is first set up, the distance from the patient's position to the chart must be measured and then the size of the test letters adjusted properly. Table 5–3 gives the size of the 20/200 test letter for different test distances. The 20/200 letter is easy to measure due to its size, so it is usually used for calibration. If it is the correct size, the other letters on the chart should be correct, assuming that the chart was manufactured properly.

The size of the 20/200 letter should be periodically checked after being initially set up. If the position of the projector is changed, the

Table 5–3. Size the 20/200 (6/60) letter should be with the chart at the different indicated distances.

Distance from patient		Size (vertical height) of 20/200 (6/60) letter	
Feet	Meters	Inches	Millimeters
10	3.05	1.75	44.3
11	3.35	1.92	48.8
12	3.66	2.09	53.1
13	3.96	2.26	57.4
14	4.27	2.44	62.0
15	4.57	2.62	66.5
16	4.88	2.79	70.9
17	5.18	2.97	75.4
18	5.49	3.14	79.8
19	5.79	3.32	84.3
20	6.1	3.49	88.7
21	6.4	3.66	93.0
22	6.71	3.84	97.5
23	7.01	4.01	101.9
24	7.32	4.19	106.4

projector screen is changed, or the tube of the projector is moved, the size of the letters will change, causing the acuity measurement to be in error.

In determining the acuity, the patient should be comfortably seated. Normally monocular (one-eye) visual acuity is taken first. It is best if the examiner holds the cover paddle to assure that the patient does not press the cover paddle against the eye, as this will cause temporary blurred vision when the paddle is removed. Also, if the patient holds the paddle, the tendency is to peek around the paddle and use both eyes. As the examiner holds the paddle and watches the patient, the patient should be asked to keep both eyes open and to read the smallest row of letters that can be seen. The patient is told not to squeeze the eyelids closed (should not "squint"), as this will change the results. After the patient reads the smallest row, the next-smallest row of letters should be read even if the patient must guess. Usually patients can read one or two rows beyond what they initially indicated, but must be encouraged to do so. They should read down the chart until the majority of the letters in a row are missed. The acuity is then recorded for that eye as, for example, 20/30 if they were able to read all the 20/30 row and none of the 20/25 row. If they were able to read all the 20/30 row and two letters out of seven in the 20/25 row, this can be recorded as $20/30^{+2/7}$. If the same chart is always used in the office, it could be recorded just as $20/30^{+2}$. If, however, they read all the 20/30 row except one letter, it can be recorded as $20/30^{-1/7}$ or $20/30^{-1}$.

If the patients' vision is so poor that they cannot read any letters on the chart, the patients can be moved halfway between where a patient is normally positioned and the chart. For example, if the chart is set up to be used at 20 feet, patients can be moved to 10 feet. In this case, the 20/200 letters become 20/400 or 10/200, the 20/100 become 20/200 or 10/100, and so forth. Other distances can be used with proportioned changes in the acuity values.

After the acuity in one eye is recorded, the cover paddle is moved to the other eye and the procedure repeated. Next the paddle is removed and the test is repeated binocularly. It is best always to measure the acuity in the right eye first, then the left, and finally binocularly, so that the same system is always used. This prevents confusion in remembering what to record. Usually the acuities will be recorded as follows: O.D. $20/30^{-1}$, O.S. 20/40, O.U. $20/30^{+2}$, where O.D. is the abbreviation for the right eye, O.S. for the left, and O.U. for both eyes.

In addition to measuring the visual acuity at distance, the acuity at near can also be measured. The same procedure holds as for distance except the chart is usually printed on a card that the patient holds at the reading distance. Most near point charts are made to be held at 40 cm

(16 in) and should be held at that distance from the patient's eyes. In addition, it should be assured that the chart is well illuminated.

The visual acuity is usually measured with no correction and with the patient's normal spectacles or contact lenses at both distance and near. At each visit after contact lens fitting the patient's VA is usually measured with the contact lenses on and then with the contact lenses removed and the spectacles on.

CORNEAL CURVATURE

The contour and curvature of the cornea are of importance to the contact lens practitioner since the contact lens fits directly on its surface and can change its shape. Due to the complex geometry of the cornea it is quite difficult to obtain accurate data of the entire surface, and clinically the most common procedure is to measure only central curvature. Readings are sometimes taken of peripheral regions that give an indication of the peripheral curvature, but these are usually not very accurate. More elaborate techniques can be used, such as photokeratoscopy (PEK), to determine the shape (topography) of the cornea.

Keratometry (Ophthalmometry)

The main function of the keratometer or ophthalometer is to measure the radius of the central area of the cornea. The cornea is treated as a mirror from which a set of patterns called mires is reflected. By an optical system the pattern is doubled and, with proper alignment of the mires, the curvature can be determined.

To use the instrument properly it must be accurately adjusted and calibrated. The eyepiece should be sharply focused for the operator. This is accomplished by turning the instrument on and either holding a white card up in front of the instrument or shining a penlight in the instrument from the end where the patient is positioned (Figure 5–1). Then, looking into the eyepiece of the instrument, one should see black crosslines. The eyepiece should then be rotated counterclockwise to its most extended postion (the crosslines are blurred), and then slowly rotated clockwise until the crosslines just come into focus and no further. This adjusts the instrument for the examiner's eye and should be repeated for each individual in the office who uses the instrument. If only one person uses it, one need only check periodically to be sure the eyepiece has not been accidentally rotated. When adjusting the eyepiece as well as when using

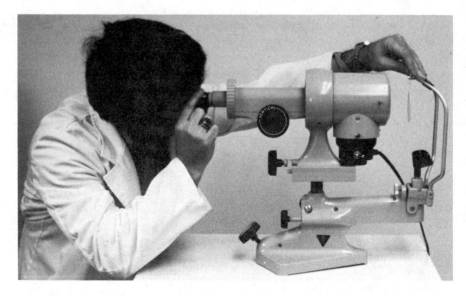

Figure 5–1.   Adjusting the eyepiece to focus the crosslines. A white card being held before the instrument so the lines can be visualized

the instrument to take a measurement, both eyes of the examiner should be kept open.

Next the instrument should be checked to determine if the readings are accurate. This is accomplished by clamping a steel calibration ball of known radius onto the instrument (Figure 5–2). The keratometer is adjusted so that the patterns (mires) on the front of the instrument are reflected from the calibration ball into the telescope of the instrument so they can be seen by the examiner looking through the eyepiece. This is done by adjusting the vertical height of the instrument by the knob directly in front of the examiner (Figure 5–3). The knob that unlocks the instrument body allowing it to be rotated (Figure 5–3) must also be loosened before the instrument can be raised or lowered. The leveling sight on the side of the instrument should be in alignment with the ball to obtain the approximate height. Once the proper height has been reached, the instrument can be rotated laterally so that the mires (Figure 5–4) are in the center of the field of view. By fine adjustment of the vertical and horizontal controls the crosslines should be in the center of the lower right circle of the mire. Once this alignment is achieved, the locking knob is tightened. Next the mires are focused by rotating the knob below the eyepiece of the instrument. After they are in sharp focus the measurement of the ball can be taken. This is done by rotating the

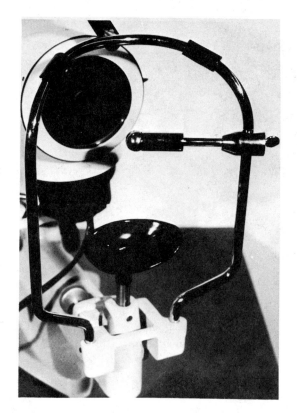

Figure 5–2. Using a calibration ball to check the accuracy of the keratometer

drums (dials) with the scales positioned to the side and in front of the eyepiece. The drum on the left side moves the mire seen on the left side. The drum is rotated until the plus sign on the left mire is superimposed on the plus sign on the center mire (see Figure 5–4a). The mire on the right side controls the movement of the top mire image and it should be rotated until the minus sign on the top mire is superimposed on the minus sign on the bottom mire. Once this is completed, the reading can be taken from the scale on the drum. Where the steel calibration ball is being measured, both readings should be the same and should equal the dioptric value (radius) of the calibration ball, which is commonly 42.50 D (7.94 mm). If it reads some other value, the instrument is out of adjustment. The measurement should be taken several times to be sure it is not a measuring error. When the instrument is out of calibration, it can be corrected by setting the mires in proper alignment and then loosening the set screws on the shaft of the drum between the drum and the body of the instrument using a small Allen wrench. The drum can then be

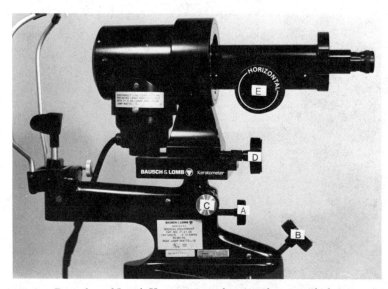

Figure 5–3.   Bausch and Lomb Keratometer showing the controls for (a) movement of the chinrest up and down; (b) movement of the body of the instrument up and down to position the mires in the center of the field; (c) lock to release the instrument body so it will rotate laterally to position the mires; (d) knob to focus the instrument; and (e) one of the drums to align the mires and take the reading

rotated to read the proper value and the screws retightened. It should be checked again to be sure it has been properly adjusted.

Another procedure is just to compensate for the reading error each time the instrument is used. For example, if the reading for the horizontal meridian (left drum) is 42.75 D when it is supposed to be 42.50 D, then, if an eye is measured at 45.00 D, it is actually 44.75 D.

The above calibration assumes that if an error exists, it will be equal over the whole dioptric range of the instrument. This may not be true, and if one wants to be very accurate, steel calibration balls of different radii, ones with long as well as short radii, can be measured to determine the accuracy over the whole range. If the instrument is accurate at 42.50 D but not at 41.00 D, for example, then a graph must be drawn with the actual radius value versus the value read with the keratometer. This graph can then be referred to each time an eye is measured to determine the actual radius. Usually the error is reasonably the same over the whole scale, and this degree of accuracy is not required.

When taking a reading of the patient's cornea, it is important to have the patient comfortably seated before the keratometer, chin in the chinrest and forehead secure against the headrest. It is also helpful to

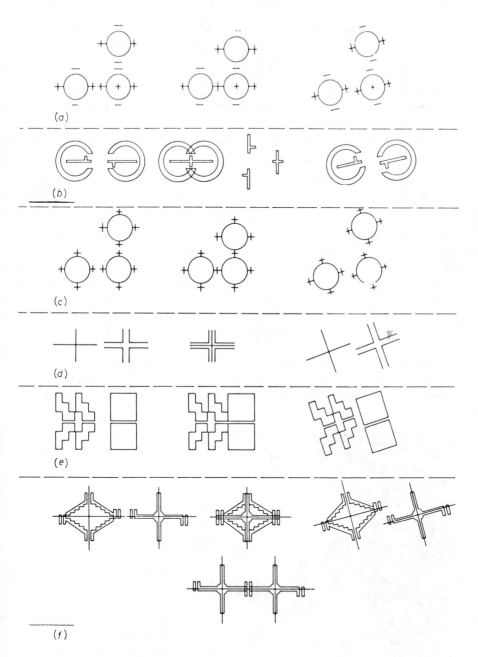

Figure 5–4. Mires used in different instruments. Shown separated on the left, properly aligned for measurement (center), and when off axis (right). (a) Bausch and Lomb; (b) American Optical CI; (c) American Optical CLC; (d) Zeiss; (e) Haag Streit

have the patient grasp the instrument in front of the chinrest to prevent any movement of the head (Figure 5–5). If the patient is not perfectly still, it may be difficult or impossible to obtain an accurate reading because with each movement the mires will go out of focus. The headrest can be adjusted forward or backward for patient comfort by the knob in front of the chinrest (knob just above the patient's fingers in Figure 5–5).

It is also important that the patient maintains accurate and steady fixation, for otherwise the mires cannot be focused. If the fixation is in the wrong direction, a peripheral rather than a central portion of the cornea will be measured. To ensure proper fixation, patients are instructed to look directly down the center of the telescope objective where a reflection of their own eye acts as the fixation point.

Once the patient is properly positioned in the instrument, the mires are positioned in the center of the field of view as previously described, the mires should be brought into sharp focus and be kept in focus during the measurement. If the cornea is spherical, the reading is taken the same as on the calibration ball. Many corneas are toric, however. With a cornea that has the major meridians at 180° and 90° the procedure is still the same except the readings on the two drums will be different. If the corneal toricity is at some other meridian, the horizontal lines of the plus signs of the mires will not line up (Figure 5–4). Before the reading can be taken, the body of the instrument must be rotated until the horizontal bars of the plus signs form a straight line. The instrument is grasped between the eyepiece and the measuring drums and rotated as

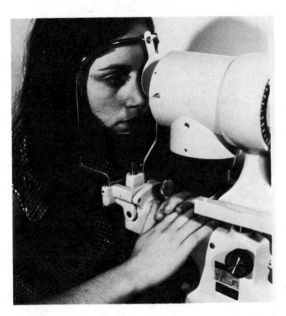

Figure 5–5.   Patient properly positioned in the keratometer

the examiner views the mires. Once they form a straight line, the power drums can be rotated to give the proper superimposition of the mires in both meridians. The power in each meridian is read from the power drums, and the axis of each meridian is read from the axis scale surrounding the instrument just in front of the power drums (Figure 5–3). There are indicator lines in the horizontal and vertical meridians where the axis is to be read. The findings are recorded by giving the power and axis closest to the horizontal first and then the one closest to vertical, for example, 44.00 @ 165; 45.25 @ 075. The dioptric values can be converted to milli- meter values by using a table (see Appendix I).

Readings should be at least double checked on each eye for accuracy. An average is taken to the nearest 0.12 diopter unless the two readings are significantly different, in which case they should be repeated. The repeatability of the instrument is ± 0.12 to ± 0.25 D, therefore, variations in this range are expected. A change in readings of 0.25 diopter from one visit to the next cannot be considered significant.

The above technique of taking K-readings was for the Bausch and Lomb Keratometer. Another commonly used instrument is the American Optical CLC Ophthalmometer (Figure 5–6). It operates on the same prin- ciple except the lateral positioning and focusing of the mires is by move- ment of a joy-stick on the base of the instrument in front of the examiner.

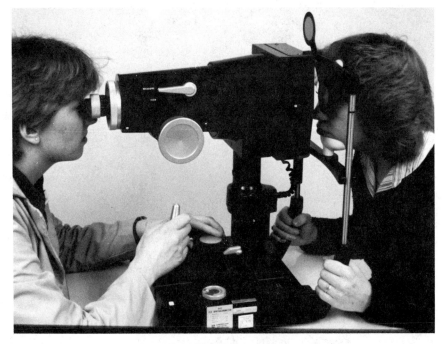

Figure 5–6.   American Optical CLC Ophthalmometer

The vertical positioning is via the wheel on the base of the instrument in front of the joy-stick. In the CLC, the mires representing the vertical meridian are plus signs instead of minus signs as in the B&L unit.

There are several other models of keratometers or ophthalmometers in use around the world. Basically they are similar in use; the manufacturers' manuals can be consulted for particular differences.

Occcassionally a patient is encountered who has either an extremely flat or steep cornea that falls outside the scale of a particular keratometer. The range of radii that most instruments can measure can be extended in such cases by placing a spectacle trial lens over the objective of the telescope by using either a special holder (Figure 5–7), taping it in place, or holding it by hand. A plus lens will extend the range to read steeper corneas and low minus for measuring flatter corneas. Commonly 1.25 D lenses are used. A graph should ideally be drawn for the instrument with the lens in place by measuring a series of calibration balls in the appropriate range. It would show the actual radii against one on the drum to which reference can be made whenever the supplementary lens is used. Practically, just using the standard chart is usually acceptable (Appendix III).

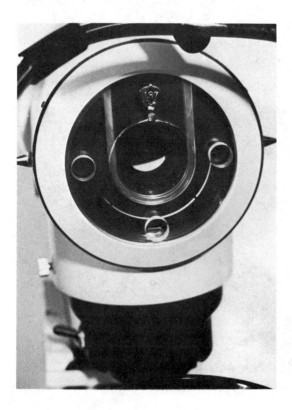

Figure 5–7. Special holder for spectacle trial lens mounted on the front of the keratometer (holder by H. D. Inns)

Peripheral Keratometry

In an attempt to obtain a better clinical picture of the corneal topography, different procedures for measuring various points across the cornea have been devised. One of the simplest methods is to use a movable fixation point (Figures 5–8 and 5–9). By knowing its distance from the center of rotation of the eye and the amount the target is moved, the approximate peripheral postion of the cornea being measured can be determined by simple geometry. This value is indicated on a scale of the instrument. Since the mires are usually reflected from a relatively large area of the cornea, normally comprising a zone of 2.2 to 3.5 mm in diameter, a change in fixation resulting in the second reading 1 to 2 mm to the side of the first does not mean that a whole new area of the cornea is being measured. The second measurement overlaps the area of the first and is just shifted slightly to the side. It cannot thus be assumed that the peripheral reading gives the curvature at a specific point. Because of this, as well as other optical problems, it is not possible to determine true corneal topography with most instruments. The main clincial advantage offered by this procedure lies in confirmation that the central keratometer reading has actually been taken from the steepest point on the cornea. This may be

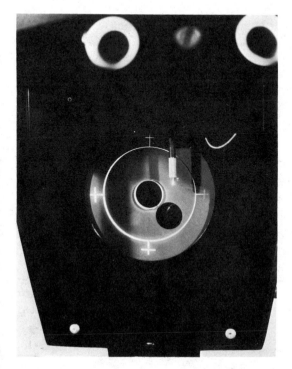

Figure 5–8. Patient's view of CLC Opthalmometer showing movable fixation point used to direct the patient's fixation to the side so that peripheral corneal readings can be taken

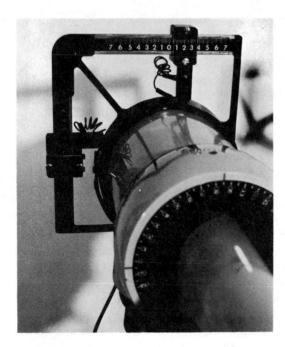

Figure 5–9. View of topogometer mounted on the keratometer showing the scale indicating horizontal and vertical fixation changes

important if the steepest part of the cornea, called the corneal apex, is decentered. Peripheral readings can also give an indication of the rate of flattening of the cornea from the apex toward the periphery.

When taking peripheral readings, the fixation position, as well as the actual dioptric values and axes, must be specified.

Keratoscopes

In order to obtain a qualitative determination only of the corneal contour a keratoscope can be used which in its simplest form consists of a flat disc with concentric rings and a sight hole in the center, widely known as Placido's disc (Figure 5–10). By holding this before the patient's eye so the rings face the patient, their reflection off the cornea can be seen when looking through the sight hole. If the cornea has a normal spherical contour or nearly so, the rings will be uniform and concentric. If a relatively large amount of regular astigmatism is present, the reflected image will be oval. If the cornea is distorted, as with keratoconus, corneal injuries, or irregular astigmatism, the rings, too, will appear distorted. If the apex is decentered, as often occurs in keratoconus, the center of the

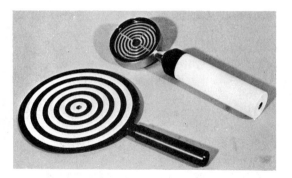

Figure 5–10. Placido's disc on left and on internally illuminated keratoscope on the right

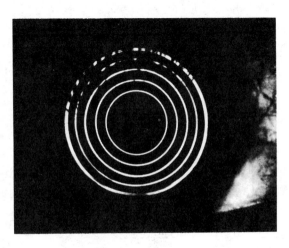

Figure 5–11. Keratogram of the cornea taken with a photokeratoscope

reflected pattern will appear displaced with respect to the center of the cornea. An internally illuminated keratoscope (Figure 5–10) is a modern modification of Placido's disc.

Photokeratoscopes

The basic principle of Placido's disc has also been utilized to determine the contour of the cornea by photographing a reflected image of a concentric pattern so that a keratogram (Figure 5–11) can be obtained. By knowing all the constants of the instrument and measuring the separation of the rings on the photograph, the radius of the cornea at the point of reflection can be calculated. The target of original keratoscopes consisted of a flat surface, but this introduced several errors and complications. In an endeavor to overcome these problems and to photograph a larger area of the cornea, photokeratoscopes were designed with concentric rings in different planes.

The operation of the instrument is similar to that of a keratometer (Figure 5–12). The eyepiece must be accurately focused for the examiner. The patient is positioned with the head securely against the headrest. The patient's head must be turned to the side in order to get the cone of the instrument close enough to the eye. To photograph the right eye, the head must be turned to the left. If difficulty is encountered with the cone hitting the forehead, the patient needs to move the chin forward on the chinrest. Adjusting the height of the chinrest can also be helpful.

The patient is asked to fixate on a cross in the instrument, and the examiner aligns the instrument using the joy-stick (Figure 5–13). The joy-stick is moved until the dark spot seen in the eyepiece is centered in the rings reflected from the cornea. The rings are brought into sharp focus by rotating the knob on the joy-stick. When in focus, the rings should appear continuous and clear. With the rings focused and centered, the patient is instructed not to blink and the photograph is taken by

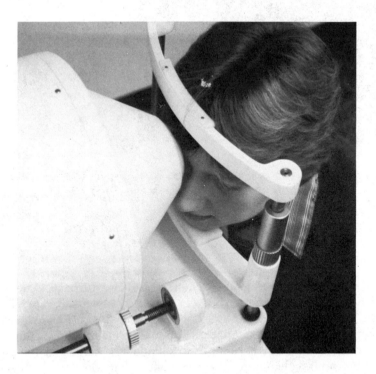

Figure 5–12.   Patient positioned in a photoelectric keratoscope (Wesley-Jessen, Inc., PEK)

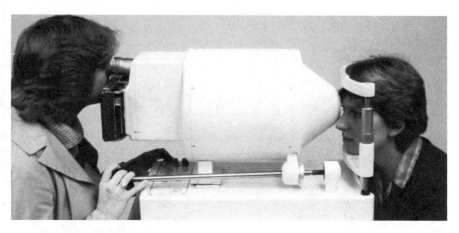

Figure 5–13.   Photoelectric keratoscope

depressing the exposure button. The keratogram (the photograph) can be analyzed by the company and/or kept in the patient's file for future reference and comparison. The data can be used to help determine the initial lens to be fitted on the patient and to follow corneal changes with photos being taken at different times.

EXTERNAL EXAMINATION

Prior to fitting contact lenses, the lids, conjunctiva, cornea, anterior chamber, and related structures must be carefully examined for abnormalities. Gross examination can be performed with a penlight and/or magnifying glass to detect major anomalies. In order to examine the eye in adequate detail, however, a slit-lamp biomicroscope is required.

Slit-Lamp Biomicroscopy

The slit-lamp biomicroscope consists of a controlled light source, the slit-lamp for illuminating the structure under consideration, and a binocular microscope for viewing, the biomicroscope (Figure 5–14). By convention this instrument is usually called either a slit-lamp or biomicroscope, but not by both names. The illumination system has adjustments to control the width and height of the light beam, to rotate the slit from a vertical to a horizontal position, to change the angle of the slit about the axis of the lamp housing, and to vary the angle of the slit in relation to the

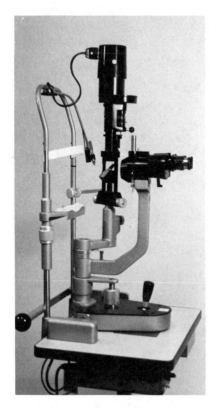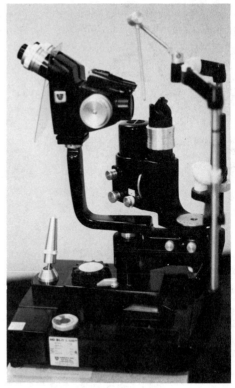

Figure 5–14.　Biomicroscopes

biomicroscope. These adjustments are necessary to examine the eye adequately. There are also auxiliary filters available. Usually a red-free (green) filter is present, which can be used to show blood vessels in greater detail, and a cobalt filter (dark blue) is used to highlight staining by the dye fluorescein better than with just white light. The slit mechanism must be of such precision that a very narrow, uniformly illuminated slit of light can be formed. If there is dust or dirt in the system or the bulb is not properly positioned, a uniformly illuminated slit is not possible.

The biomicroscope must be of good optical quality, binocular, and have several different magnifications. It should have adjustments for the examiner's refractive error, such as eyepieces that focus, and an adjustable separation of the eyepieces for different interpupillary distances. The microscope should also pivot so the eye can be viewed at different angles.

The slit image and the biomicroscope must be focused at the same point if fine detail is to be seen. The slit beam and biomicroscope should pivot about the same point and both should move as a unit so that different parts of the eye can be viewed. This movement is controlled by the joystick.

There are many different techniques for using this instrument, based on different illumination arrangements. One of the common illumination systems is called direct illumination, wherein the beam of light and the microscope are focused on the structure being examined. If the beam of light is fairly narrow, it is called a parallelopiped (Figure 5–15), and if very thin, an optic section (Figure 5–16). The optic section is used to determine the depth of defects in the cornea. If the light beam is positioned beside the object being examined, then this is called indirect illumination (Figure 5–17). Another type of illumination is where the light beam is placed on the limbus. This is called sclerotic scatter. This type of illumination is used to detect corneal edema created by the wearing of contact lenses.

The slit lamp requires considerable instruction, experience, and professional judgment. It is beyond the scope of this text to go into these

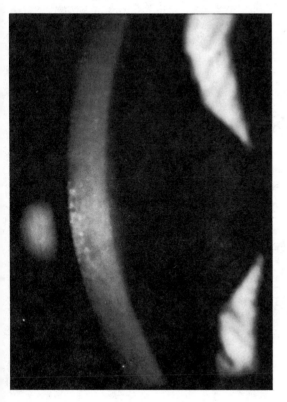

Figure 5–15. A parallelopiped illumination of the cornea

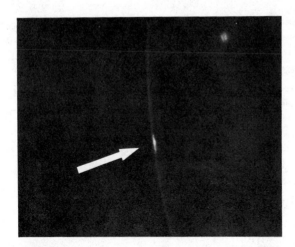

Figure 5–16. An optical section of the cornea with a small scar present

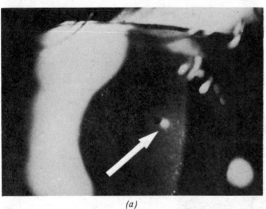

(a)

Figure 5–17. Embedded foreign body (a) viewed with direct illumination and (b) viewed with indirect illumination where beam is positioned behind the object being examined

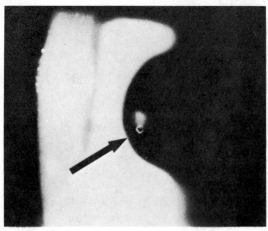

(b)

details in any further depth, but the assistant or technician should have a basic understanding of this important instrument to understand the terminology used by practitioners and to explain its function to patients.

Use of Stains to Examine the Eye

Sodium fluorescein is the most commonly used stain. It will highlight disruptions of the epithelium and conjunctiva, since any damage to the cells allows the stain to enter the intercellular spaces or the cells when their membranes are ruptured.

Fluorescein is available impregnated in paper strips (Figure 5–18) or in solution. The paper strips are preferred since they are easy to use and are less prone to contamination. When fluorescein solution is necessary, it comes packaged in unit dose packets that are discarded after each use. Fluorescein solution is a good medium for bacteria called *Pseudomonas aeruginosa* to grow. This organism can quickly destroy the cornea.

To use the paper strips, they must first be removed from their individual wrappers. Care must be taken not to touch the orange part of the strip, which is the fluorescein. The fluorescein is moistened with a drop of irrigating solution or buffered saline (as used with hydrogel lenses). Hard lens wetting solutions, other viscous solutions, or ones containing benzalkonium choloride should not be used on fluorescein strips. Also be careful not to touch the tip of the solution bottle to the fluorescein as this will contaminate the bottle. To be most effective, use only a small drop of solution on the strip and shake excess solution off before touching it to the eye. Place a sufficient quantity of fluorescein on the eye, but do not add excess solution.

To instill fluorescein, have the patient look down with the eyes, firmly hold the upper lid, and lay the flat side of the fluorescein strip against the upper conjunctiva (Figure 5–19). Do not rub the strip back and forth across the eye or hit the eye with the sharp edge of the strip. Avoid any irritation that will cause increased tearing. After the strip has been removed, a few blinks will spread the dye evenly over the cornea and conjunctiva.

An alternate method of instilling fluorescein is to have the patient look up as far as possible; then, holding the upper lid firmly and pulling the lower lid away from the eye, the flat side of the moist fluorescein strip can be laid against the lower conjunctiva. This method is preferred if the patient is apprehensive, for if the patient tries to squeeze the lids closed the eyes will roll upward. If this happens when the fluorescein strip is

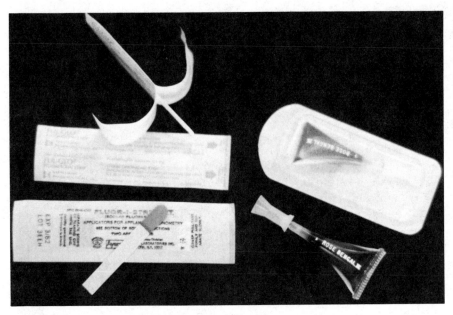

Figure 5–18.   Fluorescein strip and unit dose of rose bengal (right)

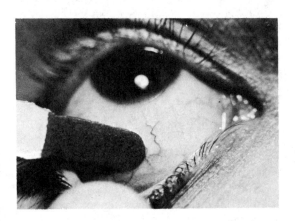

Figure 5–19. Instilling fluorescein using a sterile, moistened fluorescien strip

being touched to the upper conjunctiva, the strip may be scraped across the cornea, causing damage and staining of the cells. If the eye rolls up when the fluorescein strip is being placed on the lower conjunctiva, the cornea will not be touched.

After the fluorescein has been instilled, the eye should be examined, using ultraviolet light or with the blue cobalt filter over the light source of the slit lamp. The ultraviolet (UV) light causes the fluorescein to fluoresce a bright green. If there is no damage or anomalies of the cornea or conjunctiva, only the tear film will show this green fluorescence. If the epithelium has been damaged—scratched, for example—the damaged cells will absorb the fluorescein and will be seen as a bright area of fluorescence, which is called staining.

Since the fluorescein stains the tears, it will be found where the tears flow. For example, the natural flow of the tears is through the puncta of the lid into the nose. Thus, patients may find fluorescein on their handkerchief after blowing their nose. The patient should be warned ahead of time that this is normal. Also, if there is some excess tearing and the tears flow out over the lid, the patient will have the yellow-orange stain on the face. This is easily washed off with water. Avoid excess fluorescein, which can get on the patient's clothing although it will normally wash out without leaving a stain.

Once in the eye, the fluorescein is normally allowed to be washed out by the normal flow of the tears. In some cases, it is desirable to rinse the fluorescein away. This is true when a hydrogel lens, which absorbs fluorescein, is to be placed on the eye. This is accomplished by using an irrigating solution. The patient is asked to hold a towel against the side of the face and to look down with the eyes as far as possible. Then the upper lid is firmly held up and away from the eye (Figure 5–20). A strong stream of the irrigating solution is sprayed under the upper lid from the nasal to the temporal side. The patient is next asked to look up as far as possible and the lower lid is pulled down. The lower cul-de-sac is likewise rinsed out.

Rose bengal is another stain that can be used in the eye. It is a reddish-purple stain that colors degenerating and dead cells not stained with fluorescein, but does not penetrate abraded areas as fluorescein does. Rose bengal may be used either as a paper strip or a unit dose solution. If the solution is used, it is instilled as any ophthalmic solution. The patient is asked to tilt the head back slightly and to look up as far as possible. The examiner then pulls the lower lid away from the eye and instills a drop of the solution into the lower cul-de-sac (Figure 5–21). The lower lid is gently released and the patient is asked to blink. Only a small drop should be used, to prevent excess solution from spilling out onto the cheek.

Lid Eversion

In addition to examining the anterior structures of the eyes normally visible, the conjunctiva covering the underside of the lids (the palpebral

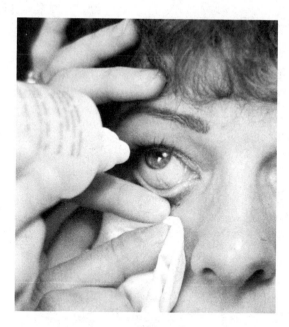

Figure 5–20. Irrigating the eye to remove excess fluorescein

conjunctiva) should be examined. The lower lid can simply be pulled down by placing the finger near the lower lid margin and pulling it down.

To examine the palpebral conjunctiva of the upper lid, the upper lid must be everted. This is easily accomplished by grasping the lid margin with the thumb and forefinger while placing a stiff object such as a cotton applicator against the upper lid above the tarsal plate (Figure 5–22). The lid margin is then lifted out and up so that it folds over the cotton applicator. Once the lid is folded over, the cotton applicator can be removed and the everted lid held in place by holding the lashes against the bone of the orbital rim (Figure 5–23). The palpebral conjunctiva can then be examined using a penlight with or without a magnifier or in greater detail with the biomicroscope. Anomalies such as foreign bodies, infected meibomian glands, deposits, and conjunctival papillae (raised areas) are looked for. It is helpful in detecting some of these problems if fluorescein is instilled prior to lid eversion. The lid should not remain everted any longer than necessary because the palpebral conjunctiva will dry in a few minutes, causing discomfort and tearing. When the examination of the palpebral conjunctiva is completed, the patient is asked to look up and blink, which will cause the lid to return to its normal position.

Sometimes it is necessary to look further up into the upper cul-de-sac, for example when there is a foreign body in the eye or a contact lens has been dislodged and is high up into the upper cul-de-sac. To do this

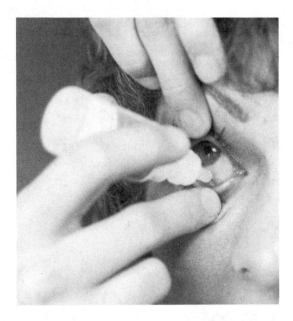

Figure 5–21. Instilling ophthalmic solution into the lower cul-de-sac

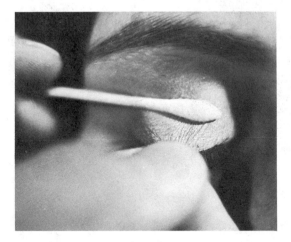

Figure 5–22. Placing cotton applicator above the tarsal plate to evert the upper lid

one of the specially designed devises for this purpose may be used (Figure 5–24). The lid is everted onto one of these devices and then the device is used to roll the lid on up and away from the eye (Figure 5–25). This is often referred to as double eversion.

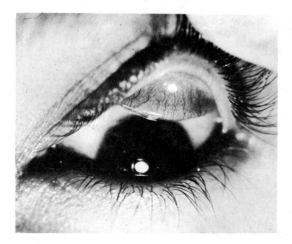

Figure 5–23. Lid everted for examination of the palpebral conjunctiva

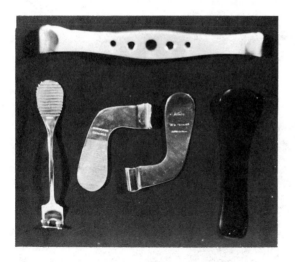

Figure 5–24. Differently designed devices to evert the lid

TEAR FILM EXAMINATION

Tear Film Break-up Time (BUT)

One of the tests of the quality of the tear film is the break-up time. The tear film should remain uniform over the corneal surface for some time following a normal blink. If it quickly breaks up and becomes discontinuous, then the epithelial cells will dry and become damaged. Likewise, problems with the wearing of contact lenses can occur with short break-up time, such as drying of the lens surface, deposit formation on the lens

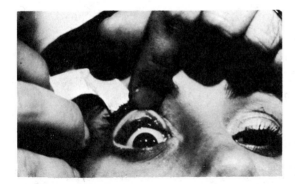

Figure 5–25. Turning the upper lid up farther than the normal single eversion

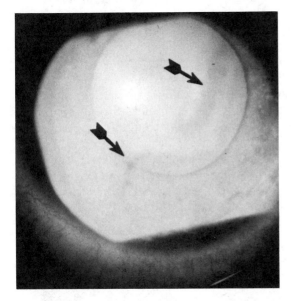

Figure 5–26. Break-up of the tear film

surface, poor tear exchange causing discomfort, and other problems. A short BUT indicates a problem with the mucoid layer of the tear film.

The BUT can be rather easily measured. A small amount of fluorescein is instilled as previously explained. The patient is asked to blink a few times and then not to blink and to stare straight ahead. The corneal surface is viewed with a moderately wide beam of light with the biomicroscope using the cobalt filter before the light source. The time from the last blink until the first appearance of a break in the tear film is measured with a stopwatch. The break in the tear film will appear as a small dark spot or streak (Figure 5–26). The average break-up time is 20 to 25 seconds with a BUT of less than 10 seconds being a potential problem. Some patients may have a BUT of a minute or longer.

When performing the BUT test, do not hold the lids open as this will decrease the measured BUT. The BUT will also decrease on repeated measurements. It should not be done immediately following contact lens wear or after other tests such as tonometry or lid eversion where the cornea or eye has been touched. Any abrasions or irregularities of the cornea will cause a break in the tear film at that point.

Schirmer Tear Test

The quantity of tears normally produced can be measured with this test. The test consists of a short strip of filter paper with a small notch near one end (Figure 5–27). The strips come sealed in plastic envelopes, so they are sterile. Before opening the envelope, the paper strip should be bent at a right angle at the notch. The envelope is then opened, being careful not to touch the strip near the bent end. On removing the strip, the bent end is placed under the patient's lower lid.

Before placing the paper strip under the lid, the patient should be seated comfortably and told that the test is to measure the amount of tears produced and will not be painful, but may be mildly irritating. The patient should look up slightly and the bent portion of the strip gently placed under the lower lid to the nasal side of the middle of the lid to avoid touching the cornea as this will cause reflex tearing giving invalid results. The patient may blink normally with the strip in place and may gently, but not forcibly, close the eye during the test. Both eyes can be tested at the same time.

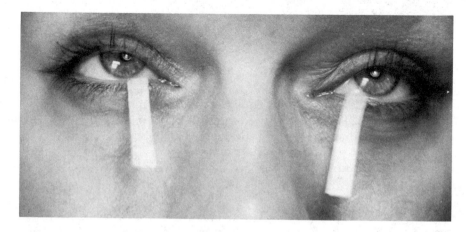

Figure 5–27. Schirmer tear test strips

The time the strip is placed in the eye is noted and it is left in for 5 minutes. Upon removal the length in millimeters of the paper strip from the notch that is moistened is measured. This value is recorded. The normal finding is 15 mm or more of moistened strip, with a decrease in those patients over 40 to between 10 and 15 mm.

Ocular Smears

The tears and surface of the conjuctiva may contain certain cells whose presence can indicate the existence of a given reaction or disease process. For example, a patient may have a "red" or "blood-shot" eye due to an allergy, bacterial infection, viral infection, or just from a mechanical irritation. A study of the cells present in the tears may help diagnose the problem.

To obtain a sample of cells a sterile cotton-tipped applicator can be used. The procedure is explained to the patient prior to taking the sample. The patient should be told the procedure is slightly irritating and uncomfortable but not painful. The patient is asked to look up and the lower lid is pulled down. The dry cotton-tipped applicator is wiped over the lower bulbar conjunctiva, down into the lower cul-de-sac, and onto the palpebral conjunctiva (Figure 5–28). The applicator should be slid across the surface and not rolled. Avoid the lid margins so that skin cells are not collected.

After the smear has been taken the cells must be transferred onto a clean microscope slide. The cotton-tipped applicator is rolled across the slide, not wiped across. If the slide is held such that a reflection can be seen from the surface, the smear is visible. Experience will soon indicate the pressure required to make the transfer.

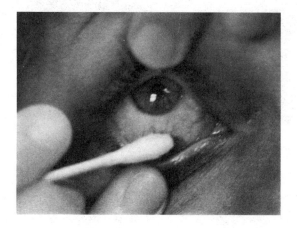

Figure 5–28. Method for taking a smear

Once the cells are transferred to the slide, the smear should air dry for 30 to 60 seconds. Now it is ready to be stained so that the cells can be identified. The staining procedure consists of three steps (Figure 5–29). The three solutions used are commercially produced to stain blood smears.[1] The slide is repeatedly dipped in the first solution, a fixative, for a total of about 5 seconds. It is then removed and the excess solution is allowed to drip off. It is then repeatedly dipped in the second solution, a stain, for another 5 seconds. The same procedure is repeated for the second dye. The slide is then rinsed under a slow-running stream of water from a faucet for a few seconds. Next it is allowed to air dry. This may be speeded up by using a hair dryer. Now the slide is ready to inspect with the microscope.

The position of the cells on the slide should be located using the low-powered objective on a regular student or laboratory light microscope. Finding the cells on the slide can be simplified if circles have been drawn with a grease pencil or if serological slides having two circles drawn on them are used. Once the cells are located, they can be inspected under higher magnifications.

There should always be epithelial cells present. These are normal cells that are sloughed off the cornea and conjunctiva. They will be larger than any other cells present and have irregular shapes. The main portion of the epithelial cells will be stained a light purple, with the nuclei stained

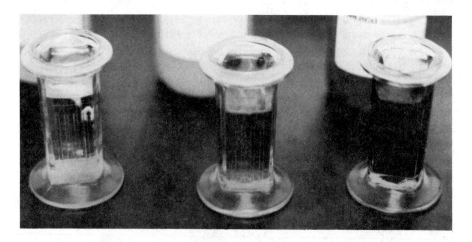

Figure 5–29. Clinical set-up for staining smears showing the three solutions, slides, and microscope

----

[1]Diff-Quik Staining procedure, Harleco Brand Product, Dade Division, American Hospital Supply Corp., P.O. Box 520672, Miami, FL 33152.

very dark (Figure 5–30). If no cells are present on the slide, this indicates the procedure was not properly performed.

Some common cells found in the smears of patients with conjunctival inflammation are the polymorphonuclear leukocytes (PMNs), also called neutrophils. These cells have a segmented nucleus that stains purple, with the surrounding portion of the cell, the cytoplasm, staining pink (Figure 5–31). If numerous PMN cells are found, then a bacterial infection is suspected. Young PMN cells, indicating a recent onset of the inflammation, have c-shaped nuclei, with the older cell nuclei segmented.

A cell similar in appearance to the PMN cell is the eosinophil. It commonly has a bilobed nucleus and is the same size as the PMN. The obvious distinguishing feature of the eosinophil is the prominent reddish or orange granules in the cytoplasm that make this cell stand out from the others. Eosinophils indicate an allergic reaction. Basophils, similar

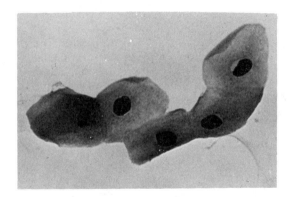

Figure 5–30.   Epithelial cells in a smear

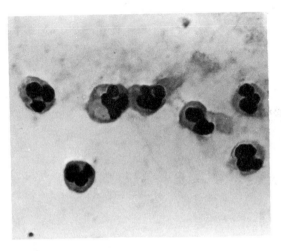

Figure 5–31.   Polymorphonuclear nentrophils showing the lobulated nucleus, normally showing 3 to 5 segments

cells with a multilobed nucleus and large, purple staining granules that tend to obscure the nucleus, are rarely found in smears.

Lymphocytes are another cell type commonly found. These are easy to identify because they are small cells made up almost wholly of a dark staining nucleus. There is only a slight amount of cytoplasm surrounding the nucleus (Figure 5–32). Smears showing a large number of lymphocytes, even if some PMN cells are present, strongly indicate a viral infection.

Monocytes are similar to lymphocytes in appearance except they are larger and have more surrounding cytoplasm. In addition, the nucleus is horseshoe shaped. Monocytes are precursors to the macrophage (Figure 5–33), which is a large cell with poorly defined nucleus and debris in the cytoplasm. Macrophages ingest other cells and debris accompanying inflammaion.

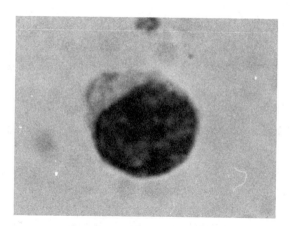

Figure 5–32. A lymphocyte showing the prominent nucleus and scant cytoplasm

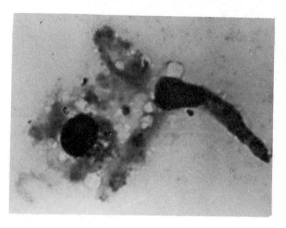

Figure 5–33. Degenerating macrophages

MEASUREMENT OF OCULAR DIMENSIONS

The Lids

The separation of the lid margins between blinks with normal, relaxed distance gaze is called the palepbral aperture. The measurement of this lid separation can be used as a guide in contact lens fitting. When making this measurement, one must be careful to take the measurement with the lids in the normal, relaxed position and not cause the patient to squeeze the lids down. If a millimeter rule, often referred to as a P.D. stick, is used, do not hold it too close to the lids since if it touches the lashes or if patients think you may hit the eye with it, they will tend to close the eye. Refer the patients' attention to an object such as the acuity chart at eye level in front of them, telling them just to relax. The examiner should also be at eye level with the patient so that erroneous measurements will not be made. Closing one eye, the examiner should measure the lid separation in the middle of the lid opening in millimeters (Figure 5–34). It may be better to estimate the lid separation, particularly if the patient is apprehensive, by comparing the lid position with respect to the corneal diameter. Then, by measuring the corneal diameter, lid separation can be determined. The normal separation is about 7 mm to 13 mm, with the average approximately 10 mm.

The position of the lid margins with respect to the cornea may be more important in fitting than the acutal palpebral aperture size. Therefore, the position of the upper lid margin in relation to the upper limbus and the lower lid margin to the lower limbus with the patient relaxed and looking straight ahead should be noted in the patient's record. This

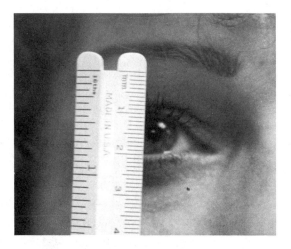

Figure 5–34.   Measuring the palpebral aperture

position is best estimated rather than actually measured. The findings can be recorded with respect to the millimeters separation of the lid margin from the limbus. For example, if the lower lid margin is at the lower limbus, the finding would be zero. If it is 1 mm below the lower limbus, it would be recorded a -1; if above the lower limbus by 2 mm, it would be $+2$. The same notation would be used for the upper lid. Another method of recording the lid position is to draw a circle on the record representing the limbus, and then draw lines at the appropriate positions indicating the lid margins.

The tension of the lids can be quite important in the positioning and comfort of the contact lenses. There is no clinical method for actually quantifying lid tension, although an estimate can be made. To make the estimate, lightly grasp the upper lid between the thumb and index finger and gently pull the lid away from the eye. The lid tension can be described as loose, average, or tight. Quite often elderly patients will have very loose, flacid lids while others—for example, some Orientals—may have fairly thick, tight lids.

The patient's blink rate can also be important in estimating the patient's ability to wear contact lenses. An unusually low blink rate may make the wearing of contact lenses difficult. Knowing the rate prior to fitting can also be useful after the patient starts wearing lenses to determine if the rate has changed.

To obtain an accurate blink rate, the patient should not be aware that you are doing it. It is best to determine the rate while you are just carrying on a normal conversation during the case history. The normal blink rate is 10 to 15 blinks per minute. The completeness of the blink is also important. If the lids are only partially closed on a blink, the patient may have difficulty wearing contact lenses.

Corneal Diameter

The corneal diameter can be important in determining the size of the lens. It is often referred to as the visible iris diameter (VID) since the outside diameter of the colored portion of the eye, the iris, is what is actually measured and not the cornea. The two are very nearly the same.

The visible iris diameter can be measured with a millimeter rule by having the patient look straight ahead and the examiner holding the upper lid open with one hand. The rule is then held up near the cornea and the measurement made with the examiner directly in front of the patient's eye (Figure 5–35).

Another method of measuring the corneal diameter is to have a reticule, a millimeter scale, in the eyepiece of the biomicroscope. Other

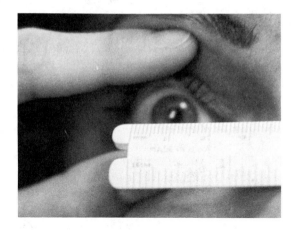

Figure 5–35. Use of a millimeter rule to measure corneal and pupil diameter

methods using special optical devices also designed to measure the interpupillary separation can be used. Such accuracy usually is not necessary.

The average horizontal diameter is about 11.7 mm, with a common range of diameters of 11.0 to 12.5 mm. The vertical dimension, usually not measured, is about 1 mm smaller.

Pupil Size

The diameter of the pupil can be helpful in indicating the type and size of contact lens to be fitted. It can also be used to predict visual problems the patient may experience such as blur from the lens edge under low light conditions.

The pupil diameter should be measured under average light conditions since if you shine a bright light in the patient's face to take the measurement, a falsely small pupil diameter will be found. The actual measurement can be taken using the same procedures as explained for corneal diameter measurements.

The normal pupil size is 3 to 6 mm, with less than 3 mm under average lighting being small and over 6 mm being large. Elderly patients will commonly have small pupils.

CORNEAL SENSITIVITY

The sensitivity of the cornea, that is, the ability to know when an object touches it or to feel pain, is of interest since a contact lens rests on this tissue. If the cornea is not sensitive prior to fitting, special instructions may be required since the patient may not "feel" a problem as a normal patient would.

A gross qualitative test for sensitivity is to take a small whisp of cotton and lightly touch the cornea. When the cotton touches the cornea, the patient will blink when sensitivity is near normal. If the cornea has lost most of the sensation, the blink reflex will not be forthcoming.

A more quantifiable test is to use an aesthesiometer, which is a nylon monofilament in a holder such that the length of the filament can be varied (Figure 5–36). The shorter the filament, the stiffer it is, and thus the more force that must be applied to get it to bend. The test consists of having the patient look up slightly and, with the filament relatively long, say at 6 on the scale, bring the tip up and touch the cornea until there is just a slight bend in the filament. If the patient does not blink or feel the filament, shorten it, say, to 5, and repeat. Do this until you obtain a response. Patients are instructed to look up so that they cannot see you bring it up to the eye. You want them to respond to touch, not your hand movement. The filament should touch the cornea about halfway between the center of the cornea and the limbus. The filament should contact the cornea at a right angle so it does not slide on the cornea surface. The result can be recorded as the number on the scale or converted to grams per square millimeter using the chart provided with the instrument.

To obtain more accurate measurements, the instrument with the filament can be mounted on a biomicroscope and the procedure done under magnification. Other complicated research devices have also been devised to measure the sensitivity.

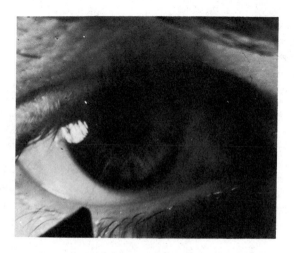

Figure 5–36. Use of a monofilament to measure corneal sensitivity

Although corneal sensitivity is not routinely measured by most practitioners, for patients where there is a question about the sensitivity level, it should be determined.

CORNEAL THICKNESS MEASUREMENT

The corneal thickness change with the wearing of contact lenses is important because this is a direct measurement of the corneal swelling or edema, one of the major problems with contact lens wear. Until recent years this measurement was not possible. Now there is an attachment for the biomicroscope called a pachometer which measures the cornea thickness (Figure 5–37). An optic section, a narrow beam of light passing through the cornea, is set up. With the pachometer on the biomicroscope, the optic section is optically split in half. The lower half of the beam can be moved independently on the top half (Figure 5–38). When the front

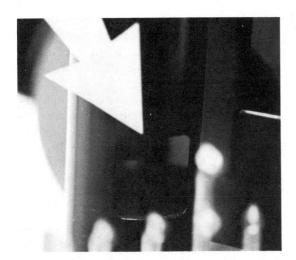

Figure 5–37. The Haag-Striet Pachometer, which consists of rotating glass plates that go in front of the microscope and a beam splitting eyepiece

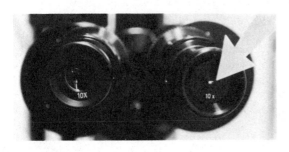

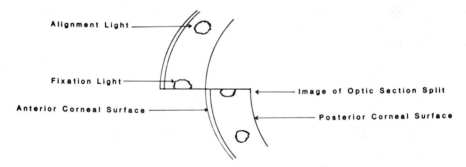

Figure 5–38. View of the split optic section as seen through the pachometer showing the setting when the measurement is taken

of the lower half of the beam is aligned with the back of the top half, then the corneal thickness is measured from the scale.

Even with the above instrumentation, it is difficult to obtain the very accurate thickness measurements needed. To overcome some of the problems, the Electronic Digital Pachometer[2] has been divised (Figure 5–39). Optically it works in the same way except the readings are recorded electronically, there is electronic calibration, and statistical calculations of the readings are printed out for the patient's records. It also has special fixation and alignment lights.

Most practitioners do not have a pachometer due to the cost and lack of flexibility of the instrument. To obtain accurate readings the biomicroscope should not be used for routine examinations as the calibration will be lost. These instruments are increasing in popularity, however, and are common research tools. Knowledge of the technique is helpful in understanding research reports and conversing with others in the field.

PHOTOGRAPHY

It is helpful in many cases to photograph anomalies of the eye for the patient's record so that any changes that might occur as a result of the wearing of a contact lens can be determined. There are several photographic arrangements that can be used. The simplest is just a normal 35 mm single reflex camera with a close-up lens, extension tubes, bellows, or a macrolens. All of these devices are available at camera shops and

---

[2]Manufactured by Dicon Ophthalmic Instruments, 7540 Trade St, San Diego, CA 92121.

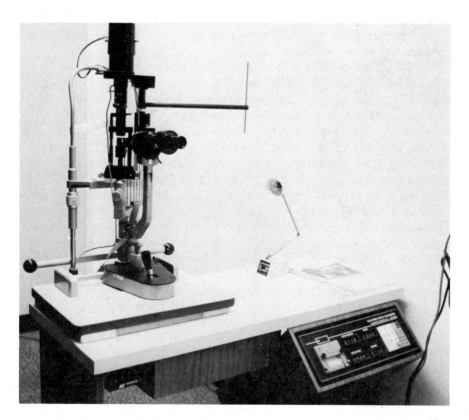

Figure 5–39.   Electronic pachometer

are designed to take close-up photographs. The close up lens is just a plus lens which screws on to the regular camera lens. It is relatively cheap and easily put on and taken off the camera. The extension tubes fit between the regular camera lens and camera body. They have the same advantages as the close-up lenses. The macrolens is more expensive as it replaces the normal camera lens. It is easier to use and has a greater range and better optics. With all of these devices, the camera is usually held within a foot or two of the patient, focused on the eye, shutter speed and aperture set as when taking normal photographs. The instruction manual accompanying the camera should be consulted if you are not familiar with it as each camera operates slightly differently. It is important when taking photographs in this manner that the patient holds very still. It helps if the head is against the headrest of the ophthalmic chair. Likewise, you must hold the camera very still.

The least expensive method is to take color slides, which usually give greater detail than black and white photographs. If immediate results are desired, a Polaroid camera is necessary, but the cost is high compared to that of slides.

One of the problems of taking close-up photographs of the eye is having enough light. To overcome this problem, a flash can be used. Figure 5–40 shows a 35 mm reflex camera with extension tubes and a small, round flash unit under the camera lens.[3] Other flash units designed for close-up photography can be used. Depending on the camera and type of film used, it may be necessary to place a neutral density filter over the flash unit if too much light is provided. When fluorescein patterns are photographed, a dark blue filter such as an Eastman Kodak filter X8779, Wratten filter 47, or Rosco 37 filter over the flash unit and a yellow filter such as Tiffen #1 yellow or Wratten 8 filter over the camera lens is necessary. As for the type of film to be used, if only white light photographs are to be taken, a daylight type film such as Kodachrome ASA 25 can be used. For fluorescein pattern photographs, it may be necessary to use a higher-speed film such as Kodak Ektachrome ASA 200. To obtain the proper exposures it is best to experiment with a test roll of film.

Close up photographs can be taken with equipment like the Photoeaze unit[4] (Figure 5–41). This consists of the 35 mm camera, a bellows for close-up focusing, two flash units, and a wire frame for proper focusing. A problem with close-up photography is that the camera must be held very still and accurately focused. The wire frames that attach to the front of this unit are placed against the patient's face, holding the camera at

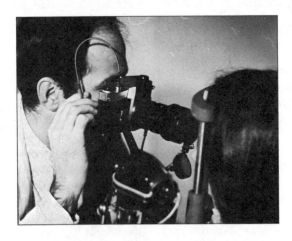

Figure 5–40. A regular 35 mm camera with extension tubes and a Foto-Flash unit for taking photographs of the eye

[3]Lester A. Dine Electronic "Foto-Flash," Lester A. Dine, Inc., 2080 Jerico Turnpike, New Hyde Park, NY 10041.
[4]Photoeaze Mfg., Inc., 241 E. 10th. St., New York, NY 10003.

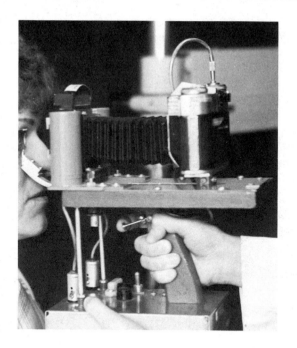

Figure 5–41. A Photoeaze unit with bellows, two flash units, and a frame for proper focusing

the proper distance from the eye and helping to hold the camera still. Different-sized frames can be attached to the front of the camera with the area of the eye or face being photographed corresponding to the size of the frame.

To obtain high magnification, detailed photographs of the eye, a photobiomicroscope must be used. Figure 5–42 shows the Nikon photobiomicroscope. In this case the flash unit is in the optics of the slit lamp and the intensity of the flash is controlled by the dial on the flash control box. The higher the dial number, the greater the intensity flash. If a low magnification photography is being taken, a low intensity flash is needed and the setting should be on one. If a high-magnification, optical section photograph of the cornea is taken, a high-intensity flash, say the highest setting of 4.0, is used. A table is provided with the instrument giving the recommended flash settings depending on the area photographed and the film being used. To obtain a photograph with this unit the desired view is obtained with the biomicroscope, the flash intensity is set, and the shutter disc just below the camera is pulled down to bring a mirror into the optics of the microscope. The shutter disc is squeezed to take the photograph. One must keep an accurate log of the photos taken so that they can be properly labeled and filed when returned from the developer. The log should contain the patient's name, date, structure being photo-

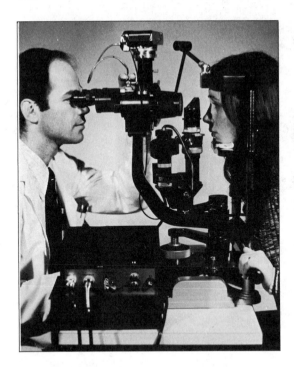

Figure 5–42. Nikon biomicroscope equipped with a camera and flash unit

graphed described in enough detail to be able to identify the photograph, the magnification used, and the flash intensity setting.

With any of the photographic systems, it is important that one read the instruction manual supplied with the camera to understand how it operates, how to load and unload the film, and other general principles. To obtain good photographs one must practice by taking a few rolls of photographs, experimenting with the equipment.

INDICATIONS AND CONTRAINDICATIONS TO CONTACT LENS WEAR

There are many factors that determine whether a particular patient will be a suitable contact lens wearer. Many of these are physical factors determined by the patient's health, ocular anatomy, and visual status. Others depend on motivation, occupation, personality, or the handling of the case. All such factors have to be taken into account in order to assess whether a patient should be encouraged or discouraged from being fitted. Professional judgment is always involved in determining if a patient should be fitted. The following are a few of the considerations.

Patients with moderate to high refractive errors are usually better candidates than those with very low ones. A means of judging if the refractive error is significant enough in terms of a patient's visual requirements is the amount of time spectacles are actually worn. If used all and every day, then the patient will most likely wear the contact lenses. Likewise, if they are worn only part-time, then the chances of successful contact lens wear are reduced, regardless of the refractive error, unless there are strong self-conscious reasons for not wearing spectacles.

The patient should be motivated to wear contact lenses. If they are sought because of encouragement by a family member or friend instead of personal desire, the chances for long-term, successful wear are reduced. From the outset, the patient should be willing to spend the time and have the financial resources to be fitted and should be available for proper follow-up care.

Some patients are involved in activities for which contact lenses would be advantageous and recommended—for example, sports, especially those involving bodily contact. In certain occupations spectacles may be in the way, easily knocked off the face, not allow sufficient peripheral vision, or become fogged up due to continuous change of atmospheric environment.

For certain pathological, medical, and surgical conditions vision is ideally corrected with contact lenses, specifically keratoconus and irregular corneas since contact lenses provide a spherical, uniform refracting surface allowing improved vision over spectacles. Aphakia is another condition for which contact lenses have definite optical advantages. They may also be used to protect the cornea and prevent the drying of the eye that occurs with lid injuries. Prosthetic or cosmetic lenses can have decided psychological advantages as well as act as a visual aid as in cases where the iris is missing (aniridia).

Contraindications

There is a relatively large number of conditions and individual reasons where contact lenses are contraindicated or will at least diminish the chances of successful wear.

The patient must be willing to take the time necessary to care for the lenses, keep a consistent wearing schedule, and realize what is involved in their upkeep. On the other hand, should a patient be unable to wear lenses, this should not be blamed on lack of motivation or psychological reasons until all other causes have been eliminated. Too many patients have been held accountable for failure when in fact a poor design or fitting was responsible.

Those who are extremely nervous or impatient may not be good candidates.

Patients in poor general health may experience many problems with contact lenses. The elderly could have difficulty in handling lenses, with placement and removal difficult, and motivation may be lacking. Even young patients may find manipulation a problem because of some physical deformity or fear of the lenses. Extended wear may be the only solution if acceptance can be demonstrated to be satisfactory.

There are many different pathological conditions that contraindicate contact lenses. Moderate to severe cases of diabetes are an example since the cornea is more prone to edema and abrasion than normal. Healing tends to be slow, which makes the patient more prone to infections. Those who are able to control the condition with diet or oral medication can usually be fitted without consequence, but patients taking daily insulin injections are safer wearing spectacles unless there are overrriding reasons requiring contact lenses.

Other endocrine disorders may also contraindicate contact lens fitting. Patients going through meopause might have substantial changes in the quality and quantity of the tear film, making wear uncomfortable. Women may prudently be advised to defer the initial fitting during pregnancy since endrocine imbalances can cause corneal edema, discomfort, and adaptation problems. A patient wearing contact lenses prior to pregnancy, on the other hand, should be allowed to continue unless edema or other problems develop, at which time wearing should cease until termination of the pregnancy. Women who begin taking birth control medication may produce symptoms brought on by water imbalance, corneal edema, or change in tear chemistry similar to pregnancy. Far more blame for contact lens problems has been attached to the taking of birth control medications than is warranted, however. Hyperthyroidism is another condition that may adversely affect tolerance.

Chronic respiratory disorders sometimes make the wearing of contact lenses difficult. Hay fever, asthma, sinusitis, and similar conditions may cause conjunctival injection, tearing, light sensitivity, and general discomfort that is aggravated by the lenses. If possible, the condition should be cured prior to fitting or the patient warned of likely discomfort. The patient must be advised that wearing may have to be restricted or discontinued during acute attacks.

Certain allergies may bring about similar symptoms that will make the wearing of contact lenses difficult during an attack. Patients may complain of discomfort with their lenses while receiving treatment, even when no physical signs can be seen.

There are several disorders of the lids that could create problems for the potential contact lens patient. Chronic lid infection is aggravated by contact lenses and should be eliminated before fitting. If the patient has a history of repeated lid infections, contact lenses may increase their frequency and thus be contraindicated.

Any active corneal infection must be cured prior to fitting. If there is a history of recurring infections, extra care must be taken to ensure that contact lenses do not cause increased occurrence. The patient should know that the practitioner must be consulted as soon as any symptoms appear since the condition could be made worse with lens wear. Contact lenses may have to be discouraged altogether in some such cases.

Patients with decreased tear flow and corneal involvement may have difficulty wearing corneal or hydrogel contact lenses. Here, too, some lenses provide protection against corneal drying.

Patients with blood vessels in the cornea from a previous injury or infection are not good candidates since any irritation or edema created by contact lenses may reactivate the condition and cause it to progress. Any such patients fitted must be followed closely. Special caution must likewise be taken with those who have a very insensitive cornea as severe corneal damage could occur before the patient is aware of it.

Patients persistently exposed to airborne foreign matter, chemicals, or other industrial or environmental hazards may not be suitable for contact lenses or may require special protective spectacles or goggles to wear when in such atmospheres.

It goes without saying that any cases of iritis must be cured prior to contact lens fitting. This condition has a tendency to recur, and the patient should be aware of the possibility so as not to relate it to the wearing of contact lenses.

Patients with cosmetically noticeable strabismus ("crossed eyes" or "walleyed") will usually find that the appearance is more noticeable with contact lenses than spectacles. Such cases are best discouraged from wearing contact lenses.

There are many individual circumstances and conditions that can contraindicate the prescribing of contact lenses. The practitioner must evaluate these in the light of knowledge of the physiology and pathology of the eye, thus arriving at a decision as to the practical feasibility of contact lens wear for the particular patient.

PATIENT CONSULTATION

Prior to fitting a contact lens, the practitioner, technician, or assistant should discuss with the patient what is involved in both fitting and wearing lenses. Many patients have misconceptions and unwarranted fears that must be alleviated.

The procedures pertaining to the initial examination and follow-up care should be explained in terms of the estimated number of visits necessary and the cost. Symptoms likely to be experienced during adaptation should be described, such as what to do if a foreign body gets under the lens in a dusty environment. Proper lens care must be stressed from the outset, and no patient should be left under the misconception that once fitted there will be no further bother. It must be pointed out that contact lenses require as much if not more attention than spectacles.

Some patients are afraid that contact lenses may cause permanent ocular damage. It should be made clear that they are quite safe with reasonable care and that harm does not normally occur since the eye is sensitive and severe pain occurs long before permanent damage. Patients may also express fears of lenses becoming lost behind the eye, and the fact that this cannot happen must be explained with patience and understanding.

The patient must be fairly presented with the negative aspects as well as the advantages of contact lenses during the initial discussion. The patient should be made aware of problems that may subsequently occur and should not become unhappy after being fitted because of misconceptions. One should always give unbiased advice in the interest of the patient and not allow his or her judgment to be influenced by commercial or publicity pressure.

Folowing the initial examination and fitting, one should again take time to explain the type of lens fitted, its advantages for the patient, and the reason why it was selected. It must be impressed that due to many individual variations and needs, different types of lenses are required for different patients. This will help lay people understand that what has been done is in their best interests and avoid doubts regarding suitability if friends are later found to have been fitted with different lenses.

REFERENCE

1. Borish, IM. Clinical refraction, 3rd edition. Chicago, Ill.: Professional Press, 1970.

6

CONTACT LENS FITTING PROCEDURES

To fit a patient with contact lenses successfully and to evaluate the patient's progress adequately, professional skill, judgment, and understanding are required. Likewise, a coordinated effort by the practitioner and assisting personnel is a must if success is to be achieved. The assistant often has greater patience and is more adept at performing certain tasks during the fitting procedure than the practitioner. Patient education, placement and removal of lenses, inventory control, and lens ordering are important aspects of fitting often performed by assistants in the office. In order to be able to execute these tasks successfully, the assistant should understand the basics of prescribing and fitting contact lenses. This chapter is intended to cover some of the basics but it is not within the scope of this text to fully explain contact lens fitting.

There are three criteria basic to contact lens fitting. First, the patient must achieve good visual acuity. The definition of good acuity will vary from patient to patient. An individual with 20/20 acuity with spectacles should expect nearly the same acuity with contact lenses, thus 20/20 or better is considered as good for that patient. Yet, someone with corneal distortion and 20/200 best corrected acuity with spectacles may obtain 20/60 with contact lenses. For this patient, 20/60 is excellent acuity.

A second criterion is patient comfort. If the lenses are not comfortable, they will be rejected.

The third criterion concerns the health of the eye. The patient must be examined periodically during the adaptation period and then at regular intervals of 6 months to a year for daily-wear patients. For extended-wear patients (those sleeping with their lenses) and others with special problems, more frequent follow-up examinations are required. Just because the patient sees well and is comfortable does not mean that all is well. Corneal edema, corneal and conjunctival changes, infections, and other problems can occur without the patient's knowledge.

Many different kinds of contact lenses, lens designs, and fitting techniques are used to achieve this success. One fitting technique or lens material might achieve success with one patient but a different procedure may be required with another. No one technique is right or wrong, the important thing being the achievement of the above criteria.

FITTING PROCEDURES

Although practitioners have individual contact lens fitting preferences, they follow one of three general fitting procedures. All involve ocular measurements but one does not include placing contact lenses on the eye prior to the ordering lenses from the laboratory and the third is dispensing lenses from an in-office inventory.

Direct Ordering Procedure

With this technique, data gathered during the preliminary examination as described in the previous chapter are used to determine the lens type and dimensions to be ordered. For example, the spectacle refraction and keratometer readings are used to determine the lens base curve and power. With rigid lenses, the lacrimal lens effect must be taken into account as described in Chapter 3. The size of the lens and optical zone are determined based on the measurement of the palpebral aperture size, position of the lid margins, corneal diameter, pupil diameter, and lid tension. With this procedure, contact lenses usually are not placed on the eye prior to ordering. The first lens placed on the eye is the one ordered for the patient.

This technique has the advantage of not requiring diagnostic lenses in the office and decreasing the office time required at the fitting visit. The disadvantage is the inability to determine how a lens will perform on the eye just from the ocular measurements. Due to complicated lid geometries and forces, peripheral corneal shape variations, differences in tear chemistry, and other factors, the fit cannot be evaluated.

Diagnostic Fitting Procedure

Lenses with a general range of base curve radii, diameters, and powers are often maintained by practitioners. From these diagnostic sets a lens can be placed on the patient's eye and evaluated. The initial lens is often determined by the same procedure as for direct ordering. A lens from the diagnostic set with the closest predicted fit is placed on the eye. If properly designed and finished, the lens should be reasonably comfortable on the patient. The fit of the diagnostic lens may be evaluated immediately to determine how close it is to the desired fit. Before a final evaluation is made, the patient should wear the lens approximately 30 minutes. This allows time for tearing to subside. In the case of hydrogel lenses, tears can stabilize with the fluid in the lens.

If the initial lens does not perform properly, a second lens is chosen based on the performance of the first. It is then evaluated and the procedure repeated until the desired performance is achieved. Both lens design and different lens materials can be evaluated. Optical performance can be determined by refracting over the lens and testing the visual acuity. Often the exact lens to be ordered is not available in the diagnostic set, but based on the performance of the diagnostic lens, the final lens can be determined.

Many people in the contact lens field use the term "trial lenses" instead of diagnostic lenses. This should be avoided since it implies to the patient that fitting is no more than trial and error. Actually it is a planned diagnostic procedure. Lenses placed on the eye are determined and evaluated by scientific and clinical principles.

After each diagnostic lens is used, it must be thoroughly cleaned and then placed in a soaking solution or disinfected depending on the type of lens used. A set of contamined diagnostic lenses could spread an ocular infection from patient to patient.

Fitting from Stock

Theoretically, the best way to fit contact lenses is from a large stock of lenses maintained in the practice. This is similar to the diagnostic fitting procedure except many more lenses are available. Thus, the proper lens is in the office set and does not have to be ordered. This will allow a practitioner to evaluate a lens that has the correct power required by the patient. If the lens performs properly, it can be immediately dispensed to the patient. One advantage of this method is that the lens evaluated in the fitting will be worn by the patient and problems of quality control, where the lens ordered from the laboratory may have dimensions different from the diagnostic lens, are avoided.

Another advantage of this method is that the patient receives the lenses at the time of fitting. One to three weeks delay to obtain the lenses from the laboratory is avoided. Patients often prefer having their lenses immediately. This is a factor in good patient relations. Another advantage allows lost or damaged lenses to be replaced immediately from the office stock.

The main disadvantage of stock fitting is the cost of the large inventory that must be maintained. This can be prohibitive unless the contact lens practice is large. Some manufacturers offer special consignment programs. Large stocks of lenses are provided the practitioner on a "rental" basis at a fraction of the lens cost. Each time a lens is used, it is then replaced at the full cost. A disadvantage is that once the lens vial is opened, it cannot be returned and must be paid for. Another related disadvantage of stock fitting is the rapid development of the contact lens field. If there is a large investment in a stock of lenses, they can become outdated in a few months due to new and better materials and designs on the market. It now becomes quite expensive to replace the stock. This can be avoided, however, by having a return policy with the laboratory which allows for full refund or replacement.

Another criticism of the stock fitting procedure is that the practitioner may be influenced to use a less than ideal lens since it is in stock rather than ordering the better lens.

RIGID LENS FITTING PRINCIPLES AND TECHNIQUES

Many different specifications of the lens to be ordered or dispensed to a patient must be determined. Some of these include the total diameter, optic zone diameter, base curve radius, peripheral curve radii, power, center thickness, tint (color), and type of material. The initial lens to be placed on the cornea is determined from the data obtained during the preliminary examination. The lens must then be placed on the cornea, evaluated, and then removed. This is repeated until the desired lens specifications are determined.

Rigid Lens Placement and Removal by the Assistant

Prior to placing a rigid corneal contact lens on a patient's eye for the first time, the patient should be informed that the lens might cause mild discomfort but should not be painful, and also that some tearing will occur and the lens may be felt when blinking. The procedure you will follow should be explained to the patient before actually putting the lens on the eye. This information allows the patient to be more cooperative during the procedure. It also helps put the patient at ease. The patient should be told to look straight ahead, keeping both eyes open and looking at a distant object. The upper and lower eyelids are held open and then the lens is gently placed on the eye. Next, have the patient look down, at which time the lids are released. Following this, the patient should continue looking down into the lap for a few minutes because the lens will be more comfortable with downgaze than when looking around. After a few minutes, the patient will be able to look straight ahead with relative comfort. If the patient is particularly apprehensive, go through the procedure once without actually placing the lens. That is, hold the lids, having the patient fixate in the proper position, and so forth.

After explaining the procedure to the patient, actually place the lens on the eye. First, be sure to wash your hands and thoroughly rinse off all the soap. It is best to use a soap that will not leave a residue and is not abrasive. Examples are Nutragena and Ivory. Remove the lens from its container and rinse the soaking solution off with water, saline, or the solution used on the lens for placement. With PMMA and some of the newer gas-permeable lenses, a wetting solution is used. If one of the solutions formulated for both soaking and placement is used, the lens does not need to be rinsed. Chapter 9 can be consulted about solutions. Once the lens is adequately moistened with the proper solution, it is ready to be placed on the cornea.

The patient is instructed to look straight ahead at a predetermined object across the room—for example, the largest letter on the acuity chart. Place the index finger of the left hand, if standing to the patient's right side, over the eyelashes of the upper lid. Be sure your hands and the patient's lids are dry. Solution on the lids or hands makes them very slippery. The lid should be brought up and held firmly against the rim of the bone above the eye (Figure 6–1). The lid should be held tightly enough so that the patient cannot close it. This is important because if the patient blinks and closes the eye about the time the lens is placed on the cornea there will be discomfort as the lid hits the lens and the lens may be dropped. This will cause the patient to lose confidence and become more apprehensive. While placing the lens, the forearm should be firmly resting on the patient's head (Figure 6–2). This prevents the patient's head from moving backwards while the lens is being placed on the cornea. Even if there is some movement, the hand will move with the patient's head. It also gives the hand more support.

The moistened lens should be resting on the tip of the index finger of the right hand (Figure 6–1). Be sure not to have excess solution on the

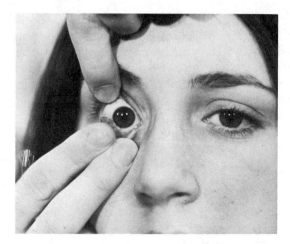

Figure 6–1. Placement of a corneal contact lens while properly holding the lids

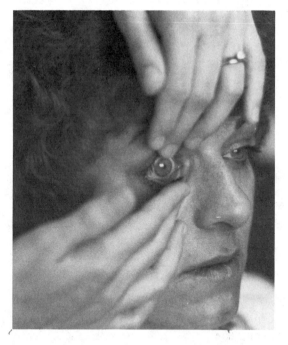

Figure 6–2. Resting the forearm on the patient's head and hand holding the lens on the cheek so if the patient moves the head, your hands will move also.

lens or your fingers. The lower lid is gently pulled down by the second finger of the same hand with this hand held against the lower cheek for support (Figure 6–2). The lens is held to the side of the patient's eye, out of sight, until it is ready to be placed on the cornea. This prevents the patient from becoming apprehensive and trying to back away. Directing the patient to look at the distant object, quickly bring the lens in front of the patient's eye and gently touch it to the cornea. Since the lens is moist, it will stick to your finger until it touches the patient's cornea, at which time it will adhere to the cornea. It is best to have a good light on the patient so you can see when the lens touches the cornea. Also stand beside, not in front of, the patient when placing the lens. This makes it easier to see when the lens is brought to the cornea and gives better control over the head movements of the patient. Do not hold the lens 2 or 3 inches in front of the eye prior to placing it on the cornea and then slowly bring it toward the eye. This will make the patient very apprehensive, causing blinking, rolling up of the eyes, and moving the head back. Keep talking to the patient during the procedure; tell the patient to look straight ahead at the chart and to keep both eyes open. Keep the patient busy thinking about what is being said and not what is being done.

Once the lens has been placed on the cornea quickly move the finger away but keep ahold of the lids. Have the patient look down, then slowly release the lids. Be sure to have the patient continue to look down for a few minutes.

A lens is placed on the left cornea in the same manner, except that you reach across the patient's face (Figure 6–3). Be sure not to block the view of the right eye when doing this (Figure 6–4).

The following summarizes the steps in the placement of a rigid corneal lens.

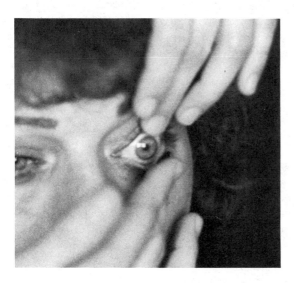

Figure 6–3. Correctly placing a lens on the patient's left eye while working from the right side

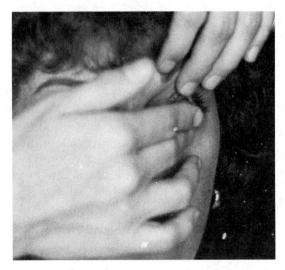

Figure 6-4. An improper method of placing a lens on the left eye because the hand obscures the view of the right eye. The patient cannot hold fixation

1. Explain procedure to patient.
2. Wash and rinse hands thoroughly.
3. Remove lens from storage and rinse.
4. Apply proper solution (wetting or combination).
5. Place lens on tip of the index finger.
6. Dry fingers which will hold lids.
7. Have patient fixate a distant object.
8. Rest left forearm on patient's head.
9. Rest right hand on cheek with lens off to the side out of view.
10. Hold lid up with index or second finger of left hand.
11. Hold lower lid down with second finger of right hand.
12. Quickly and gently place lens on cornea.
13. Have patient look down in reading position (keep head up).
14. Slowly release the lids.

Sometimes when the lens is being placed on the cornea, the eye will turn upward. The lid may not be held firmly enough or, due to excessive tearing, the lens will become decentered onto the sclera and slide under the lids. The lens then must be recentered or removed. The patient is assured that there is no harm with the lens off center; in fact, it may be more comfortable since there is less lid sensation. The lens must be located. Again, rest the left hand on the patient's forehead and right hand on the cheek. The lids are pulled away from the globe and, if necessary, the patient is asked to look in different directions to locate the lens. Once the lens is found, the patient is asked to look in the opposite direction of the lens position—for example, down if the lens is above the cornea (Figure 6–5). The index finger is placed at the lid margin and lifted above the edge of the lens. By gently pushing the lid margin back against the globe above the lens, the lid margin is used to push the lens back onto the cornea. If the lens is below the cornea, the same procedure is used except the patient looks up and the lower lid margin is used to slide the lens back onto the cornea. If the lens is off to the side of the cornea, the patient is asked to look in the opposite direction. One index finger is placed on the upper lid margin and the other index finger on the lower lid margin beyond the edge of the lens (Figure 6–6). The lens is then moved back onto the cornea, using both lid margins.

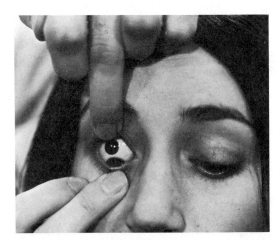

Figure 6–5. Recentering a displaced corneal lens

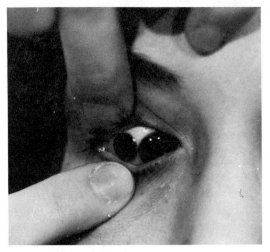

Figure 6–6. Recentering a lens displaced laterally

For removal, the patient is instructed to look straight ahead. Place the index finger of one hand at the upper lid margin directly above the lens and the index finger of the other hand at the lower lid margin directly below (Figure 6–7). By keeping the margins tight against the eye, the lids are then brought together, expelling the lens. If the fingers are placed back from the lid margins, the lids will roll away from the globe, sliding over the surface of the lens instead of hitting the edge, and the lens will not come out (Figure 6–8). With this technique, a lens can be removed virtually without the cooperation of the patient. For this reason, as well as the rapidity with which removal is possible, this procedure should be perfected.

Other methods (see Chapter 10) such as the lid-scissor technique

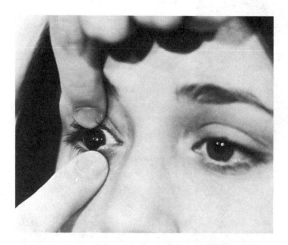

Figure 6–7. Removing a contact lens using the index fingers on the lid margins

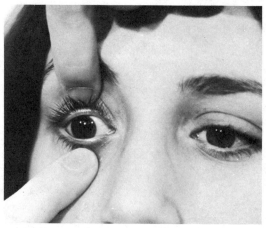

Figure 6–8. Incorrect position of the fingers on the lid margins for removal

are usually taught the patient but can be used by you. They require more cooperation of the patient than the method described.

Fluorescein Pattern Evaluation

Once the lens has been placed on the cornea and the tearing has subsided, the fit of the lens can be evaluated. The most common and easiest way to visualize the lens fit is to use sodium fluorescein to stain the tears. The fluorescein strip is moistened with irrigating solution and gently laid against either the superior or inferior conjunctiva (see Chapter 5), being careful not to add excess solution to the eye or irritate the eye. To evaluate the fit, an ultraviolet lamp, also called a black light, is held close to the eye (Figure 6–9). These usually have a magnifying lens to give better visibility. Alternately a biomicroscope can be used with the dark blue cobalt filter in place. Under the ultraviolet light, the yellow-orange fluorescein dissolved in the tears becomes a bright green. It is best seen in a darkened room. The staining should be viewed immediately after instillation of fluorescein as it will quickly be washed away by the tears.

The edge of the lens, and consequently the lens position, can be quickly ascertained. There should be a bright band of fluorescein stained tears around the edge of the lens that corresponds to the peripheral curves

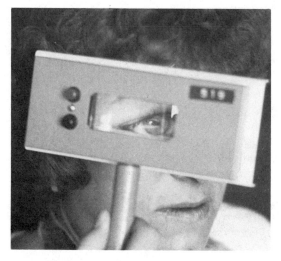

Figure 6–9. A black light being used to evaluate a fluorescein pattern

of the lens. There may or may not be fluorescein pooling in the center of the lens depending on the relation of the base curve radius to the corneal radius.

Overall Lens Diameter

The overall diameter of the lens to be used is based on the size of the palpebral aperture (lid separation), position of the lid margins in relation to the cornea with straight-ahead gaze, pupil size, effect of the lid forces on lens position, and other factors. For example, if there is a very small palpebral aperture a small lens is usually used. Likewise, if there is a very large aperture with the upper lid margin above the upper limbus, a small lens may also be used. This lens must stay centered over the pupil by fluid forces of the tears and a large lens would be too heavy and tend to slide down on the cornea. On the other hand, if the upper lid margin covers part of the upper cornea, a relatively large lens may be used so that the upper lid covers part of the lens and holds it in position. The power of the lens may also be a factor in using a given lens diameter since the weight and positioning of the plus and minus lenses are quite different. Only by evaluation of lenses on the eye can the proper size be determined for an individual patient.

Most rigid corneal contact lenses range from a small diameter of about 7.50 mm up to about 11.0 mm, with most lenses from 8.0 to 9.5 mm.

Optical Zone Diameter

The optical zone is the portion of the lens that corrects the patient's vision. It must be large enough to cover the patient's pupil. Since a contact lens moves on the cornea with blinking and eye movements, it must be large enough to keep the pupil covered with these lens movements. If the secondary curve of the lens moves in front of the pupil, the patient may see a doubling of objects (called diplopia). More common is the complaint of blurring or scattering of light from this region of the lens or lens edge. This is called flare and most commonly occurs in low-illumination conditions such as with night driving or at the movies when the pupil enlarges.

The optical zone on the majority of rigid lenses is from about 7.0 to 7.5 mm but may be as small as 6.0 mm to as large as 9.0 mm depending on the lens design.

Base Curve Radius

The radius of the back central region of the lens is chosen to give the proper fit to the cornea. The base curve radius (BCR) of most rigid corneal lenses is approximately the same as the corneal radius as determined by the keratometer reading, that is, with in ±0.20 mm (±1.00 D). The desired radius in this range depends on the lens diameter, optical zone diameter, type of lens being fitted, and the anatomy of the patient's cornea and lids. For example, the larger the lens and the optical zone diameters, the flatter the base curve must be. If the lens has a 8.0 mm OAD and 7.0 mm OZD, the base curve may be fitted 0.25 to 1.00 D steeper than the cornea. On the other hand, if the lens is a 10.00 mm OAD with an 8.5 mm OZD, it may be fitted 1.00 D flatter than the cornea. Lenses that are too steep or flat by as little as 0.25 to 0.50 D may result in corneal swelling, improper lens position, and discomfort.

The base curve radius can be evaluated by properly instilling fluorescein after the patient's tearing has subsided. If the lens has a longer radius than the cornea and fits too flat, a dark area will be seen in the center of the lens with fluorescein pooling in the periphery (Figure 6–10). When the base curve radius is too steep, tears will pool in the center of the lens (Figure 6–11). Lenses that are too flat will move excessively on blinking and may not stay well centered. Steep lenses will usually center better and may have insufficient movement.

With a spherical base curve lens on a toric cornea, an irregular fluorescein pooling will be seen. If the base curve of the lens is the same as the flat corneal meridian, there will be no pooling in this meridian but pooling will occur in the extremes of the other meridian. In the case of with-the-rule toricity the dark band of no fluorescein pooling is horizontal, with pooling at top and bottom (Figure 6–12). If the base curve

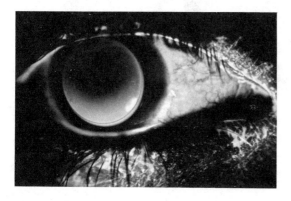

Figure 6–10. Fluorescein pattern showing a flat fitting rigid corneal contact lens

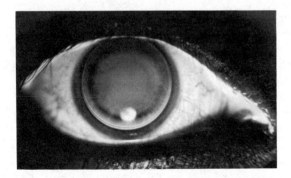

Figure 6–11. Fluorescein pattern showing a steep fitting rigid corneal contact lens

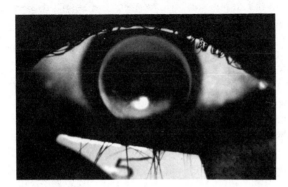

Figure 6–12. A spherical base curve lens on a with-the-rule toric cornea. The base curve radius equals the flat (horizontal) radius of the cornea

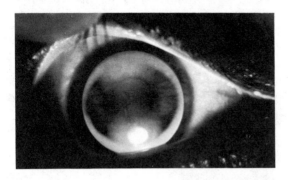

Figure 6–13. A spherical base curve lens fitted steeper than the flat meridian on a with-the-rule toric cornea

radius is made steeper, central pooling can be achieved but harsh bearing of the lens on the cornea occurs near the periphery of the optical zone in the horizontal meridian (Figure 6–13). In order to achieve a uniform fit, a toric base curve lens must be used.

Peripheral Curves

The peripheral curves are added to the lens geometry to increase the exchange of tear fluid under the lens with each blink. Without such exchange, corneal edema and discomfort would develop. Both the proper selection of the base curve radius and peripheral curve radii are required to give this exchange.

The widths (PCW) and radii (PCR) of peripheral curves are dependent upon the lens diameter, optical zone diameter, and anatomy of the patient's cornea. Comparing a large and small lens, the large would have a wider peripheral curve with a shorter radius, the small lens a narrow peripheral curve with a longer radius. Thus, the general rule is the narrower the peripheral curve, the longer the peripheral curve radius. For example, a 8.0 mm OAD lens with a 7.30 mm optical zone may have a peripheral curve with a radius of 2.0 mm flatter than the base curve radius (if the BCR is 7.50 mm, the peripheral curve radius is 9.50 mm). On the other hand, if the lens diameter is 9.7 mm with a 7.3 mm OZD, the peripheral radius may be only 0.7 mm longer than the base curve radius (if the BCR is 7.50 mm the peripheral curve radius may be 8.20 mm).

Of course the shape of the cornea is a factor. If the periphery of the cornea flattens rapidly, a flatter peripheral curve is required. This is determined by evaluating the fluorescein pattern. A definite green band of fluorescensce should be visible around the periphery of the lens.

A peripheral curve that is too flat may cause the lens to move excessively, not stay centered over the pupil and decrease the comfort. A peripheral curve that is too steep will not allow tear exchange, resulting in corneal swelling and discomfort. Little to no fluorescein pooling will be seen at the edge of a lens with a steep peripheral curve.

The radii and widths of the peripheral curves vary considerably. The widths may be as narrow as 0.10 mm to as wide as 1.5 to 2.0 mm. Of course the peripheral curve region can be divided into two or more curves. The radii of the peripheral curves may be as little as 0.5 to 0.7 mm flatter than the base curve to as much as 4 to 5 mm flatter.

Blends between the base curve and peripheral curve are often used to obtain a gradual transition between the two curves. This may increase the comfort and prevent corneal disruption by the junction.

Thickness

If a lens is made thicker than necessary, it will be heavy and unlikely to stay centered on the cornea. This is a common problem with plus lenses. In addition, a thick lens will often not be as comfortable, due to the lid irritation from the lid hitting the lenses.

With rigid gas-permeable lenses, the amount of oxygen transmitted through the material is dependent on the thickness. Thus, as the thickness is reduced the oxygen transmission is increased.

If a normally rigid lens is made quite thin, say 0.04 to 0.08 mm, it will bend quite easily. These, as well as lenses from some new materials, have been called semisoft. The advantages of such thin lenses is the reduced weight, better centration, and, in the case of oxygen permeable lenses, increased transmission. There can be disadvantages, however. One is that the lens may not be as durable. In addition, the lens will tend to flex when placed on the eye and not correct the corneal astigmatism like the thicker lens will. In some cases, this may be an advantage, but in many it is not (see Chapter 3). Of course only moderate to high minus lenses can be made this thin as it is physically impossible to make a plus lens with such a thin center.

The center thickness of a lens will vary with the lens power and diameter. Plus lenses will have center thickness of about 0.15 to 0.20 mm for very low plus up to 0.50 to 0.60 mm for high plus lenses (+ 12.00 to + 17.00 D range). With plus lenses, the limiting factor in center thickness reduction is the edge thickness (see Chapter 2). The edge cannot be made much thinner than 0.10 mm or it will be uncomfortable and tend to chip. For minus lenses, standard center thickness is 0.10 to 0.15 mm. Lenses with center thicknesses less than 0.10 mm are often termed ultrathin and may be as thin as 0.04 mm. Only lenses of more than − 2.50 D can be made this thin. With the higher minus lenses, even with very thin centers, the edges become relatively thick and must be thinned by proper manufacturing or modification. Center thicknesses can be calculated in the office or determined by computer programs by the laboratories.

Power

The power of a lens is determined by the patient's refractive error and the relationship of the base curve radius to the cornea curvature (see chapter 3). For a given patient and lens fit, the power cannot be varied. It must be taken into account, however, in the fitting process as a moderate to high minus lens will perform on the eye differently than will a low minus lens. Likewise, plus lenses will not center and move on an eye like minus lenses. This is due partially to the difference in thickness and weight but also to the shape of the lens in relation to the lid forces. The minus lens is thicker at the edge than the center, and when the lid is over the lens it acts as a wedge with the thick part under the lid (Figure

6–14). The force of the lid tends to pull the lens up and holds it. With a plus lens, the opposite occurs. The thick part of the lens is in the center so the lid force tends to push the lens down. For this reason, lenticular designs are often used with plus lenses (see Chapter 2).

Most lens powers will be from − 20.00 D to + 20.00 D. Common lens powers for myopia patients are in the range of − 1.00 to − 8.00 D and hyperopic patients up to + 8.00 D. Aphakic patients are usually + 10.00 to + 20.00 D. Of course, unusual cases will fall outside of these ranges.

Lens Material

The polymer (plastic) from which the lens is to be made must be determined. The oxygen-permeable materials offer the advantage of less corneal swelling and should be used where possible, but certain limitations exist with these materials. For example, special design lenses such as toric base curves, prism ballast front surface cylinder, and bifocals may not be available. With some patients surface coatings of tear film components may occur with the newer polymers, causing frequent blurring of vision and the need for repeated cleaning during the day. Changing solutions can help minimize this problem.

Some of the new polymers are not as stable as polymethylmethacylate (PMMA). The base curve may flatten or warp, particularly with cellulose acetate butyrate (CAB) lenses. PMMA-silicone combination polymers and rigid silicone lenses, on the other hand, appear as stable

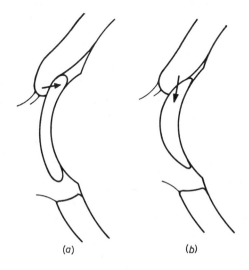

Figure 6–14. (a) Minus lens held up by upper lid; (b) plus lens forced down by upper lid

(a)   (b)

as the conventional PMMA lenses. Thickness may be a factor as CAB lenses are usually thicker than PMMA or PMMA-silicone lenses. CAB lenses resist breaking better than the other materials, however. Another factor is cost. PMMA lenses are less expensive than others. Development of additional polymers should increase the choice of lenses.

As can be seen, the type of material to be used for a particular patient depends upon the patient's prescription, likelihood of developing edema, tear film characteristics, sensitivity, and other factors. Table 6–1 summarizes some of the properties of these materials.

Tints

Often contact lenses are lightly tinted so that they are easier to find if dropped. The tint should be chosen to match the patient's eye color, but should not be dark enough to change the patient's eye color. If they were

Table 6–1.   Properties of some rigid lens materials.

Property	PMMA	CAB	PMMA-silicone	Silicone
Oxygen permeability	Poor	Fair	Fair	Good
Stability	Good	Poor	Good	Good
Resistance to heat	Fair	Poor	Poor	Good
Surface wettability	Good	Good	Good	Good only with a surface treatment
Resistance to breakage	Good	Excellent	Good	Fair
Scratch resistance	Fair	Fair	Fair	Fair
Flexibility	Low	Medium	Low	Medium
Ease of modification	Easy	Difficult	Easy	Not possible (loses wettability)
Disinfection	Chemical	Chemical	Chemical	Chemical or heat

dark enough to markedly change eye color, they would be too dark to wear indoors or for night driving.

Tints are usually specified as #1, #2, or #3, with #1 being the lightest. Sometimes halftones are available, that is, a shade between #1 and #2. Some laboratories may use letters, as A, B, and C. Since the tints are pigments all the way through the lens, specifying tints for thick lenses such as high plus or prism ballast lenses must be considered carefully. A #1 tint is very light with a thin minus lens, but quite dark with a + 15.00 D lens. A #2 tint in a + 15.00 D lens may be so dark it can hardly be seen through. Occasionally, #3 tints are prescribed for outdoor uses only, such as when playing golf. Common colors are blue, green, brown, and gray. Gray is a neutral color and can be used on most eye colors.

Some new lens polymers may only be available in clear or limited shades.

Writing Prescriptions

Once the lens design and material are decided upon, the complete prescription must be written. This prescription must be in the patient's record so that the lenses can be verified when they are received from the laboratory. This information is used on subsequent visits to determine if any lens variations have occurred and as a reference in case a lost or damaged lens must be ordered. Unless lenses are fitted from a large office stock, the order must also go to the laboratory to be filled.

An order should include the following lens dimensions: base curve radius, optical zone diameter, peripheral curve radius or radii, peripheral curve width(s) blends if any, overall diameter, front optical zone diameter (if a lenticular lens is used), center thickness (in some cases edge and junction thickness), carrier radius (if a lenticular design), tint, and type of material.

Figure 6–15 is an example of an order for a spherical single vision lens. All the lens dimensions are given in millimeters except the power, which is in diopters. With a single vision spherical lens of this type, the front optical zone diameter is usually not specified since the whole front surface is one radius and constitutes the front optic. Likewise, the edge thickness is not usually specified. There is no junction thickness, carrier radius, or lens series in this case.

Figure 6–16 is an order for a plus lenticular design. In this case only one peripheral curve was used, and thus it is specified under the secondary curve on the order. The edge and junction thicknesses are specified. In this case since the edge is thicker than the junction, it is a

CONTACT LENS ORDER FORM

PATIENT NAME _____ DATE _____

ADDRESS _____ PHONE _____ DATE WANTED _____

LENS SPECIFICATIONS

	BC	SCR	SCW	PCR	PCW	BLEND	DIA	OZD	FOZD	POWER
O.D.	7.60	9.20	0.5	12.0	0.2	light	8.80	7.40		-3.00
O.S.	7.75	9.35	0.5	12.0	0.2	light	8.80	7.40		-3.25

	c.t.	e.t.	j.t.	carrier R	tint	series	manufacturer	Lot no.	type of polymer
O.D.	0.12				#1 blue				PMMA
O.S.	0.11				#1 blue				PMMA

Other specifications:

Laboratory _____ Date ordered _____ Ordered by _____

Date received _____ Received by _____ Verified by _____

Figure 6–15. Lens order for a single vision spherical lens

CONTACT LENS ORDER FORM

PATIENT NAME _____ DATE _____

ADDRESS _____ PHONE _____ DATE WANTED _____

LENS SPECIFICATIONS

	BC	SCR	SCW	PCR	PCW	BLEND	DIA	OZD	FOZD	POWER
O.D.	8.27	9.00	0.95	12.0	0.1	light	9.60	7.50	7.70	+16.00
O.S.	8.10	8.90	0.95	12.0	0.1	light	9.60	7.50	7.70	+15.75

	c.t.	e.t.	j.t.	carrier R	tint	series	manufacturer	Lot no.	type of polymer
O.D.	0.41	0.20	0.13	10.0	clear				PMMA
O.S.	0.40	0.20	0.13	10.0	clear				PMMA

Other specifications:

Laboratory _____ Date ordered _____ Ordered by _____

Date received _____ Received by _____ Verified by _____

Figure 6–16. Lens order for a plus lenticular lens

minus carrier lenticular design. This creates an upward force on the lens by the upper lid and helps hold the lens centered. The carrier radius to give the desired edge thickness has been specified. Often this calculation is left up to the laboratory.

When writing an order to be sent to the laboratory, all the necessary lens data must be included to avoid delays. The patient's name and the date of the order are also recorded. When ordering the lenses from the laboratory by telephone, fill out the order form before calling to be sure all data are specified. After all lens specifications are given, the laboratory personnel taking the order should read them back to be sure they have understood the order properly. It is a waste of time and money as well as poor patient relations to wait for a lens to arrive from the laboratory to find it is incorrect due to poor communications between the office and laboratory.

HYDROGEL LENS FITTING

Hydrogel lenses can be fitted by the ocular measurement, diagnostic lenses, or stock lenses techniques. As with rigid lenses, the use of diagnostic or stock lenses is usually preferable.

Overall Diameter

Most hydrogel lenses are about the size of the cornea (12.5 to 13.5 mm) or larger (up to about 16 mm). Hydrogel lenses smaller than the diameter of the cornea are difficult to keep centered and may be uncomfortable.

The limbal designed hydrogel lenses (12.5 to 13.5 mm) are most often used. They just cover the limbus and move about ½ to 1 mm on each blink when properly fitted. On some patients, lenses of this diameter will not stay properly centered over the cornea, and a larger lens must be used. When a lens decenters and its edge is across the periphery of the cornea, it may irritate the corneal epithelium and cause staining.

With larger lenses, often called paralimbal or semiscleral, the lens edge is a millimeter or more beyond the limbus onto the conjunctiva. The conjunctiva is relatively soft, allowing the edge of the lens to settle into this tissue. When this happens, the lens may stop moving or the soft conjunctiva may move with the lens. In either case tear exchange under the lens is stopped, causing build-up of metabolic waste products and resulting in wearing difficulties. Therefore, the proper fitting of these lenses is critical.

An advantage of larger lenses is that they will center over the cornea better than the smaller lenses. Likewise, they are not decentered or lost from the eye as easily as the smaller lenses. Since the edges are under the lids and out on the conjunctiva, dust and debris are less likely to get under the lens to cause discomfort. Therefore, the larger lenses may be chosen for the patient who will be around dusty environments and those taking part in contact sports.

Optical Zone Diameter

The optical zone of a hydrogel lens is usually considerably larger than that of a rigid lens. It is not unusual to have 9 to 11 mm diameter back optical zone on hydrogel lenses. Since they are relatively soft they tend to conform to the shape of the cornea; therefore, only narrow peripheral curves are required. This is a visual advantage since the optical zone will remain over the pupil even with considerable lens movement.

The size of the usable optic of hydrogel lenses is usually limited by the front optic diameter. Even moderate minus prescription (– 3.00 D or more) must be made in lenticular form to minimize edge thickness. Any plus lens must be made in lenticular form to minimize center thickness. The greater the lens power, the smaller the front optic zone. With high prescriptions, the front optic may be as small as 7.5 mm.

Many manufacturers have set optical zones for their lenses. Those with very large back optics must be fitted with longer base curve radii than those with the smaller zones. A lens with a large optic zone may be used for those patients with very large pupils to prevent visual disturbance from the periphery of the lens.

Base Curve Radius

To obtain the desired lens movement, the base curve radius is the variable most often used. A lens should move ½ to 1 mm on each blink and will slide down 1 mm on upward gaze. This assures enough movement to exchange some tears under the lens preventing a build-up of waste products of metabolism and debris.

The lens movement and fit is best evaluated with the biomicroscope. After the lens has been placed on the cornea and allowed to settle for 15 to 20 minutes, the movement is determined by looking at the edge of the lens. If it is moving excessively, a steeper lens is required. If no movement is occurring, a flatter (longer radius) lens is tried.

The initial lens placed on the cornea is determined by taking into account the corneal curvature (keratometer reading), lens diameter, back optic diameter, lens thickness, and water content. The larger the lens diameter, the flatter the base curve must be.

Hydrogel lenses are fitted from about 0.3 to 1.5 mm flatter than the patient's keratometer reading. If the lens has a small diameter and back optic zone it will be fitted with a steeper base curve, say only 0.3 to 0.5 mm flatter than the cornea. A larger lens with a very large optic zone might be fitted 1.0 mm flatter than the cornea. In all cases, adequate lens movement of ½ to 1 mm is desired.

The softness and flexibility of the lens can affect the base curve radius chosen. A very thin lens or a high water content lens may have to be fitted steeper than thicker or lower water content lenses of the same dimensions. Thin or high water content lenses of a given base curve radius will fit a wider range of corneal curvatures than stiffer lenses because the thin lens will flex easily to take the shape of the eye. Lower water content lenses (30 to 45 percent) of standard thickness (0.10 to 0.20 mm) may require base curve radius steps in 0.2 to 0.3 mm intervals in order to be properly fitted. Very thin or high water content lenses may only have to be manufactured in 0.5 to 0.6 mm steps. In fact, some manufacturers only provide one base curve radius in the ultrathin lenses, assuming that it will fit the majority of patients.

Thickness

The thickness of hydrogel lenses is important since most of the oxygen supplied to the cornea comes through the lens. Therefore, the thinner the lens, the greater the oxygen supply. The first hydrogel lenses were quite thick, 0.3 to 0.5 mm, and caused considerable edema. Later, more clinically acceptable minus lenses were 0.12 to 0.20 mm thick. Still, significant edema occurs with some patients. Recently even thinner lenses, 0.04 to 0.08 mm thick, are being used. These do not cause significant edema in the majority of patients.

One must consider not only the center thickness but also the thickness in the periphery of the lens. A lens with minus power will be thicker in the periphery. If the front optic is quite large, the peripheral portion of the lens may be so thick that cornea swelling may occur under that portion of the lens.

The thinner the lens, the softer and more flexible it is. It tends to take the shape of the cornea, and will not move as much on a blink as thicker lenses. There is not as much lens bulk for the lid to hit.

There are two disadvantages of thin lenses; handling difficulty and fragility. It is extremely important to teach the patient proper handling, placement, and removal techniques.

The trend in hydrogel lens fitting is toward thinner lenses. Of course plus lenses are all going to be relatively thick, creating more physiological problems.

Power

The power required in a hydrogel lens can be determined by the spectacle lens correction or by refracting over a diagnostic lens. Since a well-fitted hydrogel lens does not create a lacrimal lens effect, the power of the contact lens should be the same as the spectacle lens. If the spectacle lens is over 4.00 D the power of the lens at the corneal surface must be calculated (see Chapter 3). The residual astigmatism should be the same as the spectacle astigmatism. For example, if the patient's spectacle correction is $-3.00 -0.50 \times 180$ and a -3.00 D hydrogel lens is used, a refraction over the lens should give plano -0.50×180. In practice, the spherical equivalent power, -3.25 D, might be given.

Both the calculation of the required power as well as the refraction over diagnostic lenses should be performed. If they do not compare very closely, the power and fit of the lens should be reevaluated.

Material

There are many hydrogel materials. The water content, elasticity, and durability vary. Generally, the higher the water content, the more fragile the lens. For daily lens wear, water content of 30 to 45 percent is normally used. Higher water content lenses (60 to 85 percent) have greater oxygen transmission and are thus used for extended wear. Of course, with extended wear, the lens is not handled as much as with daily wear, making the problem of fragility less important.

The type of material to be used must be determined for each patient. Those prone to edema may require high water content, thin lenses while the patient who is rough in handling the lens may do better with a lower water content, thicker lens.

Writing Prescriptions

The writing of a hydrogel lens prescription follows the same form as with rigid lenses. The base curve, diameter, power, and thickness must be specified. Likewise, the manufacturer and type of material must be specified. Many manufacturers have predetermined optical zones and peripheral curves that cannot be varied. In addition, the lens thickness may be set within a company's given lens series. That is, they may provide a range of diameters and base curves in standard thicknesses and a second series in thin lenses. One must become familiar with the lens specifications and limitations of the manufacturers used.

7

INSPECTION AND VERIFICATION

The most carefully fitted lens will not be satisfactory if the lens ordered is not manufactured to specifications or not properly finished. When lenses are received from the laboratory, they should be carefully verified to determine if the parameters are as ordered and carefully inspected for quality of the surface, edge, and polymer. In addition, lenses previously fitted to patients must be periodically verified to determine if the dimensions have changed. Likewise, patients coming to your office wearing lenses fitted by others must have them measured and inspected.

There are several different techniques available to verify each lens dimension. The most common techniques will be explained.

RIGID LENS INSPECTION AND VERIFICATION

Lens Diameter

The easiest parameter to inspect is the overall size (OS) or overall diameter (OAD), which is specified as the greatest linear distance across the lens and given in millimeters.

V-channel Gauge. One of the quickest methods of measuring the overall size is to use a plastic or metal V-channel gauge as shown in Figure 7–1. The lens is placed concave surface down in the gauge at the wide end of the channel. That end of the gauge is raised so that the lens will

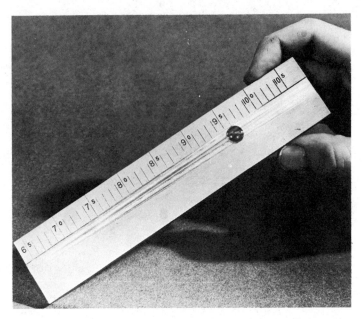

Figure 7–1. V-channel gauge to measure overall lens diameter

slide down the channel by gravity until it stops. The diameter is then measured from the scale along the channel. The gauge and lens must be dry and clean. This permits the lens to slide freely and eliminates the possibility of the surface or edge being scratched. The lens should never be pushed down the V-channel gauge since it may bend, causing it to go further and giving an erroneously small diameter reading. The overall size should be checked about four times, rotating the lens 45 degrees between each measurement. The lens should measure the same in each meridian unless a design other than round was ordered. If the lens is not round, the largest and smallest diameters should be recorded.

Hand Measuring Magnifier.   A 7x to 10x hand-held measuring magnifier (Figure 7–2) can be used to measure the diameter. The lens is placed on the flat surface of the magnifier, held in place by the index finger, and then the magnifier is held before the eye toward a light source (Figure 7–3). The diameter is assessed by use of a measuring reticule (Figure 7–4), and the lens should again be looked at to ensure that it is round.

Projection Magnifier (Shadow Graph).   Another method is to use a projection magnifier (Figure 7–5). The lens is placed in a light beam and

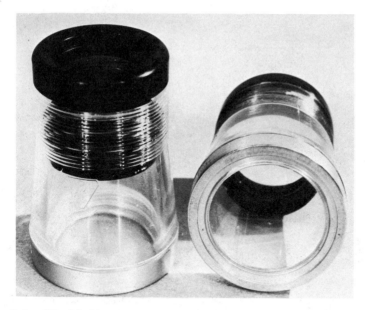

Figure 7–2. Hand-held measuring magnifiers to measure lens diameter, optical zone diameter, and peripheral curve widths

the shadow of the lens projected onto a screen which has a scale. By means of the scale, the diameter can be measured.

Tolerance. The lens size should be within ±0.05 mm of that ordered in all meridians.

Back Optical Zone Diameter

Hand Measuring Magnifier. The greatest linear distance across the back optical zone can be measured with a hand-held magnifier (Figure 7–2). The lens is placed on the front surface of the magnifier, held toward a light source, the edge of the optical zone lined up with the zero point on the reticule scale, and the back optical zone diameter (OZD) read. When there is a sharp, distinct junction between the central optical portion and the peripheral curves, this determination is easily made. If the junction between the curves is blended and thus blurred, it may be quite difficult to measure. The junction between the curves is easier to see if the hand magnifier is moved around, across an area of illumination. With very heavily blended lenses it is never easy to measure the optical portion

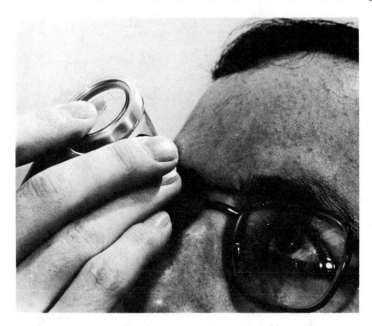

Figure 7–3.   Measuring magnifier in use

with any degree of accuracy. With a blended lens the back optical zone should be measured from the inside edge of the blend since this is the portion of the lens through which the patient will have good vision. The laboratory will usually work the optical diameter before the lens is blended, however, so that the measured value will be less than specified. When measuring the optical portion it should be examined in several meridians to be certain it is round. Poor fabrication techniques of the secondary curve often result in an oval zone. It is perhaps best to order all lenses without blends, inspect them, and then if a blend is desired, it may be carried out in the office. A heavy blend will usually cover up a poor secondary curve fabrication. One should be concerned about its accuracy if a laboratory will supply only blended lenses.

Lenses manufactured with: (1) a spherical base curve radius and a toric peripheral curve; (2) a toric base curve and a spherical peripheral curve; or (3) a toric base curve and toric secondary curve where the differences in curvature of the major meridians are not the same will result in an oval optical zone. Therefore, if one of these designs is ordered, an oval optical zone should be recorded. If a lens is ordered with spherical base curve and peripheral curves but on inspection is found to have an oval optical zone, the fabrication of the peripheral curve is faulty. If the

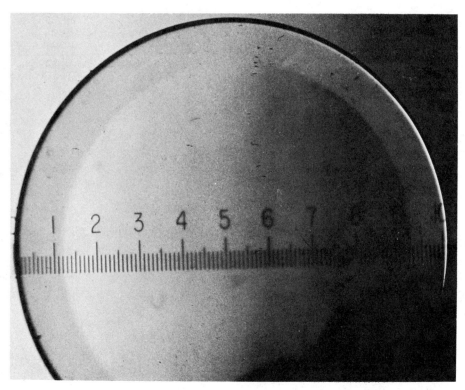

Figure 7-4. Contact lens viewed through hand-held magnifier. The reticule (scale) is visible as well as the overall lens diameter, optical zone, and peripheral curve

difference in the two meridians of the optical zone is greater than 0.10 mm, the lens should be rejected.

On lenses that have a lenticular design, as with high plus or minus powers, the front zone should also be measured. The same method as used for the optical zone diameter can be applied. Care must be exercised not to confuse the anterior optical portion with the posterior or with the junction of the posterior secondary and tertiary curve. The presence of an anterior optical zone can be verified by viewing the front surface of the lens with reflected light, preferably under high magnification. If an anterior junction is present, it will be seen when the lens is slightly tilted. If the presence of an anterior junction has been verified but cannot be distinguished from the posterior, either the anterior or posterior junction can be marked with a fine felt-tipped pen to show its position so that it can be identified with a hand magnifier.

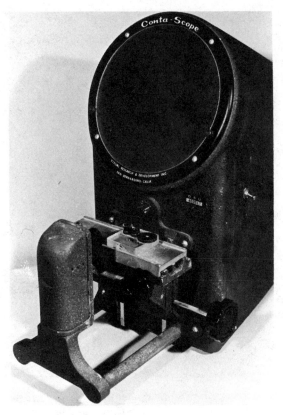

Figure 7–5. One of the available projection magnifiers to measure overall lens size, optical zone diameter, and peripheral curve width and to inspect edges

Projection Magnifier. The optical zone can be measured using a projection magnifier. The lens is placed in the light beam and a shadow of the lens projected onto a screen that has a scale on it. Again, if the lens is blended it is difficult to locate the junctions.

Tolerance. The optical zone diameter should be manufactured to a tolerance of ± 0.10 mm. If a medium or heavy blend is present, it is difficult to make accurate determination of the optical zone diameter and greater tolerance must be allowed, normally ± 0.20 mm.

BLEND

When the transition or junction between two curves is altered either by the addition of a very narrow curve or a series of curves of some intermediate radius, the lens is said to be blended. Specification of the amount of blend present is difficult because the beginning and end of the blended area is not easily delineated and the radius of the blending curve cannot be determined. Customarily the blend is specified as either light, medium, or heavy. With a light blend, it is possible to see the area of the blend as it is relatively narrow—approximately 0.10 mm wide. With a medium blend the transition zone is increasingly difficult to see. With a heavy blend it is usually impossible to determine the width of the blend with any accuracy as there is a wide blurred area of 0.30 mm or more.

Hand Measuring Magnifier. The blend is normally inspected using a hand magnifier. Its width can be estimated by the scale. The blurred area of the blend can often be seen by moving the head and the magnifier back and forth while viewing the lens against a background which is evenly illuminated.

Projection Magnifier or Microscope. The projection magnifier can also be used to identify a blend, but does not offer any advantage over the hand magnifier. Junctions or blends can further be seen by means of the stereomicroscope with approximately 40x magnification and with specular reflection of the light source from the lens surface.

Tolerances. It is not possible to give tolerances to which blends must conform due to the difficulty in measuring a blend, and the fact that they can vary from being imperceptibly light to very heavy. There is no way to quantify a blend. When ordering blended lenses from a laboratory, it must be remembered that by adding a blend, the effective back optical portion is reduced and the optics ruined over the extent of its width. Since many laboratories specifiy the OZD before blending, the resultant lens will have a smaller optical area than originally wanted, with the consequence that the patient may have physical and visual problems. Allowance must therefore be made for this.

PERIPHERAL CURVE WIDTHS

The widths of peripheral curves can be measured with the hand measuring magnifier in the same way as the back optical zone. If the junctions of the curves are blended, the widths will be difficult to determine, and with heavy blends, practically impossible.

When only one peripheral curve is present, the width is one-half the difference between the back central optic diameter and the overall lens size. For example, if the back optical zone is 7.50 mm and the overall size is 9.50 mm, then the peripheral curve width is 1.0 mm. When inspecting a lens it should be confirmed that the sum of the measured value of the back central optic diameter and twice the value of the peripheral curve widths equals the overall size. If several peripheral curves are present, the same procedure can be used. For example, if the overall diameter is 9.50 mm, the optical zone diameter 7.50 mm, and the tertiary curve 0.20 mm wide, the secondary curve width on a tri-curve lens should be 0.80 mm.

An alternative method for measuring the peripheral curve widths is to use a projection magnifier. The lens is placed in the light beam so that its image is projected on to the screen containing the reticule. The widths of the curves can be verified using the reticule.

Tolerance. Laboratory tolerances for peripheral curve widths are ±0.05 mm for a lens without or with a light blend, and ±0.10 mm for lenses with medium or heavy blends.

BASE CURVE RADIUS

The base curve radius (BCR), or radii in the case of toric lenses, is an important parameter in terms of both optical and physiological performance. The BCR is the radius of the central posterior surface and is specified in millimeters.

Optical Microspherometer (Radiuscope). The most common and one of the most accurate methods of measuring the BCR is to use an optical microspherometer, for example, a radiuscope. The radiuscope is basically a microscope with an eyepiece and objective. It has been modified to accurately measure the distance between two focal planes (Figures 7–6 and 7–7). To measure the BCR of a contact lens, the lens is floated on a small drop of water in the depression of the holder on the stage of the microscope (Figure 7–8). The water greatly reduces the reflection of the light from the front (convex) surface of the lens. The lens should be clean and dry before being placed on the holder. If there is a drop of water on the back surface of the lens or if the surface is dirty, the image used to make the measurement will be blurred, distorted, or incorrect. When handling the lens, be careful not to bend or distort the lens since it may take some time for the lens to return to its original shape. In the meantime, an erroneous reading will be obtained. When the lens is floated on the holder, only a minimum amount of water should be used. If there is too much, the lens will tend to move while the measurement is being taken, making an accurate reading difficult. The lens should be allowed

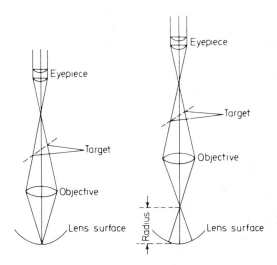

Figure 7–6. Diagram of the optical principle of the radiuscope

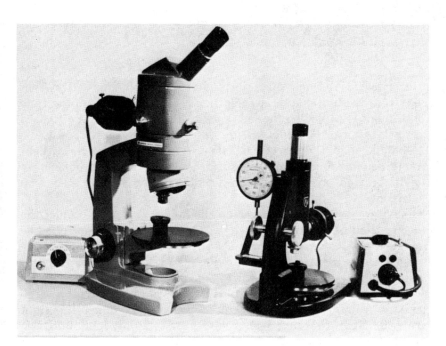

Figure 7–7. Two models of American Optical Radiuscope. The one on the left has an internal scale. The earlier model, on the right, has an external dial

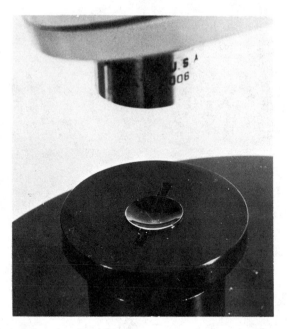

Figure 7–8. A contact lens floated on the lens mount in position to measure the base curve radius.

to settle for several seconds before the reading is started. This will prevent an inaccurate reading due to any additional settling, between the time the instrument is zeroed on the lens surface and the microscope focused on the aerial image. The effect is greatest when an excess of water is used. A bubble under the lens or too little water in the lens holder without effectively neutralizing the convex surface can also cause problems resulting in blurred or double outlines of the target and confusion in measurement.

Once the lens has been floated on the holder and placed under the microscope, the instrument is turned on. The brightness is controlled by a rheostat. It should be turned only about halfway up. Turning it to the brightest setting will just shorten the bulb life. With the American Optical Co. instrument be sure the aperture slide which is between the bulb housing and the body of the instrument is positioned with the large aperture in front of the light beam to prevent occluding the light (Figure 7–9). Next, the stage is moved (Figure 7–10) by hand until the spot of light, viewed without looking in the microscope, is centered on the contact lens. Then, looking through the instrument, it is aligned to give the brightest image. The microscope is then racked up to at least 10 or 12 on the scale seen in the instrument or as high as it will go. This is done by turning the coarse focusing knob located near the base of the instrument (Figure 7–11). It is the larger-diameter sleeve nearest the

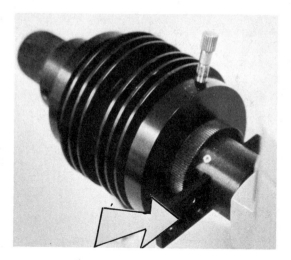

Figure 7–9. The bulb housing of the radiuscope with the arrow indicating the aperture slide, which must be positioned with either the large or small aperture in front of the light beam

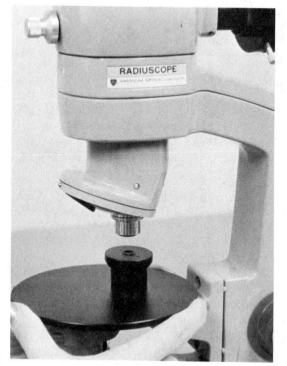

Figure 7–10. Moving the stage to position the lens directly under the objective and light beam

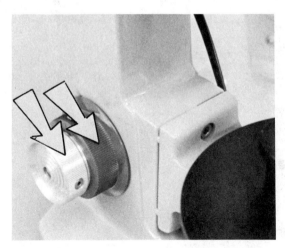

Figure 7–11. Base of radiuscope showing the focusing knobs. The right arrow indicates the course focus, the left the fine focus

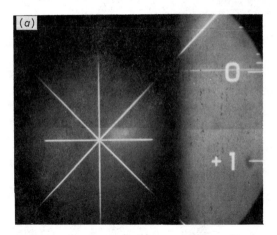

Figure 7–12. (a) Lens surface image of radiuscope pattern

body of the instrument. The smaller inner knob is for fine focusing. Now the instrument is focused slowly downward with the coarse focusing knob until the spoke pattern comes into focus. This is the image of the pattern reflected from the concave lens surface and is called the aerial image (Figure 7–12c, d). The stage on which the lens is mounted is moved until the spoke pattern is centered in the field of view or aligned with the reference marks, depending on the instrument used (Figure 7–12d). The microscope is now focused downward and the image of the bulb filament will come into view (Figure 7–12b) but is ignored. The microscope is moved father downward until the spoke pattern is again in focus. This is the image of the pattern on the lens surface, which may also reveal scratches or dirt. This pattern is brought into sharp focus with the fine

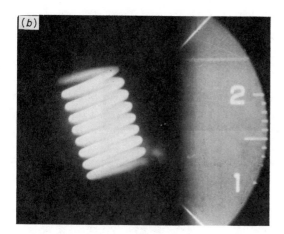

Figure 7–12. (b) Appearance of bulb filament seen as microscope is focused up from the surface image toward the aerial image

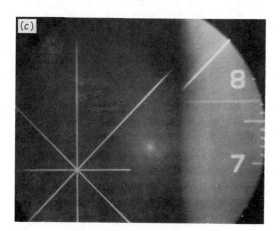

Figure 7–12. (c) Aerial image not properly aligned

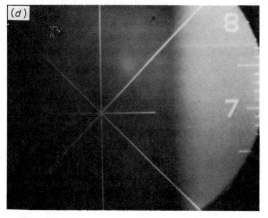

Figure 7–12. (d) Aerial image properly centered with reference line

focusing knob (Figure 7–12a). The measuring dial is set at zero. The method of zeroing the dial and its position varies with different instruments. For the American Optical instrument the small knob on the left side (Figure 7–13) moves the index line so that it can be placed through zero. In some cases the lens may be too low for the line to be moved up enough to go through zero. In this case the index line is placed on +1 or +2 on the scale and this value is then added to the final reading. The small knob on the front of the instrument is to focus the scale and index line.

Once zeroed the microscope is focused upward, using the coarse focusing knob, past the image of the filament to the second spoke pattern (the aerial image). The fine focus should be used to get the image in as sharp a focus as possible. It is best just to look at one of the spokes near

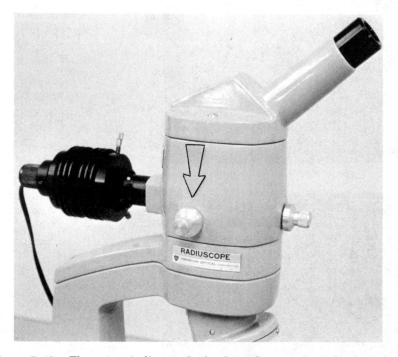

Figure 7–13. The arrow indicates the knob used to set the index line on zero. The similar knob to the right is to focus the scale

the center of the pattern and focus it until the edges of the spoke are as sharp as possible. The other spokes should also be in sharp focus if the base curve is spherical. At this point the value on the dial is the radius of curvature (BCR) of the lens.

If the contact lens is warped or has a toric base curve, all the spokes of the aerial image will not come into focus at one time. If this is the case when the aerial image is brought into focus the first time, one of the spokes should be focused as clearly as possible. If a single spoke does not come into focus, the lens mount should be rotated until only one spoke is in focus. Then proceed to zero the instrument on the lens surface as with a spherical lens. All the spokes of the surface image will be in focus at one time even though the lens is toric. When the microscope is then focused upward to the aerial image, a reading is taken when the first spoke appears in focus. This is the radius of the steepest meridian (Figure 7–14a). The microscope is then focused farther upward until the spoke 90° from the first one is in sharp view (Figure 7–14b). The reading at this point is the radius of curvature of the flattest meridian of the lens.

The accuracy and calibration of the radiuscope should be checked periodically by using thick back surface buttons with known radii. The buttons can be placed on the stage and do not need to be floated on water (Figure 7–15).

The radius of curvature can easily be determined to an accuracy of ± 0.02 mm if care is taken in making the measurement.

Keratometer or Ophthalmometer. A second method commonly employed to measure the BCR utilizes a conventional keratometer or ophthalmometer. The same principle applies when measuring the curvature of the cornea (see Chapter 5) except a special lens holder is required (Figure 7–16). The holder consists of a clamp that mounts it to the headrest of the instrument, a depression to hold the lens, and a front surface mirror. The lens, which must be clean, is floated on a small drop of water cancave side up. The keratometer or ophthalmometer is focused on the reflected mires and aligned in the same manner as when measuring the cornea. Alignment of mires and the dioptric power reading on the drum are noted and the power converted to millimeters of radius using the index for which the keratometer or ophthalmometer is calibrated. There is a slight difference in the conversion from diopters to millimeters between corneal and BCR readings due to the fact that a concave and not convex surface is measured. A conversion table is given in Appendix IV.

If the lens is warped or toric, the mires will appear the same as the cornea with astigmatism. The keratometer or ophthalmometer can be rotated to measure the radii in the major meridians. It is simpler to rotate

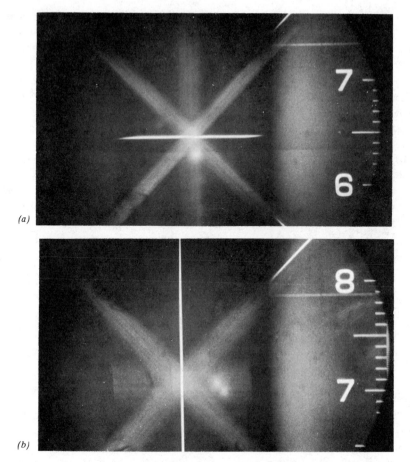

(a)

(b)

Figure 7–14. (a) Radiuscope pattern as it appears with a warped or toric lens; (b) spoke in meridian 90 degrees from the one in (a) in focus

the instrument in the same manner as measuring oblique astigmatism than attempt turning the contact lens.

Other lens holders, as seen in Figure 7–17, can be used to hold the lens on the keratometer or ophthalmometer to measure the BCR, but with these devices the lens must be positioned vertically and surface tension of water is often not great enough to hold it. Other substances, such as double-faced tape, toothpaste, or clay, can be utilized but may warp the lens.

To obtain accurate readings, the instrument should be in correct adjustment and calibrated, the lens clean, no water allowed on the concave surface, and an accurate conversion table always available. One disad-

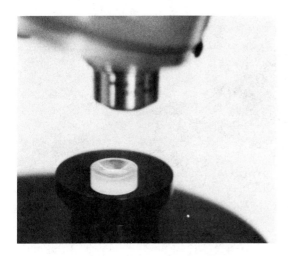

Figure 7–15. Using a back surface button to check the calibration of the radiuscope

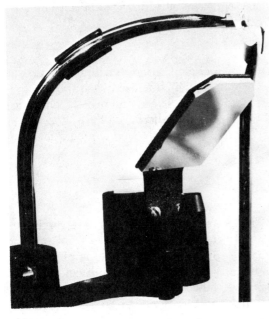

Figure 7–16. Device attached to the headrest of the keratometer to measure BCR

vantage of employing a keratometer or ophthalmometer is that the instrument is frequently found in the examining room, and if the BCR of a lens has to be checked, the patient will perhaps be in the way and have to be moved. Also, the lens holder must be attached each time, with the result that back central optic radii are not inspected as often as desired.

Other Methods. Other methods of measuring the base curve radius

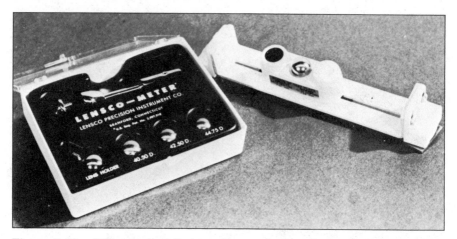

Figure 7–17. Other devices that can be attached to the headrest of the keratometer to hold contact lenses for measurement of BCR. The steel balls are used to calibrate the keratometer

have been devised. Such techniques include the moire fringe instrument (Toposcope or Lenscope); the R-C device, which is used with the lensometer; mechanical spherometers; and others. These and other techniques that have only found limited use will not be discussed here. For an explanation of these techniques, *Contact Lens Correction* can be consulted.

Front Surface Radius

If the BCR, center thickness and power of a contact lens are correct as ordered, it follows from basic optical principles that the front surface radius must be correct. Because of this and concern for the physical fit of the lens on the cornea, one usually checks the back and not the front curve. When the lens is on the eye, however, the front is the most important refracting surface because the index change at this surface is from air (1.00) to plastic (1.49). Any distortion of this surface or other poor optical quality will therefore cause greater visual loss than the same distortion of the back central optics since the back is in contact with the tear layer (index 1.336). For this reason, the front surface radius should be closely examined if questionable optics are suspected when verifying the power or if the patient has an unexplained vision problem with a lens.

Optical Microspherometer (Radiuscope). The contact lens is mounted under the microscope of the radiuscope by floating it on a special mount with a drop of water with the concave surface contacting the water as shown in Figure 7–18. A large drop of water is placed on the pedestal and the lens gently dropped on it. Be sure not to trap a bubble under the lens. The radius is measured in the same manner as the BCR. The only difference is that the surface image is higher—coming into focus when the microscope is focused downward—than the aerial image. This is the opposite from that where the BCR is measured since the latter acts as a concave mirror whereas the front surface acts as a convex one. The instrument can be zeroed on the reflected image, lower image, and then the measurement made at the lens surface, the top image. The same procedure is followed as when the base curve radius is measured, with similar conditions and problems applying.

Keratometer of Ophthalmometer. The keratometer or ophthalmometer can be employed to verify the front surface radius by mounting the lens on the same holder and mirror system used to measure the BCR except that the lens is mounted with the convex surface towards the mirror. The instrument is aligned and focused on the mires in the same manner as when a corneal measurement is made. The dioptric reading can be converted to millimeters of radius by using the index for which

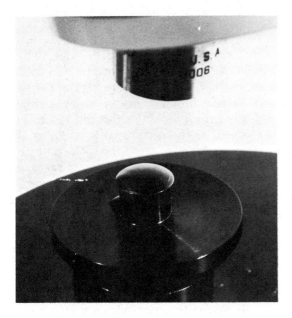

Figure 7–18. Contact lens mounted under the radiuscope to measure the front surface radius

the instrument is calibrated (Appendix IV). Special attention should be given to the quality of the reflected mires to determine if there is any distortion.

PERIPHERAL CURVE RADIUS

The peripheral curve radius is an important lens parameter for obtaining a successful fit but very difficult to check, and one must normally rely on the laboratory to furnish the correct radius, without verification. If the width of the secondary curve is 0.8 mm or more, of optical finish, and there is no blend, then there are several methods that can give a good approximation of the peripheral radius and an indication of the optical quality.

Optical Microspherometer (Radiuscope). To measure the peripheral curve radius using the radiuscope the contact lens is floated on a minimal amount of water on the lens mount in the same manner as when measuring the BCR. The microscope is then focused on the surface image, and while being viewed, the lens mount is slowly tilted and moved laterally so that the junction between the central and peripheral curve and then the edge of the lens come into view. While the lens is being moved, its angle of tilt should be changed so that the image remains in view and the amount of light reflected from the surface is maintained at a maximum. The secondary curve will be perpendicular to the axis of the microscope when the lens is positioned correctly (Figure 7–19). The radiuscope is zeroed at this point, imaged on the lens surface, and then focused upward beyond the image of the filament until the aerial target comes into focus. The first spoke pattern brought into view beyond the filament image may be the reflection from the BC since the source is often reflected from the central as well as the peripheral curve. Should this be so, it is necessary to focus upward further until the spoke pattern reflected from the secondary curve comes into focus. The gauge reading at this point will be the peripheral curve radius. If the aerial image is not positioned in the middle of the field, the stage may be moved slightly to center it. In this case, the instrument has to be zeroed on the surface again before making a final reading. The same precautions must be followed as when measuring the BCR.

The quality of the aerial image from the peripheral radius depends on the width of the curve and optical quality of the surface. A narrow band will not give as clear an image as a wide one. With a wide and true curve the aerial pattern will be sharp and distinct, and with some practice,

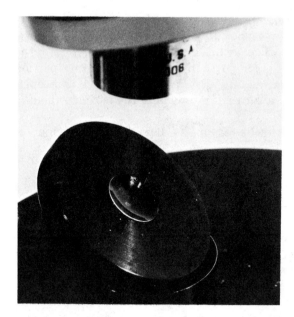

Figure 7-19. Lens positioned under the radiuscope to measure the peripheral curve radius

it is possible to assess the optical quality of the peripheral curve using this technique.

Keratometer of Ophthalmometer. These instruments cannot be used to measure the peripheral curve radius because the mires are reflected from a large area of the lens surface and thus not totally from the peripheral curve.

Use of Radius Laps. It is possible to estimate the peripheral curve radius by coating the back surface of the contact lens (using a waterproof felt marking pen), mounting it on a small button or holding it by a suction cup, and placing it for a few seconds on a rotating radius lap (see Chapter 8 for use of this equipment). If the ink is polished off toward the outer edge of the peripheral curve, the lap is flatter, that is, of longer radius than the peripheral curve. On the other hand, if the ink is polished off at the inner portion of the peripheral curve, the radius lap is steeper than the secondary curve. By using laps of different radii the one most nearly approximating the peripheral curve can be determined. Caution must be taken to make sure the lens is not left on the lap too long causing it to be blended or the peripheral radius changed. It should be on the radius lap only long enough to polish away a small amount of the ink. Excess ink can be removed with cigarette lighter fluid or benzine.

Another method is to place the lens on a metal radius lap with a layer of dye, such as fluorescein, between it and the lap. If no dye is present in the region of the peripheral curve, it matches the lap. If the outer portion of the peripheral curve has a thicker layer of dye than the inner, the peripheral radius is longer than the lap. If the inner portion has a thicker dye layer than the outer, the peripheral curve is steeper. Thus, by placing the lens on a series of radius laps, the peripheral curve radius can be estimated.

Both of these methods utilizing laps to determine the peripheral radius are time-consuming and not routinely used. The peripheral curve must be reasonably wide for these techniques to be at all effective.

Use of Lensometer, Vertexometer, or Focimeter

A lensometer can be used to determine the peripheral curve radius when it is 1.0 mm wide or more. A small aperture is used on the lensometer and the power of the lens read both through the optical zone and secondary curve portion. Since the anterior curve radius is the same for both regions, the power difference is due to the different back surface radii. This technique requires that there is only one front surface radius. Peripheral curve radii of lenticular designs, lenses with wide front bevels or aspherical front surfaces cannot be determined. Once the difference in power between the central and peripheral curve is established and the BCR known, the following formula can be applied to determine the peripheral curve radius:

$$\Delta F = (4.90) \left[\frac{100}{r_B} - \frac{100}{r_{PC}} \right]$$

or

$$\frac{100}{r_{PC}} = \frac{100}{r_B} - (0.2041)\Delta F$$

where:

r_B is the base curve radius of the lens in millimeters
r_{PC} is the peripheral curve radius in millimeters
ΔF is the difference in power in diopters between the central and peripheral portions.

This formula shows that each 0.75 D difference in power between the central and peripheral portions of the lens is equivalent to approximately 0.1 mm peripheral curve flattening. For example, if the central power is -5.00 DS and the power through the peripheral curve region -2.00 DS, the peripheral curve radius is approximately 0.4 mm flatter than the BCR.

Methods of Specifying the Peripheral Curve Radius. Usually the peripheral curve radius is specified in millimeters of radius, such as 8.50 mm. This specification is preferred since this is the actual radius of the lens surface. In some cases it may be specified in terms of millimeters flatter than the BCR—for example, that the peripheral curve is 1.00 mm flatter than the BCR. Another convention used, but one that can be confused with lens power or difference in power between central and peripheral zones, is to specify the peripheral curve as so many diopters flatter than the BCR. This has arisen from the method employed by some practitioners of specifying the base curve radius of the contact lens in terms of diopters as determined by the index to calibrate the keratometer. In this case, a peripheral curve that is said to be 10.00 D flatter than the BCR is actually 2.0 mm as expressed in millimeters. That is, 0.20 mm approximately equals 1.00 D of flattening.

Tolerance. The tolerance for the peripheral curve radius is ± 0.10 mm.

LENS POWER

The lensometer is the instrument used to determine the power of a contact lens. The procedure is generally the same as is employed with spectacle lenses, but with a few exceptions.

Most lensometers are made to measure the vertex power of spectacle lenses; thus, the stop is made for lenses with base curves of approximately 88 mm whereas contact lenses have radii of only 7 or 8 mm. The sagittal depth of the contact lens over the aperture, therefore, is much greater than with the spectacle lens. Since the lensometer measures the vertex power (back focal length) from the point corresponding to where the back surface of the spectacle lens would be, there may be a considerable difference in power due to the steep radius of the contact lens. This error is especially important with high prescriptions. Because of this problem some lensometers are equipped with a special stop to be used with contact lenses to compensate for the difference in curvature (Figure 7–20). Most practitioners specify the power of contact lenses in terms of the back vertex power, that is, the inverse of the focal length as measured from the back lens surface. In actual practice it is the power measured with the concave surface against the lensometer stop that may or may not be exactly from the back vertex of the lens for the reasons discussed. Some laboratories, however, measure the front surface vertex power and not the back vertex power. Thus, if the laboratory manufactures the lens so that the front vertex matches the power ordered but you measure it in terms of back vertex power, there will be a large discrepancy for high

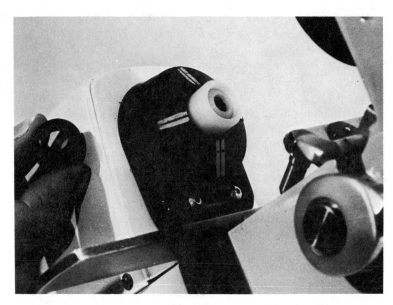

Figure 7–20. Special lens stop to hold contact lenses shown on the lensometer (white stop on the instrument) compared with the stop used for spectacles (held next to the instrument)

dioptric prescriptions and the patient's refractive error will not be properly corrected. For example, if the back vertex power of a contact lens is +16.00 D, the front vertex will be approximately 1 diopter less.

Power Measurement. First the lensometer or vertexometer should be properly adjusted. Looking through the eyepiece (Figure 7–21), it should be rotated counterclockwise until the black reference lines become blurred. The eyepiece is then rotated clockwise until the lines just come into focus again and no further. With the projection vertexometer there is no eyepiece to adjust since the image is projected onto a screen. Next, looking into the instrument the power wheel (Figure 7–22) is rotated until the mire pattern is sharply focused (Figure 7–23). The mire patterns vary with the different instruments. Some are lines as in Figure 7–23, while others are dot patterns. In any case, they should be sharply focused to take a reading. With no lens in the instrument the power should read zero. If it does not, then the error should be taken into account. For example, if it reads +0.25 D with no lens, then a lens is measured with the instrument to be −3.00 D, it is actually −3.25 D. A lens having a reading of +3.00 D will actually be +2.75 D.

After the eyepiece has been adjusted and calibration checked, lenses

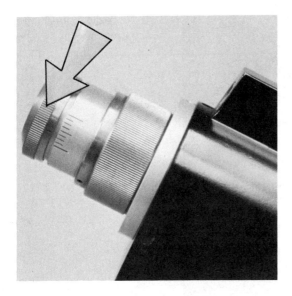

Figure 7–21. The arrow points to the eyepiece of the American Optical Lensometer, which is rotated to focus the reference lines. The lined knob to the right of the arrow rotates the reference lines.

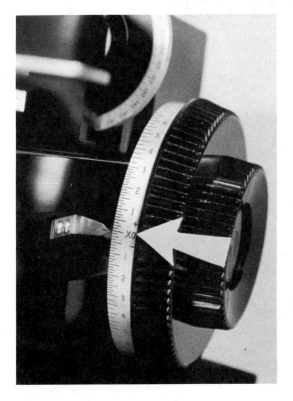

Figure 7–22. The power wheel on the lensometer set at zero diopters

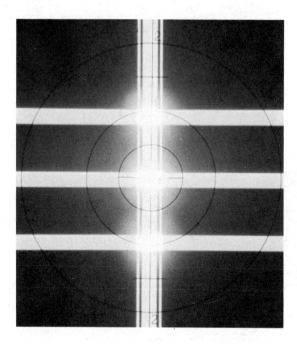

Figure 7-23. Lensometer mire pattern in sharp focus

can be measured. The lens should be dry and clean. It is then placed concave side against the lensometer stop being held centered over the stop with the thumb or index finger against the edge of the lens. Some lensometers can be tilted up so the instrument is vertical, which allows the lens to rest on the stop without being held. With the lens in place the power wheel is rotated again until the mires are brought into sharp focus (the same as in Figure 7-23). At this point the power can be read from the power wheel.

Prism. The above technique is for spherical lenses with no prism. If prism power is present in the lens, the mire pattern will be displaced, that is, not be centered in the field of view and with respect to the reference lines visible in the instrument. The amount of prism can be determined by the scale on the black reference lines. If the center of the cross falls on the one prism diopter line, the lens has one prism diopter.

To measure the amount of prism accurately, the lens must be carefully centered over the lensometer stop. If it is decentered, a false reading will be obtained because decentering any lens with power will give a prism reading. The higher the prescription the more important proper centration becomes.

A contact lens may have prism as part of the prescription or unwanted prism may be incorporated due to poor manufacturing techniques. Therefore, when verifying contact lenses it is necessary to look for prism even if it is not ordered.

Prism Ballast Front Surface Cylinders.   One use of prism is to prevent excessive lens rotation if a cylindrical prescription is incorporated to correct residual astigmatism. When the power of such a lens is determined, the lens is held centered over the lensometer stop. It is rotated until the center of the mires is directly below the center of the reference lines in the instrument. With the lens in this position the sphere, cylinder, and axis of the lens are determined. This is accomplished by first rotating the power drum in the plus power direction until the mires are blurred. Then, slowly rotate the power drum until the first line of the mires comes into focus (Figure 7–24). At this point the cylinder axis drum (Figure 7–25) must be rotated until the single line of the mire is in focus and forms a single, continuous straight line (Figure 7–26). The three lines 90 degrees from the single are out of focus. The power indicated on the power wheel is the spherical power of the lens. The reading on the cylinder axis drum is the minus cylinder axis. Next, the power wheel is rotated toward the less plus or more minus power until the three lines are in focus (Figure 7–27). This is the power in the second major meridian. The difference between this finding and the sphere power previously found

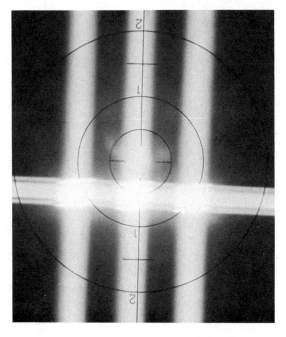

Figure 7–24. A cylindrical lens in the lensometer with the axis improperly aligned

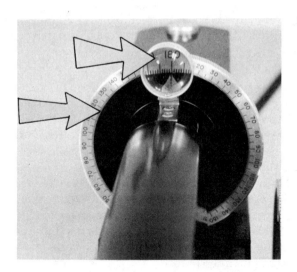

Figure 7–25. Cylinder axis wheel indicated with the left arrow and the point at which the axis is read indicated by the top arrow

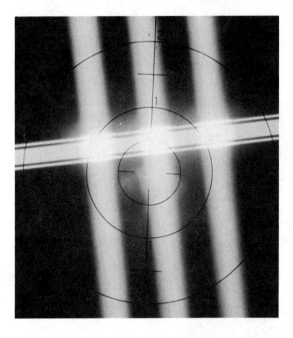

Figure 7–26. Cylinder axis properly aligned with the first major meridian in focus

is the cylinder power. For example, if when the single line is in focus the lensometer power reads −3.50 D with the axis wheel at 10, when refocusing for cylinder, when the three lines are in focus the power reads −4.25 D, the lens power is −3.50 −0.75 × 010.

When the above technique is used, the base-apex line of the prism

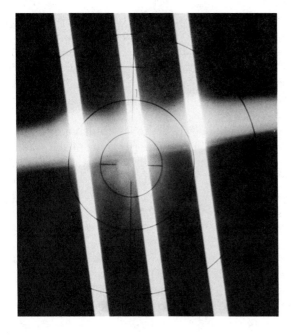

Figure 7-27. The second major meridian in focus to determine the cylinder power

is in the vertical meridian and used as the reference. In fact, the base of the prism can be marked with a permanent ink felt pen with the lens held in this position by just dotting the bottom edge of the lens. This can be helpful when the lens is placed on the eye to see how much the base of the lens rotates away from the vertical meridian.

A prismatic contact lens can also be truncated, that is, one edge of the lens cut off so that it is not round. In this case, the cylinder axis is still specified in relation to the base-apex line and so is the truncation. For example, the cylinder axis may be at 80 degrees and the truncation 20° to the base-apex line.

Toric Lenses. Lenses fabricated with a toric surface, such as a toric back central optical portion or bitoric design with toric curves on the front and back surfaces, can have a cylindrical prescription. There is, however, no base-apex line to use as reference to specify the cylinder axis. The power in each major meridian is, therefore, stated for that meridian. For example, if the base curves are 7.40 mm and 8.00 mm, the corresponding powers are written as − 6.00 D and − 2.00 D or 7.40/8.00, − 6.00/ − 2.00. The powers in the two meridians are not subtracted as in the previous example.

Tolerances. For lens prescriptions between + 10.00 D and − 10.00 D the tolerance is ±0.12 D. For powers greater than 10.00 diopters it is ±0.25 D. The limit for unwanted prism is ±0.25△ if the lens power is +10.00 D to −10.00 D and ±0.50△ is greater than ±10.00 diopters.

If a cylindrical prescription is present, the tolerance is ±0.25 D for cylindrical powers of less than 2.00 D, ±0.37 D if between 2.00 D and 4.00 D, and ±0.50 D if greater than 4.00 D. The axis of the cylinder should be within ±5° of that ordered.

Another factor that must be considered is the cumulative effect of errors in the refractive power and the base curve radius of a lens. For example, if the power is ±0.12 DS over that ordered, within the tolerance for power, and the base curve 0.02 mm steeper than ordered, but again within the tolerance for the BCR, there would be approximately +0.12 DS from the tear lens, giving a total refractive error of the lens on the patient's eye of +0.25 DS, causing a possible binocular imbalance of 0.50 diopters, and yet each lens parameter would be within the specified tolerance. The cumulative error should not exceed 0.25 D in a lens, and there should not be an error of more than 0.25 D between the two eyes.

If a bifocal segment (see Chapter 12) is present, the additional power should be within ±0.25 D of that specified. All these tolerances are set within normal clinically acceptable levels and yet are fair to the average laboratory's fabrication abilities.

OPTICAL QUALITY

In addition to checking the lens for the correct refractive power, the optical quality should be examined. When the power is checked with the lensometer, the quality of the target image should always be noted. It should be sharp and distinct with no significant degradation or doubling of the image.

Loss of optical quality can result from faults on the surface of a lens. There may be grayish unpolished areas or embedded polish in the surface. If a lens is allowed to become too hot during the polishing process due to insufficient lubricant on the pad, there may be polish burns or an orange-peel effect on the surface, appearing rough when viewed under reflected light. If the pad or polishing compound had dirt or grit present there may be surface scratches. If the tool that cuts the lens is rough or dull or if the lens is not sufficiently polished, circular ridges or lathe marks will appear on the surface (Figure 7–28). Also, if the lathe used to cut the lens is not correctly aligned, there may be a central defect that will degrade the optics.

Defects within the plastic material will cause optical problems.

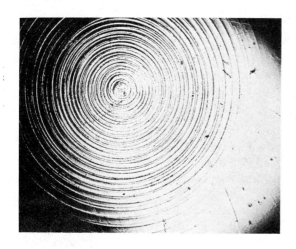

Figure 7–28. Circular lathe marks present at the center of a contact lens

There may be bubbles, striae, areas of varying index, or other inhomogeneities within the plastic.

There are several ways to inspect the lens for such optical defects other than using the lensometer. More than one method must often be employed to determine the cause of poor optics in a contact lens.

Stereomicroscope. If a lens is well illuminated while being viewed under a stereomicroscope with at least $40\times$ magnification, many of the defects will be detected. The lens should be held in the fingers or a special holder may be employed for this purpose, so that it can be illuminated from different angles. The surfaces should be inspected by specular reflection and diffuse illumination. A small, high-intensity desk lamp is a good light source.

Radiuscope. When the radiuscope is focused on a lens while the instrument is being zeroed, surface defects such as scratches are often apparent. This should alert one to inspect the surface further. With the radiuscope the lens is normally viewed under a magnification of $75\times$ (objective $5\times$ and eyepiece $15\times$). A high intensity source can be used to illuminate the lens while under the radiuscope for further inspection of the surface. This method is not as good as using a stereomicroscope because of the short working distance of the objective and the lack of space to hold and manipulate a lens under the radiuscope.

Line or Grid Pattern. Many optical defects will be detected if the contact lens is held up at arms length and a line or grid pattern viewed through the lens. The line or grid will appear wavy or distorted if the optics are of poor quality. If the lens is moved, the lines will appear to bend and change shape. This is a quick, easy test for lens quality.

CENTER THICKNESS

It is important to verify the center thickness of all contact lenses ordered because a lens that is thicker than desired will have greater mass, which may adversely affect wearing performance. A lens which is too thin may have a tendency to warp and cause vision problems.

Thickness Gauges.   Hand-held gauges or those on small stands calibrated in millimeters are routinely used to measure center thickness (Figure 7–29). Those specifically made for contact lens work have ball-bearing or rounded pedestals to minimize the possibility of scratching.

The gauges should be checked periodically for accuracy by using standard thickness plates or lenses of known thickness.

Lens Clock or Geneva Lens Gauge.   This instrument that normally measures the curvature of spectacle lens surfaces can also be employed to measure the center thickness of contact lenses. A flat surface, such as

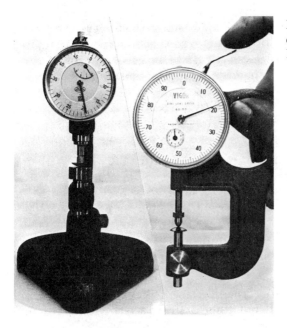

Figure 7–29. Two types of dial gauges used to measure lens thickness

a glass microscope slide, is used. The gauge is first placed on the flat surface to make sure it reads zero; next, the contact lens is placed convex surface down against the slide. The middle post of the gauge is then placed at the center of the lens with the outer two posts on the glass slide (Figure 7–30). The gauge will give a reading in diopters, which must be converted to millimeters. One diopter is equal to approximately 0.10 mm.

Optical Microspherometer (Radiuscope).   A radiuscope can be used to measure thickness by placing the lens on the mount in the same manner as that for measuring the front surface radius, but without water. There will be two images of the spoke pattern, one from the front of the lens and the second from the back surface. The instrument should be focused on the lower image and zeroed. It is then focused upward, using the fine adjustment only, until the second surface image is in focus. The distance between the images is indicated on the dial. This is the apparent thickness. To obtain the actual, the distance must be multiplied by 1.49, the index of the lens, which will give the thickness in millimeters.

The center thickness of a contact lens should be within ±0.02 mm of that specified.

Edge Contour

The shape of the edge is one of the most important parameters in terms of patient comfort and acceptance of contact lenses. It is also one of the most difficult to specify, reproduce, and inspect. Also, there has not been

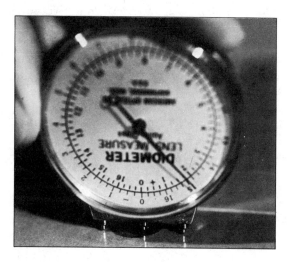

Figure 7–30.   Using a lens clock to measure the center thickness of a contact lens

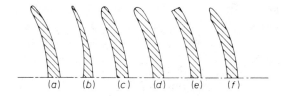

Figure 7–31. (a) Good edge contour; (b) sharp; (c) peak to near anterior surface; (d) rounded, blunt; (e) square; (f) peak of edge too near anterior surface

general agreement on the contour and thickness of the "ideal" edge. Studies and clinical experience have shown that such an edge is tapered from the front so that the peak of the apex is near the posterior surface of the lens (Figure 7–31). In actual practice, it is not possible to measure the edge thicknesses at these points precisely and it is necessary to learn to evaluate thickness and contour by looking at them. Figure 7–31 shows the configuration of commonly occurring edges, and there are several methods of inspection that can be applied.

Stereomicroscope. The stereomicroscope is the best instrument to inspect the edge contour, thickness, and surface quality. To be able to use it efficiently requires experience, and one should not be discouraged at first if difficulty is found in evaluating an edge.

The edge must first be well illuminated. A high-intensity light source placed close to the lens position gives good assessment (Figure 7–32). If a special holder is not utilized, the lens is held with the concave surface against the index finger as if the finger were the cornea (Figure 7–33), but should not be pressed against the finger tightly as this will cause the contour of the edge to be obscured. The finger acts as a reference for comparison of the edge shape. The lens is held under the stereomicroscope with the instrument focused about 5 cm above the stage (Figure 7–32); this allows room for the lens to be manipulated. When viewing the edge against the finger, the portion near the top should be looked at. The edge is inspected at different angles by rotating the fingers and then the lens to evaluate the edge all the way around. While inspecting the edge, not only its shape but any irregularities, chips, scratches, or unpolished areas should be searched for.

It is important to use the index finger as a reference point because the position of the peak of the lens edge in relation to the finger is important. If the peak stands away from the finger, as in Figure 7–34b corresponding to the profile in Figure 7–35b, the lens will be uncomfortable because the lid margin will hit this edge very abruptly. It may help in learning to evaluate an edge to remember that viewing it should be from the same position the upper eyelid takes as it approaches the lens on a blink. With this concept in mind the effect the lens edge under

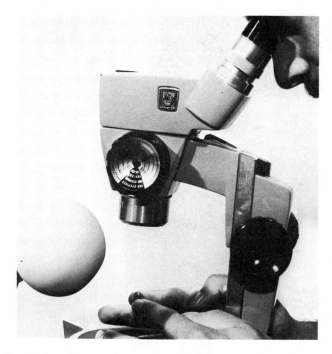

Figure 7–32.   Using a stereomicroscope and high-intensity light source to inspect the edge of a contact lens

consideration has on the lid can be judged. Discomfort from a poor lens edge is almost exculsively from lid sensation and not from corneal stimulation. The exception is a very thin edge with its peak near the cornea.

Figure 7–34a shows a good lens edge as viewed under the stereomicroscope. Note that the peak of the edge is near the finger, thus offering little resistance to the lid as it would move over the lens. Figure 7–35a gives a profile of this edge.

Biomicroscope.   The biomicroscope can be used to inspect the lens edge in the same manner as with a stereomicroscope. The lens is held against the index finger and illuminated with the light source of the instrument. The edge is then viewed through the microscope with the magnification set at the highest obtainable, usually $30 \times$ to $40 \times$.

Hand Loupe.   A small hand loupe or a measuring magnifier, viewing from the side with the scale, can be used to inspect the edge, although the magnification obtainable by this method is not great enough. In addition, there is no stereo-acuity.

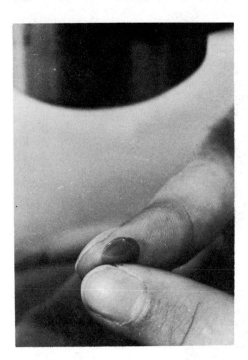

Figure 7-33. Holding the lens against the index finger so the edge can be inspected

Projection Magnifier (Shadowgraph).   A device which produces a magnified silhouette or shadow of the lens edge is one of the most commonly used techniques to evaluate edges (Figure 7-5). The lens is placed on the stage of the instrument in the light beam and its silhouette projected on to the screen (Figure 7-36). The lens can be rotated to view the edge at different positions around the circumference. The greatest advantage of a projection magnifier is that it is easy to use. Many laboratories and practitioners, therefore, employ it because they can teach technicians in a short period of time to evaluate an edge.

A major disadvantage of this instrument is that many poorly shaped edges will appear well contoured, because only the portion of the lens edge from the peak to the anterior surface is silhouetted and not the portion toward the posterior surface. The silhouette seen on the screen is not a profile of the edge as would be seen in a cross-section because the lens is a portion of a sphere and the light of the beam that would silhouette the interior portion of the edge is blocked by the portion of the lens nearest the light source. The view seen is analogous to placing an opaque lens or a bowl concave surface down on a flat surface and viewing the edge.

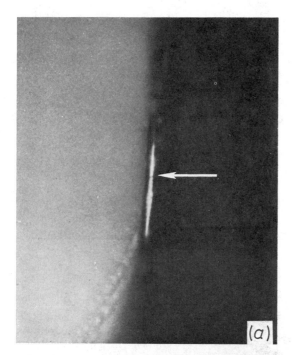

Figure 7-34. (a) Micro-
scopic view of a good lens edge
corresponding to Figure
7-35a; (b) the peak is near
the anterior surface corresponding to Figure 7-35b.
Note the dark area indicated
edge thickness between the
peak and finger. Arrows show
the position of the peak

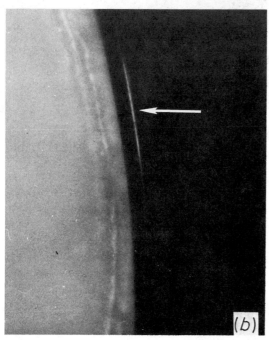

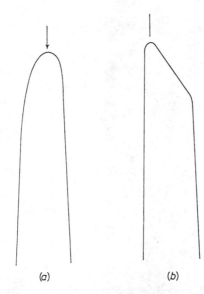

Figure 7–35. (a) Profile of a good lens edge corresponding to Figure 7–34a; (b) a poor edge with the peak toward the front surface corresponding to Figure 7–34b

(a)   (b)

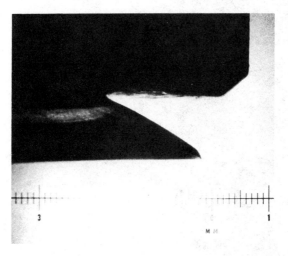

Figure 7–36. Shadowgraph silhouette showing front contour of the edge

Only the portion of the edge from the peak, where the lens or bowl rests on the surface, toward the outside convex side will be visible. Thus, two lenses with very different edge contours may appear similar if the outer portion of the edge contour is the same.

Bifocal Lenses

Several additional verification procedures are necessary with bifocal lens designs. Apart from the distance correction, the near power must be checked. This can be done by placing the reading segment over the stop of the lensometer, for which a reduced stop diameter is helpful since the near portion of the lens is relatively small. The size, shape, and position of the addition depend on the lens type. In the case of fused bifocals or where the addition is obtained by two radii on the front surface as in concentric designs, the power determined by the vertometer should conform to the refractive addition exactly as ordered. For example, if a -3.00 D distance prescription with a $+2.00$ D addition is asked for, the power through the near portion of the lens should be -1.00 D.

Where the addition is obtained by two radii on the back surface, the power read with the lensometer through the near portion of the lens is 3.18 times the effective addition on the eye. The lensometer reads lens power in air, while on the eye the back surface is in contact with the tears. With a distance power of -3.00 D, the power read through the near portion would be $+3.36$ D to give a $+2.00$ D add on the eye.

The BCR and PCR can be verified in the same manner as with single vision lenses. With bifocal designs, which obtain the near power by peripheral radii on the front or back surface, the quality of the curves should be evaluated with the radiuscope as described earlier for measuring peripheral radii. The BCR of a fused segment must be examined for warpage and aberration, particularly at the top of the reading segment because the fusing process may cause strain in the plastic. The radiuscope image should therefore be carefully evaluated at the point of junction where the higher index plastic is fused to the main portion of the lens. If there is a break in the image reflection, this indicates that the radius of the segment is different from the rest of the surface. This may be caused by uneven polishing of the back surface due to the higher-index plastic being softer than the main portion of the lens. For this reason also, the segment should be examined for scratches.

With fused bifocals, the quality of the fusing process should further be verified by holding the lens before a light source and visually examining the junction between the two plastics. If this area is blurred or doubling experienced at the demarcation line, the lens should be rejected.

When a concentric bifocal design is checked, the size of the distance and near portions is measured with a hand-held magnifier in the same way as for the optical zone diameter. In the case of an segment, it is important to verify its size, position, and height. A hand-held magnifier will clearly show the distance from the bottom edge of the lens to the top of the segment (Figure 7–37), though it may be necessary to concentrate on the center of the reticule scale in order to prevent error due to parallax. Truncation, whenever prescribed, must be evaluated independently for

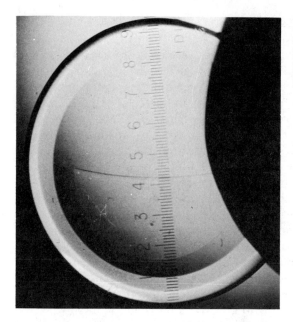

Figure 7–37. Measuring the segment height of a crescent bifocal contact lens using a hand magnifier to measure lens size

size, relative position, and finish, particularly if combined with prism, which must also be checked. Equal prismatic balance between the two eyes is important.

HYDROGEL LENS INSPECTION AND VERIFICATION

Due to the softness and flexibility of hydrogel lenses, techniques other than those used with rigid lenses are necessary to measure some of the parameters. One must be careful not to distort or damage the lens during the measurement. Numerous methods have been devised to verify hydrogel lenses and they can be measured with adequate accuracy. Due to difficulty in manufacturing and variability in quality control from the laboratory, it is important to verify and inspect these lenses in the office.

Lens Diameter, Optical Zone Diameter, and Peripheral Curve Width

It is best to keep the lens fully hydrated and in solution while taking measurements if possible. This prevents shrinking and distortion of the lens during measurement. One method of measuring the overall size and width of the major portions of a lens is to palce the lens in a wet cell and then hold a hand magnifier up to the wet cell (Figure 7–38). The overall size as well as optical zone and peripheral curve widths can then be measured in the same manner as with rigid lenses.

The lens surface can be blotted and placed on the face of the magnifier as with rigid lenses, but this technique often results in erroneous readings due to distortion and bending of the lens.

Another method is to place a scale, like the one on the hand-held magnifier, in the bottom of a wet cell, placing the lens on the scale in solution then placing the unit under a low magnification microscope (Figure 7–39). The lens dimensions can then be determined.

The hydrogel lens can also be placed in a wet cell that is placed in a projection magnifier (Figure 7–40). The scale on the screen is used to measure the diameter and zones of the magnified lens image on the screen.

The overall diameter and optical zone diameter of the lens should be within ± 0.20 mm of the values ordered.

Base Curve Radius

The base curve radius is one of the most difficult lens dimensions to measure because any bending or distortion of the lens will result in an erroneous reading. If the lens surface is blotted, then one cannot obtain a good reflected image from the surface. These problems preclude the use

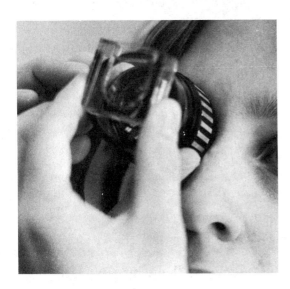

Figure 7–38. Hydrogel lens in a wet cell being held up before a hand magnifier to measure lens size

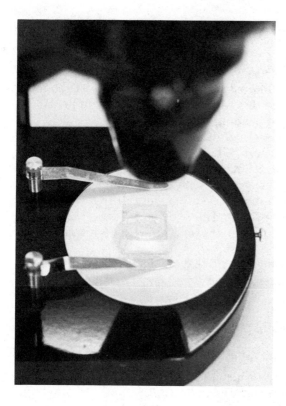

Figure 7–39. Hydrogel lens in a wet cell with a scale placed in the bottom, all under a microscope to measure lens dimensions

of the radiuscope or keratometer in the same manner as used with rigid lenses.

Templates. One of the first methods used to estimate the BCR was optical gauging. The lens is placed on a series of laps or templates of known radii. If the BCR is shorter (steeper) than the lap, a bubble may be trapped in the center of the lens (Figure 7–41a). If the lens is flatter (has a longer radius) than the lap a bubble is formed at the edge (figure 7–41b). A series of laps is required and the lens is progressively placed on them until the one where a bubble is first seen centrally is found and the one where a bubble is first formed at the edge. The middle of the range of these two laps is taken as the radius. The obvious problem with this technique is that a hydrogel lens will conform to several laps, making the actual radius difficult to determine. This is particularly a problem with the very thin and the high water content lenses, which are quite soft and flexible. Thus just placing lens on laps and grossly viewing the fit is not an accurate method.

A refinement of the template technique that can result in clinically

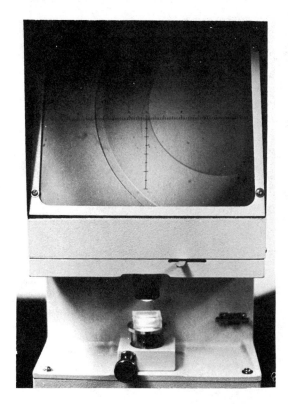

Figure 7–40. Projection magnifier used to measure lens dimensions

acceptable readings is to have the template and lens in solution. This keeps the lens hydrated and decreases lens bending due to the buoyancy of the saline solution. If the lens on the template is then placed in the light beam of a projection magnifier, the magnified image can be seen on the screen. This technique is utilized with the Soft Lens Analyzer.[1] By viewing the lens on the screen, one can determine when the lens is slightly steeper (Figure 7–42a) or flatter (Figure 7–42b) than the lap. With practice an accuracy of ±0.10 mm can be achieved. One should use saline solution in the chamber so that the lens hydration is proper. If tap water or distilled water is used, the lens will tend to swell, changing the BCR. The lens should be reasonably well centered on the lap when the measurement is taken. With smaller-diameter lenses, a metal plate with holes can be placed over the templates to help hold the lens centered (Figure 7–43). To help determine if a lens is steeper than the lap, the center of the lens can be touched with the soft tip of tweezers used to handle soft

[1]The Soft Lens Analyzer is manufactured by Hydrovue, Inc., 5327 Jacuzzi St, Richmond, Calif. 94804

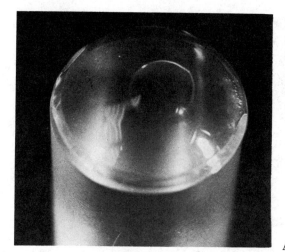

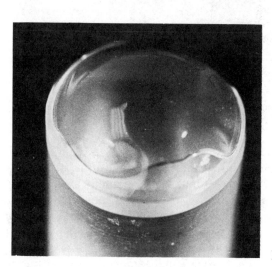

Figure 7–41. (a) A lens placed on the gauge where the lens is steeper than the gauge resulting in a central bubble; (b) the lens is flatter than the gauge with a bubble at the edge

A

B

lenses while viewing the lens on the screen. If the lens is steeper, it will be seen to give when touched. The lens should be placed on laps steeper and flatter than the one it appears to match to verify the match. This bracketing of the match is necessary as the lens may appear to match two of the laps if the BCR is actually between the radii of the laps.

The diameter of the lens can also be measured with the lens on the template by placing the plastic scale on the screen (Figure 7–44).

The saline in the trough should not be allowed to evaporate away as it will leave a residue. At the end of each day it should be rinsed out and dried. Leaving saline in the trough for more than a day would increase

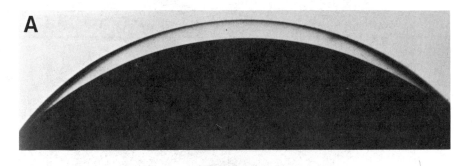

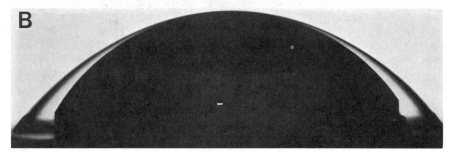

Figure 7–42. (a) Lens is steeper than the lap; (b) lens is flatter than the lap (Photo courtesy of Hydrovue Inc.)

the possibility of bacterial contamination. Preserved saline should be used to decrease the likelihood of contamination over the day's use.

Use of the Keratometer. To measure the BCR with the keratometer, the lens is immersed in saline with the concave surface toward the bottom of the chamber (Figure 7–45). Below the chamber is either a front surface mirror or a reflecting prism so that the light from the keratometer mires can be focused on the lens and the reflected image from the lens surface can be seen with the keratometer. The bottom of the wet cell must be a flat surface and of optical quality.

One of the problems with using an optical technique like this, where the lens is immersed in solution, is that very little light is reflected from the lens surface since it is immersed in saline. In air, the lens surface will reflect 3 to 4 percent of the light falling on it while in solution only about 0.1 percent is reflected. Thus the image will be quite dim. The higher the intensity of the light source of the keratometer the easier it will be to make the reading. Some keratometers have sufficient light while others may not. With the Bausch and Lomb keratometer, for ex-

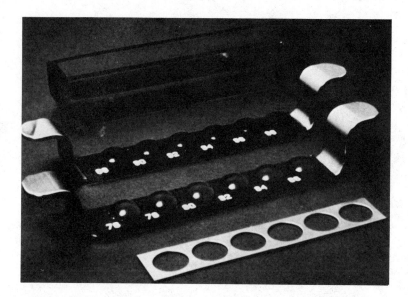

Figure 7–43.   The two template bars with radii from 7.6 to 8.6 mm and 8.8 to 9.8 mm, the metal bar to place over the templates to center the smaller diameter lenses and the trough the templates and lenses are placed in

ample, the intensity of the image can be increased by removing the diffusing filter above the light bulb and replacing the 15-watt bulb with a 25-watt bulb. It also helps to do the measurement in a dark room.

In taking the measurement, the keratometer is aligned on the lens in the same manner as when the BCR of a rigid lens is measured or when the curvature of the cornea is being measured (see Chapter 5 for use of the keratometer). Once aligned and focused, two overlapping images will be seen, one from the back surface of the lens and the other from the front surface. If the lens is a minus prescription, the image giving the steepest radius (highest dioptric reading on the instrument) will be the back surface image. For a plus contact lens the flattest radius will be the back surface. In order to be able to make the measurement, it may be necessary to place a − 1.25 D lens over the front of the telescope of the keratometer to extend the range of the instrument as explained in Chapter 5.

The system should be calibrated by placing a series of rigid lenses of known base curve radii in the chamber and measuring them. Then a graph can be drawn with the actual radius versus the measured radius. From then on anytime a hydrogel lens is measured, the graph can be consulted to make the quick conversion from the keratometer reading to the actual lens radius. The same thing can be done by formula.

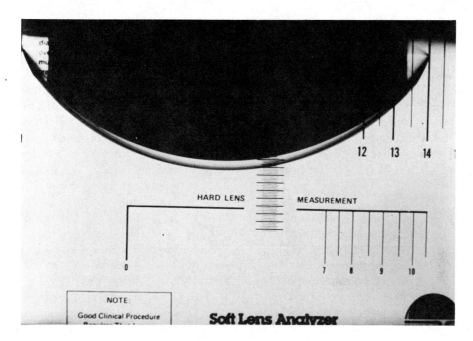

Figure 7–44. Measuring lens diameter with the lens on the template. The small vertical scale is for measuring lens thickness (Photo courtesy of Hydrovue Inc.)

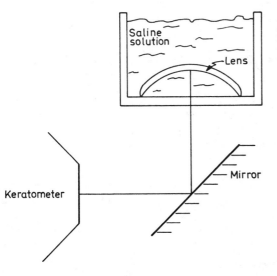

Figure 7–45. Arrangement for measuring the BCR of hydrogel lenses using a keratometer

Other Techniques.   Numerous additional procedures have been devised
to measure the BCR of hydrogel lenses. At this time, they have not
received widespread usage in the average contact lens practice, and thus
will not be explained in full detail here.

Many techniques use the basic principle of measuring the sagittal
depth of the lens over a given central chord diameter (Figure 7–46). The
lens is placed over a pedestal that has a fixed and known diameter. Then
the distance from the surface of the pedestal to the back surface of the
lens is measured. This can be done just visually. For example, one instrument, Wet Cell Radiusgauge,[2] is a modified microscope where the
lens is viewed under magnification and a central movable peg is brought
up until it just touches the back surface of the lens. The movement of the
peg is accurately calibrated so that its distance from the flat surface of
the pedestal is known and indicated on the dial controlling the peg movement. With this instrument, the lens and pedestal is in a wet cell to
maintain hydration. One of the problems with this procedure is the difficulty in determining when the peg actually touches the lens.

Other instruments such as the B.C. Tronic[3] and Soft Lens Measuring
Instrument[4] use an electrical technique to measure the sagittal depth.
The lens is blotted dry using the same procedure as when measuring
power and then is placed on the pedestal. Then the central peg or needle
is moved either automatically in the case of the B.C. Tronic instrument

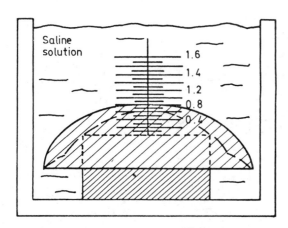

Figure 7–46. Principle of measuring the sagittal depth to determine the BCR

---

[2]The Wet Cell Radiusgauge is manufactured by Contact Lens Manufacturing, London, England.

[3]B.C. Tronic Instrument is manufactured by Laboratories Medicornea, France.

[4]Soft Lens Measuring Instrument is manufactured by Redher Development Co., California.

or manually with the Soft Lens Measuring Instrument until it just touches the lens. At this point the electrical circuit is closed and the sagittal depth is either automatically indicated or an indicator light is activated. The sagittal depth is read from a gauge on the instrument. The main difficulty with such techniques is that the lens must be in air rather than in so-lution. This often results in some lens distortion, resulting in erroneous readings. Care must therefore be taken in blotting the lens and placing it on the pedestal. This is especially true with thin and/or high water content lenses.

An ultrasound technique has also been designed to measure the sagittal depth.[5] With this instrument, the lens and pedestal are immersed in saline and the sagittal depth is determined by the reflection of sound waves from the lens surface.

With any of the sagittal depth measuring techniques, the sagittal depth must be measured very accurately as a small change in the sagittal depth makes a significant change in the radius. For example, if a 10 mm chord diameter is used, a sagittal depth of 1.58 mm is a radius of 8.70 mm whereas a sagittal depth of 1.537 is a radius of 8.90 mm. Thus the sagittal depth must be measured to an accuracy of 0.01 mm.

The sagittal depth can be converted to radius by using tables or by the formula:

$$R = \frac{S^2 + \left(\frac{D}{2}\right)^2}{2S}$$

where R is the radius of curvature, S the sagittal depth, and D the chord (pedestal diameter).

The radiuscope has also been modified to measure the base curve of hydrogel lenses. The Ultra-Radiuscope[6] is an example. The lens is placed under the objective of the instrument in a wet cell. The objective is made to be immersed in the solution to eliminate the reflection from the surface of the solution. It also has a higher-intensity light source to obtain an adequately reflected image from the lens surface. The problem of obtaining adequate intensity and seeing reflections from both lens surfaces is the same as with the use of the keratometer as previously explained. This radiuscope technique can give very accurate results. An-other technique is a projection profile procedure. The lens is placed in solution in a wet cell and projected onto a screen, for example, using a projection magnifier. The lens is positioned so that a profile image is produced on the screen and then curves of different radii drawn on the

---

[5]Panametrics, Waltham, Mass.
[6]Manufactured by G. Nissel, England.

screen are aligned with the image, one at a time. By obtaining a match between the drawn radii and lens image, the radius can be determined. One problem with this technique is the difficulty in obtaining a sharp image of the back surface of the lens that will match the curves, too. Also it is often difficult to determine which curve actually matches the surface over the small diameter of the lens. Two instruments using this technique are the Kontr-Mess System[7] and the Hydro-Marc Optical Comparator.[8]

All of the above techniques can give clinically acceptable findings if the proper precautions are followed and experience is gained using the particular system. Each instrument has certain advantages and disadvantages. The accuracy varies from as good as about ±0.02 mm to ±0.20 mm radius.

Tolerance.   The base curve radius should be within at least ±0.20 mm of the specified radius.

Power

The power of a hydrogel lens can be measured by first removing it from the solution and gently shaking the excess saline off. The lens is then placed on a lint-free tissue, and the tissue is folded over the lens and gently pressed against the lens. The lens is then picked up, moved to a dry spot on the tissue, and blotted a second time. The lens is then picked up and placed over the stop of the lensometer (Figure 7–47), being careful

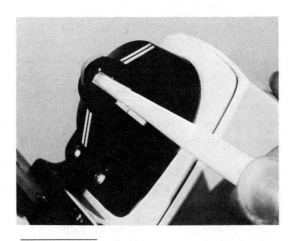

Figure 7–47.   Placing a hydrogel lens on the stop of the lensometer

---

[7]Sohnges, W. Germany.
[8]Frontier Contact Lenses, Inc., Jacksonville, Florida.

not to distort the lens. It is usually best to use the stop designed for spectacle lenses as the lens easily tends to conform to its shape. The lens power is then read in the same way as with rigid lenses. If the image is blurred and cannot be properly focused, the lens should be removed, rewetted, and the procedure repeated. The lens power should be determined in 2 to 3 minutes after the surface has been blotted because the lens will begin to dehydrate. With dehydration, the refractive index and lens shape will change causing a change in lens power. With a little practice, accurate, repeatable readings can be taken.

If the lens is toric, the sphere, cylinder, axis, and prism can be determined again in the same way as with rigid lenses. The lens surface is dried as explained above and placed on the lensometer stop. It is then rotated by rotating the stop until base down prism is read. Then the sphere and cylinder power are determined.

If the lens is truncated, the angle of the truncation should be determined. With the lens rotated to the base down position, one can determine if the truncation is perpendicular to the base-apex line—that is, if the cut off portion of the lens is horizontal. If not, the angle between the base-apex line and the truncation can be estimated by just noting the angle between the truncation and horizontal. This angle can be precisely determined by rotating the lens after making the first cylinder axis reading with the prism base down so that the truncation is now horizontal. The cylinder axis is again determined. The difference between the axis read with the prism base down and the axis with the truncation horizontal gives the precise location for the truncation. For example, a lens is positioned base down and the following prescription is found $-2.00 \ -1.25 \times 80 \ \frac{3}{4} \ \triangle$B.D. At this position the truncation is not horizontal but at an angle to horizontal (Figure 7–48). The lens is next rotated so that the truncation is horizontal, and with the lens in this position, the power is again determined. If the prescription is $-2.00 \ -1.25 \times 060$ then the truncation is 20 degrees from the base-apex line of the prism. If this is the right lens, the truncation is 20 degrees nasal of the prism base.

Another method of determining lens power is to put the lens in a wet cell which can be held against the stop of the lensometer. The advantage is that the lens is maintained hydrated and does not become distorted. There are a couple of major drawbacks to using this system. However one is that with the lens in saline solution the power actually read is considerably less than the actual power of the lens in air. Thus, a correction factor must be used. This factor can be determined by the following formula: $\text{CF} = \frac{n_L - n_A}{n_L - n_W}$ where CF is the correction factor, n_L the refractive index of the lens, n_A the refractive index of air (1.0) and n_W the refractive index of the saline the lens is in (1.336). For most hydrogel lenses (n = 1.43) the correction factor is 4.57. Thus if a power

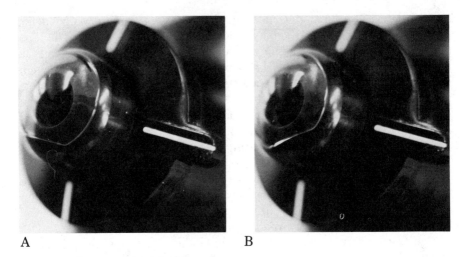

A   B

Figure 7–48. (a) Toric hydrogel lens positioned base down showing truncation at an angle to the base-apex line; (b) same lens rotated so that truncation is horizontal

of −1.00 D is read with the lens in the wet cell, the actual power is −4.57 D. Thus a small error in reading the power is multiplied by 4.57. Furthermore, it is difficult to position the lens at the stop of the lensometer. This results in additional errors, especially with high prescriptions, and the technique is not often used in clincial practice.

Tolerance. The power should be within ±0.25 D of the power ordered.

Center Thickness

The center thickness of hydrogel lenses is quite important since most of the oxygen reaching the cornea is through the lens, and the thinner the lens, the more oxygen that will diffuse through. Thickness also affects lens performance in other ways.

Radiuscope Techniques. Center thickness of hydrogel lenses cannot be measured with conventional thickness gauges or calipers due to the softness of the lens. Therefore optical or electrical techniques must be used.

The radiuscope can be used in several ways to measure thickness. One method is to blot the lens surface and then place the lens on a large uncut rigid lens that has a hole drilled in it (Figure 7–49) to give the hydrogel lens support. Another method is to place the lens on the pedestal

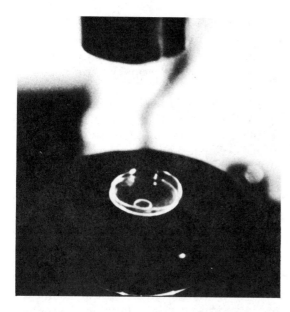

Figure 7–49. Hydrogel lens, with rigid lens support, placed under the radiuscope for thickness measurement

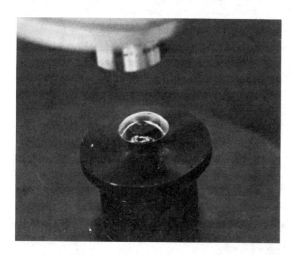

Figure 7–50. Lens mounted on the pedestal of the radiuscope for thickness measurement

used to measure the front surface of rigid lenses but without using water (Figure 7–50). The lens is then positioned under the radiuscope, centering it under the objective. The radiuscope is focused on the surface of the lens (see the previous section in this chapter on the use of the radiuscope). There will be two images of the spoke pattern quite close together, one from each lens surface. Using the fine-focus knob, accurately focus on the lower image. Set the reference line through zero or one of the numbers on the scale. Next, using only the fine-focus knob, accurately focus on the second image. The difference in the two images as read from the scale is multiplied by the refractive index of the lens, 1.43 for many of the hydrogel lenses. For example, if the distance between the two images is 0.10 mm, the actual thickness is 0.143 mm.

With thin lenses it is difficult to see and focus the two images because they are close together. One way to overcome that problem is to use an aluminum post (Figure 7–51) that is mounted on the base of the radiuscope. One-half of the post surface is polished and the other half is mildly abraded to give a diffusing surface. The contact lens is blotted and placed concave surface up on the post so that the center of the lens is on the dividing line. The stage of the radiuscope is moved until it is aligned under the objective. The spoke pattern should be centered on the line between the shiny and diffusing sides of the post. The image is accurately focused on the shiny side of the post, on the post surface through the lens. Since the lens is on the surface of the post, this is also the position of the front surface of the lens. The radiuscope is zeroed on the reference line or set through one of the numbers. Next the image on the side of the diffuse surface is focused. Only a very faint reflected image is obtained from the diffuse surface with a brighter, sharper focus from the back surface of the lens. Thus it is easier to focus on this surface since the front surface image has been diminshed. The difference between the two images is multiplied by the refractive index as before.

Another method to measure the center thickness is to place a microscope slide on the radiuscope stage, mount a post with a polished top on the stage (Figure 7–52), or use just the shiny side of the post described above. The radiuscope is focused on the surface of the slide or post without

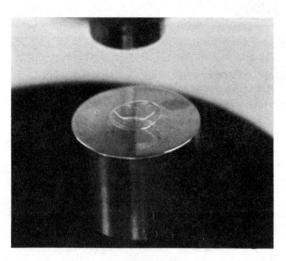

Figure 7–51. Aluminum post on which a hydrogel lens is placed to measure center thickness

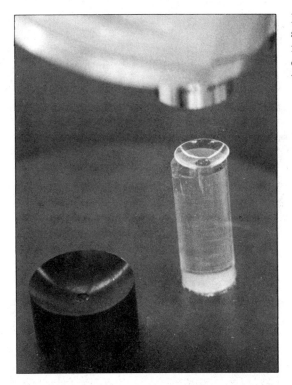

Figure 7–52. Hydrogel lenses placed on the flat, polished surface of a plastic rod on the stage of the radiuscope to measure center thickness

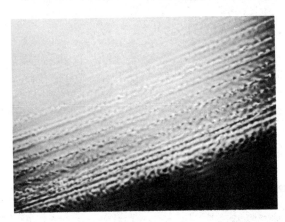

Figure 7–53. Lathe marks on the surface of a hydrogel lens as seen with phase contrast microscopy

the lens on it and the instrument zeroed or reference line set on a known value on the scale. Next the lens is blotted and placed concave surface up on the slide or post with the center of the lens on the spot on the slide or post where the image was initially focused. The spot of light can usually

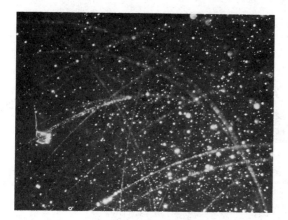

Figure 7–54. Scratches on the surface of a hydrogel lens

be seen on the surface where the lens should be placed. Be careful not to bump or jar the radiuscope or post on which the lens is placed as this will ruin the zeroing of the instrument, giving an erroneous reading or requiring repetition of the procedure. Also be careful to position the lens center precisely under the objective so the center thickness is measured and not a peripheral point. With the lens in postion focus on the back surface (top) of the lens. The distance between the mounting surface first focused on and the lens surface is the actual center thickness; no correction factor is required. This technique is simple to perform but the precautions on lens positioning and placement must be observed.

Projection Techniques. The thickness can be measured using the projection devices used to measure BCR (Figure 7–44). The thickness of the image is measured with a scale taking into account that the magnification or a conversion factor must be used. The difficulty with such a system is the problem of obtaining a sharp image of both the front and back surface of the lens from which to measure. The greater the magnification, the more accurate the reading.

Electrical Technique. The thickness can be measured by an electrical contact technique where the lens is placed one electrode and a second electrode is moved toward the center of the lens until it just touches. When it touches, the circuit is closed and a light or a resistance meter can be wired to the system to indicate this.

Tolerance. The center thickness should be within ±0.02 mm of the thickness ordered.

Surface and Edge Inspection

The surface and edge quality should be inspected on all lenses received from the laboratory. The surface should be smooth, well polished, and the edge should be even, well contoured, and free of tears. A disrupted surface can cause discomfort and also provide a niche for debris and lacrimal components to build up and microorganisms to be harbored. A small tear in the edge can be the starting point for a large tear through normal handling by the patient. The optical quality may be poor due to an inadequately polished surface. A thorough inspection of the surface and edges must be carried out routinely when patients return for follow-up care irrespective of whether or not problems are experienced. Lenses may be found to be torn or scratched or to have deposits. Frequently the patient is unaware of the problem.

Projection Magnification. To float the lens in a chamber and to use a projection magnifier is one method for inspecting both surface and edge quality. Any irregular edges, tears, lens punctures, and similar gross defects will readily be detected with this procedure. Many defects such as scratches and lathe marks will not, however, be apparent because of the low magnification and method of illumination.

Microscopes. A rather simple clinical method is to hold the lens before a biomicroscope. It can be in one of the wet cells and positioned either on a platform before the instrument or held by hand. With the lens in such a chamber, however, many surface defects will not be detected due to the small difference in refractive index between the material and the saline solution. A better method is to hold the lens in air before the biomicroscope, using a pair of tweezers. As the surface of a lens dries, numerous defects which might otherwise not be visible will become apparent, such as lathe marks, scratches, debris, and small tears. Both direct and indirect illumination should be used for the inspection with low and high biomicroscope magnification. The highest magnification will still prove inadequate in detecting some of the defects that may cause clinical problems.

A stereomicroscope, as used to inspect rigid lens surfaces and edges, can also be used for the inspection of hydrogel lenses. There are limitations as to magnification and method of illuminating with this procedure as with a biomicroscope, but many faults can nevertheless be discovered. It is possible to evaluate the shape of an edge under the stereomicroscope in the same way as rigid lenses by holding the lens lightly against the finger.

The best way to inspect a hydrogel lens adequately for material irregularities, surface defects, scratches, edge imperfections, tears, and artifacts is to use a phase contrast light microscope. A regular brightfield microscope is not adequate. Magnification in the range of $50\times$ to $400\times$ should be available.

To inspect a lens with the microscope it is best to mount the lens on an ordinary microscope slide. To do this, a couple of drops of saline are placed on the slide and then the lens is placed concave side down on the saline. A microscope slide cover slip is then placed over the lens and the lens flattened out on the slide. This allows for easy inspection over the whole lens surface, with only small adjustments in focus of the microscope. Most hydrogel lenses can be flattened repeatedly without damage or changes in lens dimensions. The only lenses that cannot be flattened are very thick lenses or some very low water content lenses. In this case a hanging drop microscope slide, a slide with a depression ground in it, can be used. The lens is placed in the depression with saline and the cover slip placed over it. With both mounting procedures, the lens is in solution and thus is maintained hydrated and can be kept on the slide for a long while for viewing.

The illumination and viewing system of the microscope should be accurately set up and adjusted according to the manufacturer's instructions. Using low magnification the lens should be scanned for any defects. Then higher magnification should be used to study the lens surface and matrix in greater detail. Special attention should be paid to the detection of lathe or similar marks that have not been adequately polished out (Figure 7–53), and to defects in the molded surface of spin-cast lenses. Scratches (Figure 7–54) due to poor polishing procedures or rough handling by the patient are easily seen with phase contrast microscopy. They may cause discomfort, form points for mucus and debris collection, and provide locations for a culture of microbes.

The region of the peripheral bevel and edge should be carefully inspected. With incorrect or incomplete finishing a rough surface may result near the edge (Figure 7–55). Part of the material may be left at the edge (Figure 7–56) to break away during wear causing irritation or discomfort. A serrated or torn edge (Figure 7–57) may result in corneal or conjunctival insult and also provide a starting point for a large tear. Red spots may also be seen as the result of a small metal particle being on the lens surface and rusting.

If the microscope has a scale on the fine-focus knob, this instrument can be used to measure lens thickness accurately. You can focus on one surface, note the scale value, and then focus on the second surface. The difference between the two readings multiplied by the refractive index is the lens thickness. The higher magnifications give more precise findings.

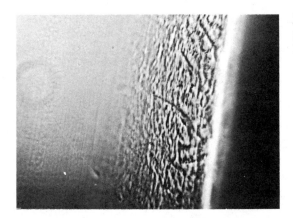

Figure 7–55. Rough surface near the edge of a hydrogel lens

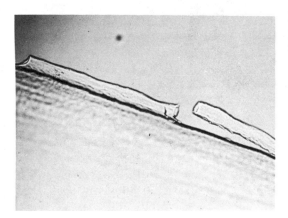

Figure 7–56. Thin pieces of polymer about to break away from the edge of a lens

Tolerance. Precise tolerances for surface and polymer defects cannot be given. One must evaluate each defect and determine if it is likely to affect lens fit, comfort, or vision. Most lenses will have fine scratches or other minor surface and edge imperfections, but lenses with rough edges, tears, deep scratches, extensive lathe marks, internal defects, and other extensive defects should be rejected.

Lens Rejection

When lenses are received from the laboratory and their specifications are different from those ordered, a decision must be made as to whether the lenses should be kept and dispensed to the patient or if they should be

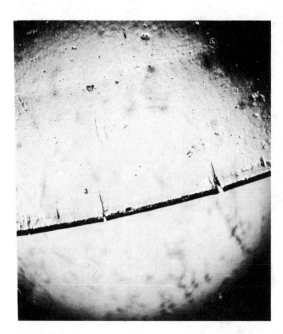

Figure 7-57. Tears in the edge of a lens

rejected. If the specifications are outside the tolerance levels previously given in the text (see Table 7–1), the lenses can be rejected. There are times, however, when greater variation from these tolerances may be accepted for a given patient where the variance will not adversely affect the lens fit and wearability. This is a professional judgment that must be made in each case.

Table 7–1. Summary of recommended tolerances for rigid lenses.

Parameter	Tolerance
Overall size	± 0.05 mm
Optical zone	
Light blend	± 0.1 mm
Medium or heavy blend	± 0.2 mm
Base curve radius	± 0.020 mm
Secondary, intermediate, or peripheral curve width	
Light blend	± 0.05 mm
Medium or heavy blend	± 0.10 mm
Peripheral curve radius	± 0.1 mm
Refractive power	
+ 10.00 D to − 10.00 D	± 0.12 D
More than ± 10.00 D	± 0.25 D
Prism power (measured from geometric center) if lens power is:	
+ 10.00 D to − 10.00 D	± 0.25
More than ± 10.00 D	± 0.50
Cylinder power	
Less than 2.00 D	± 0.25 D
2.00 D–4.00 D	± 0.37 D
Greater than 4.00 D	± 0.50 D
Cylinder axis	± 5 degrees
Toric base curve radii	
Δr 0–0.20 mm	± 0.02 mm
Δr 0.21–0.40 mm	± 0.03 mm
Δr 0.41–0.60 mm	± 0.05 mm
Δr > 0.60 mm	± 0.07 mm
Bifocal refractive power addition	± 0.25 D
Bifocal segment height	− 0.1 mm to + 0.2 mm
Center thickness	Less than ± 0.02 mm
Edges	As specified
Front peripheral curve radius	± 0.2 mm
Front optic zone diameter	± 0.1 mm
Optical quality and surface quality	No bubbles, striae, waves, inhomogeneities, crazing, pits, scratches, chips, lathe, or stone marks
Color	Pigment inert and uniformly distributed

8

MODIFICATION OF CONTACT LENSES

Lens modifications can be carried out in the office to adjust the way a rigid lens fits the eye. Such changes can be made in just minutes, saving the time and cost of returning the lenses to the laboratory. In some cases, for example the shaping of an edge, it may not help to return the lens to the laboratory, as it may come back with a worse edge than first received.

Some practitioners order uncut blanks, lenses with finished single curve front and back surfaces but with no peripheral curves or edge finish. These lenses are completed in their offices. They feel they can obtain better and more consistent results than ordering finished lenses from the laboratory.

Lens modifications are not difficult to perform if proper procedures are followed. The skills necessary can be acquired by obtaining reject lenses from a laboratory on which to practice.

There are numerous techniques used to do each modification. Examples of methods to perform the most common modifications will be given here, but other procedures may be equally acceptable. The following techniques apply to most rigid lenses except those with surface coatings or treatments, most notably rigid pure silicone lenses. These can not be modified or polished.

MODIFICATION UNIT

Only a small amount of equipment is necessary to carry out most in-office modifications. One of the basic pieces of equipment is a spindle unit, consisting of a small electric motor that can either be mounted in a portable box or in a counter top (Figure 8–1). Many practitioners prefer to have their unit mounted in the counter top together with their inspection, modification, and adjustment apparatus. The motor can be either of a constant speed of 1000–1500 rev/min, or a variable. A small motor of ⅟₂₀ to ¼ horsepower is adequate. The tools to be used on the unit can be mounted on the motor by either a spindle adapted with a male taper (Figure 8–2) or by a Jacob's chuck (Figure 8–2b). The use of tapers allows more rapid interchange of tools on the spindle unit than does the Jacob's chuck.

The unit should have a splash pan to prevent water and polish from splashing the operator and other equipment. It can be made from metal or plastic, although plastic is less likely to scratch or break a lens. The bowl must be large enough to be able to get the hands and tools down into it to work. A number of commercial units are available and one should always ascertain that the tools and unit are compatible, for example, that the tools have the proper taper for the unit or the tools have a stem suitable for a Jacob's chuck. Laboratories can advise you as to the design of specific tools.

Other tools employed in the modification procedure depend on the particular adjustment called for and will be discussed when the individual modification is explained.

POLISHES

Silvo,[1] a polish manufactured for polishing silver, is commonly used to make lens modifications. It is available from most contact lens laboratories and department or hardware stores and is supplied as a liquid.

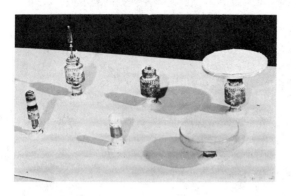

Figure 8–1. Multi-spindle modification unit with spindles mounted in table top

[1]R. T. French Co., 1 Mustard St. Rochester, N.Y. 14692

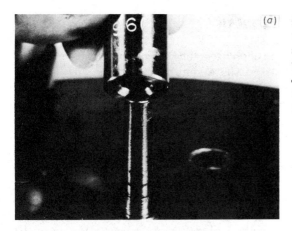

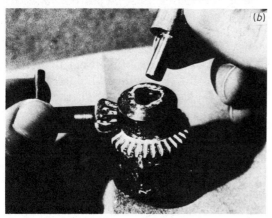

(a)

Figure 8–2. (a) A spindle unit with a tapered shaft showing a tool with a female taper being placed on it; (b) a Jacob's chuck with key, which is used to tighten the jaws against the stem of the tool

Another polish is XPAL,[2] which has been specifically formulated for polishing contact lenses and is available from most contact lens laboratories. It is supplied as a powder to which water can be added to make up the polishing solution. Some like to add a contact lens wetting solution instead of water to form a more viscous solution so that it will stay on the modification tool and lens longer. Other polishes such as tin oxide and precipitated calcium carbonate are sometimes used. XPAL is recommended for use with some of the new lens polymers since Silvo has cleaning agents that might harm the lens surface.

With most modification procedures, a moist polishing compound must be constantly used to obtain the proper polishing action and to prevent build-up of heat, which can adversely affect the lens.

---

[2]W. R. Grace and Co., Davison Chem. Dr., P.O. Box 188, Pompton Pins, N.J. 07444

OVERALL SIZE REDUCTION

Several methods can be used to decrease a lens diameter. The best method for a particular case depends on the extent to which the size is to be reduced, the number of lenses to be done, and one's preference and skill.

Use of a Razor Blade or Other Cutting Tool

The lens is mounted on a spindle by its convex surface using a double-faced tape (available from contact lens laboratories) or a low melting point dental wax (Figure 8–3). The centering of the lens is important. To prevent unwanted prism, the optical center must be at the geometrical center of the lens. To do this the optical center must be positioned at the center of the spindle on which it is mounted. One method is to dot the optical center by positioning the lens before the lensometer so that a value of zero prism is indicated and then dotting the lens. The dotting device on the instrument should be used with care taken not to scratch or break the lens. Next, dot the center of the spindle and place the lens on it so that the dot on the lens coincides with the dot on the spindle (Figure 8–3).

Another method for centration is to align the lens visually on a rotating spindle while viewing a line reflection (Figure 8–3), such as an overhead fluorescent light bulb, from the concave surface. If the reflection appears to move or wobble as the lens slowly rotates, it is not properly centered and should be repositioned slightly and checked again. This can be repeated until the image no longer moves when the lens is rotated.

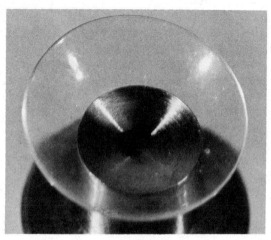

Figure 8–3. Lens mounted on a holder with double-faced tape for diameter reduction. A dot at the optical center of the lens is aligned with a dot at the center of the tool. Movement of a reflected image from the posterior surface of the lens as it is spinning can also be used to check alignment

With experience, the lens can be centered quite quickly using this technique.

The lens can also be mechanically centered on the spindle with a centering device (Figure 8–4a), having an inside taper fitting over the spindle and moved down on to the lens. As the device is lowered, the taper guides the lens to the center by edge contact (Figure 8–4b). Since the lens, however, is centered with respect to the existing edge of the lens unwanted prism will result if the optical center of the lens is not in the geometrical center. Moreover, if double-faced tape is used, the centering device will force the lens to be centered when pushed down onto the lens, but when removed, the tape will tend to pull the lens back toward its original position and will thus leave it incorrectly centered.

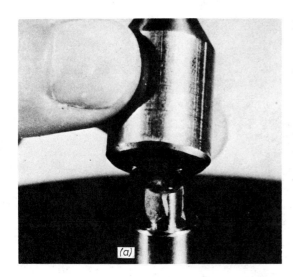

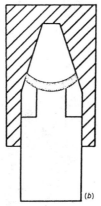

Figure 8–4. (a) Lens being centered on lens holder; (b) diagram showing angle of inside of centering device

Once the lens is mounted and centered by one of the above techniques, the diameter is cut down by holding a single-edge razor blade (Figure 8–5a), a fine file (Figure 8–5b), an emery board, a scalpel, or other cutting device against the edge of the lens as it rotates. If a razor blade is used, it should be held perpendicular to the lens edge as in Figure 8–6a or at a slight angle with the direction of lens rotation. Never angle the blade in the direction of rotation (Figure 8–6b) because the razor edge will tend to cut into the plastic, either breaking the lens or causing an uneven serrated edge (Figure 8–7b). A serrated edge will also occur if the lens is incorrectly centered or not round in the first place, if excessive pressure is applied on the razor blade, or if the spindle does not run true and thus wobbles. Light, even pressure is adequate to remove plastic if the blade is held at the correct angle and is sharp.

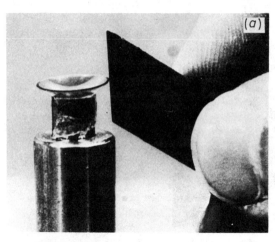

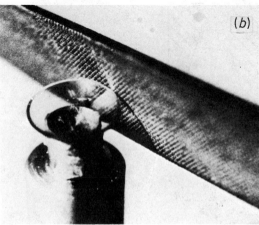

Figure 8–5. (a) Razor blade being held against the edge of the lens as it rotates to reduce diameter; (b) a file being held against the edge of the spinning lens to reduce the diameter

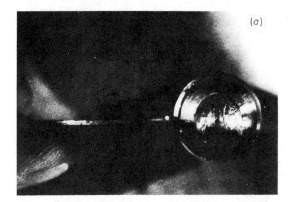

(a)

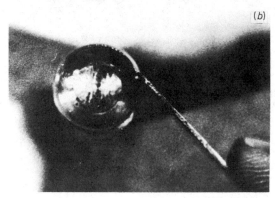

(b)

Figure 8–6. (a) Razor blade being held perpendicular to the edge of the lens in the correct manner; (b) razor blade being held at an incorrect angle. If the lens is rotated in a clockwise direction, its blade will dig into the edge, resulting in a broken or uneven edge

The overall lens size can be checked periodically by placing a hand magnifier on the lens while still on the unit or by removing the lens with a holder and using the V-channel gauge (Figure 8–8), being careful not to force the lens down too far into the channel. The lens diameter at this stage of the lens fabrication should be left about 0.2 mm larger than the final desired diameter because the process of contouring an edge will cause a reduction of diameter by approximately 0.2 mm.

This method of diameter reduction is a good technique when a large change in overall size is desired, as when starting with a large uncut lens.

Use of Abrasive Cones or Laps

Another method for reducing the lens diameter by a small amount, 0.5 mm or less, is to use an abrasive cone or concave radius lap. The contact lens is held by a suction cup, a rod with a concave surface on one end, or a spinner with a concave mounting button using double-faced

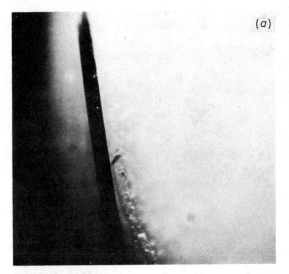

(a)

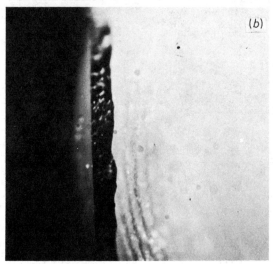

(b)

Figure 8–7. (a) Photomicrograph of lens edge after correct technique with the razor blade; (b) uneven, serrated edge caused by razor blade held at the wrong angle, excessive pressure, or incorrect mounting of lens

tape. The lens must be centered on the holder to prevent vibration when it is placed in the cone, as this could otherwise cause a rough edge, or a noncircular lens with prism. The lens is placed down into the rotating cone or concave lap (Figure 8–9a) and the grinding tool is constantly

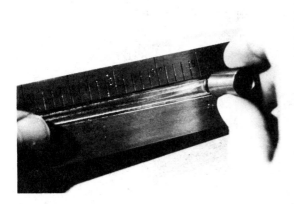

Figure 8–8. Measuring the lens diameter without removing the lens from the holder

moistened with water to prevent heat from friction and to keep the ground-off plastic from building up on the grinding tool. The lens is allowed to rotate slowly and move slightly from perpendicular in a circular fashion to increase the rate of plastic removal (Figure 8–9b). The cones or laps can be emery, crystalon, carborundum, or brass with impregnated diamond dust (600 to 1200 grade). The cones usually have angles of 60 to 90 degrees with the 90-degree cone being most commonly used (Figure 8–10a). Concave laps with radii of 6.5 to 7.0 mm can be employed (Figure 8–10b).

Other Methods

Punches or dies can also be used to cut the lens to the approximate diameter (Figure 8–11). The uncut lens is placed over an aperture to the size desired. A sleeve is next placed over the lower position of the punch to hold the lens centered and a cutting edge is then positioned over the lens through a hole in the sleeve. A sharp rap on the top of the cutting tool will cause the lens to be cut out. These punches are usually in 0.5 mm steps and the punch of the next largest size than the desired lens diameter is used. One of the previously explained techniques is then employed to obtain the final diameter.

Special cut-down lathes are used by some laboratories.

PERIPHERAL CURVE FABRICATION

In order to grind or polish a peripheral curve the lens must be mounted on some type of holder. The best method is to fix the lens on a small mounting button using sticky wax. The wax is heated by a small alcohol

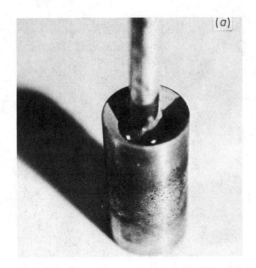

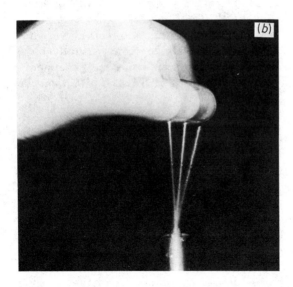

Figure 8–9. (a) Lens mounted by the convex surface on a stationary holder and placed down into the abrasive cone to reduce the diameter; (b) Lens is moved back and forth from perpendicular to increase the rate of diameter reduction

lamp and a drop is placed in the concave depression of the mounting button, which is held by a small pair of pliers or forceps. The lens is then gently set down on the wax so that it is centered over the button. The wax should have a low melting point since excess heat can affect the lens surface or warp it. To help center the lens, after is has been placed on the wax, the mounted lens is set down on a flat surface to determine if it is level. If not, the high side is gently pushed down to the correct level

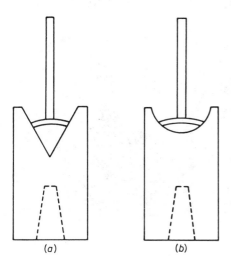

Figure 8–10. (a) Diagram showing the use of an abrasive cone to reduce lens diameter; (b) use of a concave tool

(a)   (b)

(Figure 8–12). This procedure must be performed rapidly since the wax hardens quickly.

Double-faced tape is not the best material to use to mount the lens on the button because the lens will often be warped or distorted when it is forced to conform to the radius cut on the button. When wax is used, soft wax fills in the space between button and lens and the lens thus maintains its correct shape. Even when using wax, one must be careful not to force the lens down into the wax with pressure because this may warp or distort it if the wax has started to harden. A lens can be checked to determine if it is warped while on the mounting button by placing it on the stage of the radiuscope (Figure 8–13) and then focusing on the aerial image. If all the spokes are in focus at one time, the lens is not warped. It is recommended that the lens be checked in this manner while first learning this technique because if it is warped, the peripheral curve fabricated will be toric and the back optical zone will be oval.

A lens can be easily removed from the mounting button by passing lens and button under cold water and then applying slight pressure to one side of the lens. Any excess wax left on the lens can be removed with a cleaning agent such as lighter fluid, or kerosene.

Other means of mounting lenses such as suction cups, spinners, or rods are commonly employed. The use of these methods can, however, result in the lens being held in a manner that will cause it to warp. The lens could also be held against the radius lap at an angle causing greater pressure on one side than the other (Figure 8–14) and leaving poor peripheral curve fabrication. The peripheral curve cannot be reproduced on

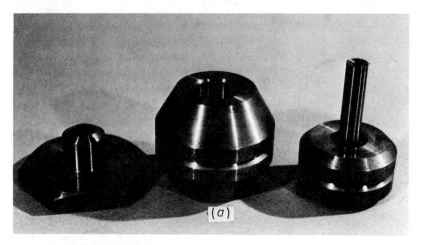

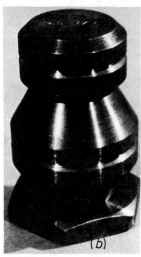

Figure 8–11. (a) A disassembled punch used to reduce lens diameter. Lens is placed over aperture in base unit (left), centering device is placed over base (center) and cutting unit is inserted through centering device. A sharp rap on the cutting unit cuts the lens out; (b) the assembled unit

a replacement lens accurately if a true, accurate curve is not produced in the first place.

The method of using a small mounting button to hold the lens while fabricating the peripheral curve is called the double rotation technique

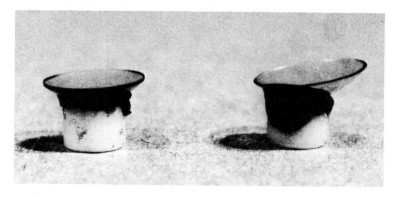

Figure 8–12.   A contact lens mounted on a button for secondary curve production. Left lens is correctly centered, the right one incorrectly

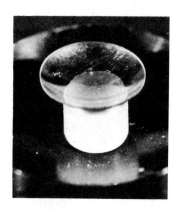

Figure 8–13. Contact lens mounted on button placed under the radiuscope to determine if it is warped

since both lens and radius lap rotate. When a lens is mounted on a rod or by suction cup, this is the single rotation technique since the radius lap is rotating.

Grinding Radius Laps

Emery tools, crystalon, carborundum spheres, or diamond impregnated radius laps with a 600 to 1200 grade can be used to rough in rapidly the peripheral curve radius. The lens is mounted on the button as explained above, placed on the spinning lap (Figure 8–15), kept moist with water to prevent build-up of heat, and moved over the surface of the lap in a figure-eight pattern. A stylus or pencil placed in the depression in the

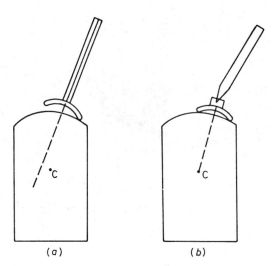

Figure 8–14. (a) Lens mounted on a rod or suction cup can result in excessive pressure on one side, causing poor peripheral curve fabrication; (b) with the double rotation technique, the lens rests evenly on the lap at all times

(a)   (b)

back of the button (Figure 8–15) is used to guide the lens. It should be pointed at the center of curvature of the lap during the polishing process.

Abrasive radius laps will leave fine scratches in the region of the peripheral curve (Figure 8–16) that must be polished out. The back optical zone diameter should be left approximately 0.2 mm oversize since the procedure for polishing the peripheral curve will decrease the zone by this amount (the peripheral curve is left about 0.1 mm narrower than the final desired width). The diameter of the optical zone or width of the peripheral curve can be checked periodically by placing the lens, still mounted on the button, on a hand-held magnifier used to measure the optic. Abrasive tools remove plastic rapidly. Measurement should therefore be undertaken after short intervals of grinding.

Polishing Laps

The use of wax or pitch radius laps to polish peripheral curves after they have been roughed in by the grinding tool provides excellent results. Wax polishing tools are easily made and used in the office. Molds are available to make the cylinders of wax (Figure 8–17). A sleeve is placed over the base of the tool and the polishing wax is melted and poured into the cylinder. When it has hardened, the sleeve can be removed by placing it in cold water or heating it slightly over a flame. The sleeve is easier to remove if it is coated with a lubricant on the inside before the wax is poured into it. There are also molds available to make several laps at a time (Figure 8–17).

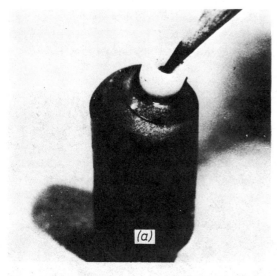

Figure 8–15. (a) Lens mounted on a button and held on a diamond impregnated bran lap for peripheral curve fabrication; (b) lens being moved over the surface of a lap in a figure-eight pattern

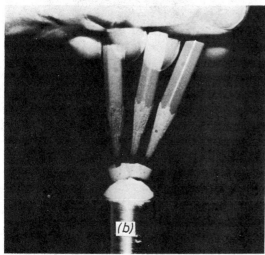

Once the cylinder of wax is made, the desired radius of the peripheral curve being fabricated is cut into the lap using a female template of the correct curve. The template is held down against the spinning wax as shown in Figure 8–18. This radius could also be cut into the wax using a lathe. Two grooves are next cut into the surface of the wax (Figure 8–18) to hold the polishing compound. Tin oxide, precipitated calcium carbonate, and commercial preparations such as Silvo or XPAL can be used as polishing compounds. A viscous material such as a contact lens

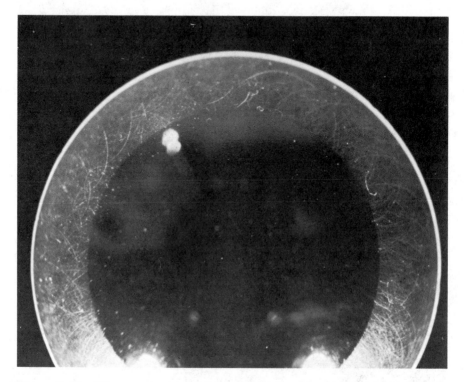

Figure 8–16.   Microscopic view of fine scratches produced by an abrasive radius lap

wetting solution, mineral oil, or glycerol may be mixed with the polishing compound to keep it on the tool for a longer period of time. The lens remains mounted on the button and is moved on the lap in the same manner as when abrasive laps are used. The polishing compound is dropped on the surface of the spinning tool as the lens is moved in a figure-eight pattern over the polishing surface. The lens surface is inspected at intervals to determine if the scratches from the abrasive tool have been polished out. A highly polished, smooth surface should be the final result.

A wax tool can be used many times by just cutting a new radius on the surface of the wax to correspond to the next desired peripheral curve radius. When all the wax has been used, a new wax cylinder can be made.

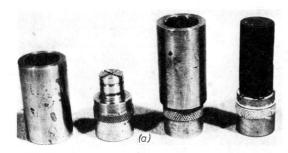

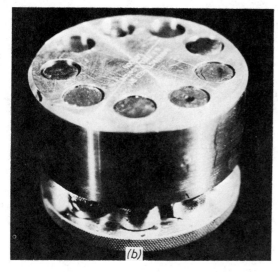

Figure 8–17. (a) Cylindrical sleeve and base to make wax laps (left). Sleeve is placed over base and filled with wax to produce the cylinder of wax (right); (b) mold used to make several wax cylinders simultaneously

Another method that can be employed to polish the peripheral curve is to make use of a plastic or metal radius lap (stainless steel or brass) covered with material such as nonwaterproof adhesive tape, or velveteen. A relatively noncompressible material such as adhesive tape produces better peripheral curve optics and a more distinct junction between curves than does a soft pad material.

When a pad material is placed on a radius lap the radius fabricated with the lap is longer (flatter) than the tool by the thickness of the pad material (Figure 8–19). For example, commonly used adhesive tape is about 0.20 mm thick. Thus, if the radius of the lap is 7.50 mm and the tape is placed on it, the radius of the surface becomes 7.70 mm. Some radius lap sets are engraved with the radius of the tool plus the tape (usually 0.20 mm longer than the radius of the metal surface) and are known as compensated radius lap sets. Others are engraved with the actual radius of the metal lap and are therefore uncompensated. When one buys or uses a set of radius laps, it must be determined if they are

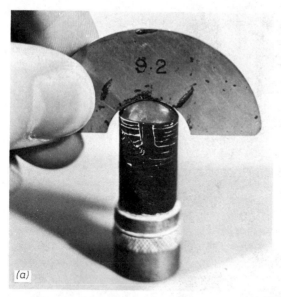

Figure 8–18. (a) Using a metal template to cut a radius on the wax; (b) grooves cut in the surface of the wax to hold the polish.

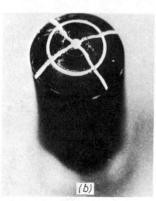

Figure 8–19. Radius (r_1) of lap is increased to a longer radius (r_2) when a pad material is placed on it. The radius increases by the thickness of the pad.

compensated or uncompensated. Laps can be checked by placing a series of female templates on the metal convex surface to find the one that matches (Figure 8–20). If the radius found is the same as that marked on the lap, the set is uncompensated. If the actual radius is steeper than marked, the lap is compensated by the difference in the two values.

Tape is placed on the lap by cutting a piece slightly larger than needed and then stretching it over the lap. Pull it tight on two sides, and then rotate the lap 90° and pull it tight again. This is repeated at different points around the lap until all the wrinkles are removed from the surface of the lap. Wrinkles must be removed or the lens will catch on them either throwing the lens off and/or breaking it. Excess tape can be cut off by holding a razor blade against the side of the lap just below the curved portion as the lap spins.

Once the pad material has been placed on the lap, polishing compound is placed on the lap and the lens is mounted on a small mounting button as previously described. With the lap spinning, the lens is moved over the surface in a figure-eight pattern as with the other techniques. Polish is continually dropped on the surface of the lap to keep it moist. This is very important with pad-covered laps because a tremendous amount of heat is produced if the pad is allowed to run dry. Since the plastic softens at about 125°C and has low heat conductivity surface defects can occur from excessive heat and spontaneous warping of the lens can occur.

When using polishing laps of any type, one must be careful not to get dirt or grit on the surface of the lap or in the polishing compound because it will produce fine surface scratches. The finish of peripheral

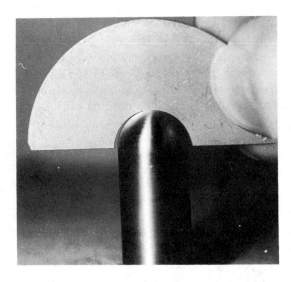

Figure 8–20. Template used to check the radius of the lap. In this case the lap is steeper than the template.

curves should be routinely examined with a microscope to be certain that this is not occurring.

Pad-covered laps can be used to fabricate peripheral curves without using abrasive laps. If one starts with an uncut lens, however, it will take longer to fabricate the curve and the final radius is usually not as accurate. If only a small change in peripheral curve width or radius is desired on a lens, the use of a pad-covered lap is the method of choice.

The rate at which a peripheral curve is being added can often be followed more easily if the back surface of the lens is marked with a water-proof felt-tipped pen. The ink will be removed as the pad polishes in the curve.

BLENDING

A lens can be blended by placing it on a polishing lap with a radius between the two curves being blended. For example, if the base curve radius is 7.50 mm and the secondary curve 9.50 mm, a radius lap of 8.50 mm can be used to blend this junction. The lens is placed on the lap in the same manner as when peripheral curves are fabricated. It usually takes only a few seconds and light pressure to blend the lens. Several intermediate radii are often used. In the above example, an 8.0 mm and 9.0 mm lap could also be used in addition to the 8.5 radius to blend the lens further. Many practitioners use a soft-pad material to obtain more complete, gradual blends but one must be careful not to distort the optics too far into the optical zone.

OPTICAL ZONE DIAMETER

The OZD is easily reduced by widening the secondary curve portion of the lens and the same methods are employed as have been described for peripheral curve fabrication. The lens is held on a lap as explained above for the secondary curve radius. The OZD can be reduced by quite substantial proportions, substance permitting. A change of 0.5 to 1.0 mm or more can frequently be achieved. A flatter secondary radius can also be introduced if this parameter is to be altered. The OZD should be checked frequently with a hand magnifier to determine the rate at which it is being reduced.

The OZD can also be increased slightly, say by 0.2 to 0.3 mm, by using a wax polishing tool with a radius equal to the BCR of the lens. The optical zone is polished in the same manner as when a peripheral curve is polished with a wax tool. Caution must be exercised when undertaking this modification since any loss in optical quality of the surface may affect the patient's vision. There must always be adequate center thickness as this will be reduced slightly. Increasing the OZD is a more difficult operation and therefore not routinely employed.

EDGE CONTOURING

The edge contour is extremely important in obtaining a comfortably fitted lens. This modification procedure should be learned even if other procedures are not routinely done because it is practically impossible to obtain consistently good edges from a laboratory. Therefore, edges of many lenses must be modified. There are several acceptable methods for obtaining consistently well-contoured edges. The key to producing a good edge is the ability to inspect it and know what changes need to be made. If this can be accomplished, then most edging methods will produce good results if the limitations of the methods are understood and a given technique is mastered.

Thinning a Thick Edge

The first step in obtaining a good edge is to start with a lens that has a reasonable edge thickness before it is shaped. The edge should be 0.12 to 0.15 mm thick before shaping. This thickness can be obtained with plus and low minus lenses by ordering the correct center thickness.

If excessive edge thickness is established in any given lens, it should be reduced before the edge is shaped. This can be done by using a concave radius lap or cone (Figure 8–21). The lens is mounted with double-faced tape on a rod or spinner by its concave surface and then placed down into the cone or radius lap so that the convex surface is against the tool. If the edge is quite thick, an abrasive tool, such as emery or diamond impregnated, can be used to grind off the excess plastic (Figure 8–22). A 90-degree cone, a 6.5 mm or a 7.0 mm concave radius lap is most commonly employed. The lens is rotated very slowly during the grinding process. A slight rocking motion of the lens away from perpendicular, as is done when the cone is used to reduce the lens diameter, will cause the plastic to be removed more rapidly. The abrasive tool must be kept moist with water.

After the excess plastic has been removed from the front edge of the lens (verified by using a stereomicroscope) a pad-covered cone or concave lap (Figure 8–22) of the same angle or radius is used to polish the lens, thus eliminating scratches left by the abrasive tool. A polishing compound

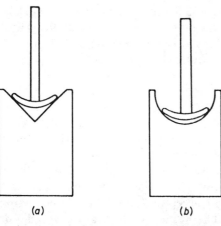

Figure 8–21. Lens held in (a) a cone or (b) concave radius lap to decrease edge thickness

(a)   (b)

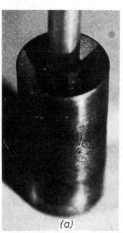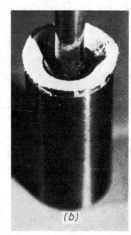

Figure 8–22. (a) Lens held in a diamond impregnated cone to decrease edge thickness; (b) Using a tape cone to remove scratches left by the abrasive cone or to decrease edge thickness slowly

(a)   (b)

is used on the pad tools. When a 90-degree cone is employed a sharp junction may be produced on the front surface. If this occurs, it may be eliminated by the use of a flatter pad-covered cone, most commonly with a 105-degree angle. The flatter the cone, the further from the edge the plastic is removed.

When removing small amounts of plastic, a pad-covered tool will be adequate. The plastic is removed at a much slower rate with a pad than with abrasive tools.

Shaping the Edge with a Flat Pad and Foam Tool

Once the edge thickness has been reduced to 0.12 to 0.15 mm the edge is ready to be shaped. The lens is mounted on a precision spinner (Figure 8–23) by the concave surface (convex surface exposed) with double-faced

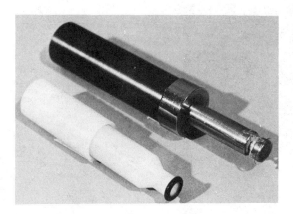

Figure 8–23. Two spinners on which lenses can be mounted for modification. The one on the left holds the lens by suction and one on the right, the more common type, holds the lens by double-faced tape

tape, at the same time ascertaining that it does not cover the edge at any point. If a small piece of tape extends over the edge, a rough spot will be produced at this point. A flat disc approximately 3½ inches in diameter covered with a pad material[3] is used. The lens is placed on the pad approximately halfway between the center and the edge of the pad such that the pad is rotating into the back of the lens. (Figure 8–24).

The pad and lens are spinning and the lens is moved back and forth on the one side of the disc (Figure 8–24) and simultaneously the angle of the spinner with the pad is varied from near parallel to the pad to about 45 degrees (Figure 8–24). The greater the angle between the spinner axis and pad, the further from the edge the plastic is being removed. This action causes the lens to be thinned from the front surface and only a few seconds of polishing will result in a correctly contoured edge.

The fact that the pad is rotating against the lens edge from the concave side may seem contrary to the action desired, but this relation with the pad gives the best tapered and contoured edge. The pad material is slightly indented by the lens edge, thus tending to roll it. The main polishing action is on the front (convex lens surface) of the edge producing the taper (Figure 8–25). A lens must never be held at such an angle that the edge is perpendicular to the pad or the main polishing action is on the back surface (concave surface). If the lens is placed on the opposite side of the pad so that the pad is rotating into the front surface of the lens, the edge will be tapered but not correctly rolled and polished at, and posterior to, the peak of the edge because the pad material does not polish this region (Figure 8–25).

If the lens is polished for too long with a flat pad or received from the laboratory with an edge that is too thin, the edge can be reshaped by

---

[3]The pad consists of polyester foam with a layer of moleskin on the surface, has an adhesive backing, and is commercially available as Dr. Scholl's Molefoam No. 35.

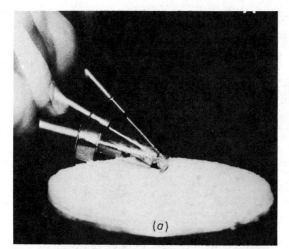

(a)

Figure 8-24. (a) Lens mounted on a precision spinner and placed on a flat rotating (clockwise in figure) pad. Angle with pad is varied from near parallel to about 45 degrees; (b) simultaneously the lens is moved back and forth across one side of the pad

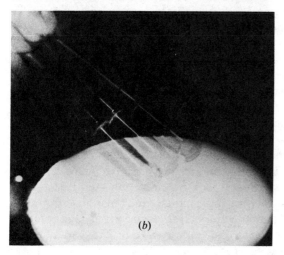

(b)

mounting the lens on a spinner by the convex surface (concave surface exposed) and placing the lens on a polyester foam polishing tool so that the tool is rotating into the posterior (concave) surface of the lens (Figure 8–26). The lens should be held so that the foam tool just touches the edge of the lens. The foam must be kept moist with a polishing compound, and the lens should be spinning through the force of the tool against it during the procedure.

By the use of a flat pad and foam tool, the edge can be correctly contoured. Edge inspection during the procedure determines the appropriate tool to be used.

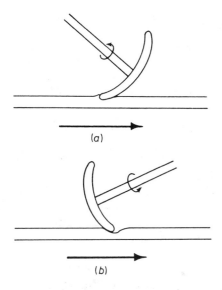

Figure 8–25. (a) Diagram of the effect of the pad material coming into the back edge of the lens in the correct manner producing a well-tapered, rounded edge; (b) effect of the pad rotating into the front of the lens resulting in a poorly shaped back portion of the edge

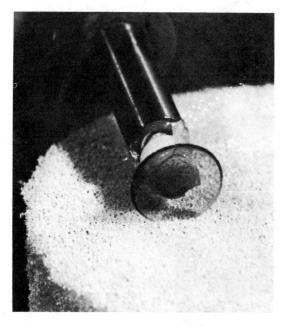

Figure 8–26. Using a polyester foam pad to polish the inside edge of the lens when it is too sharp or the peak of the edge is at the posterior surface

Using a Cutting Tool

An alternative method of contouring an edge is to mount the lens on a spindle (same as with the diameter reduction procedure) and use a cutting tool such as a razor blade or small file. A scalpel with a rounded cutting edge or a similar cutting device can also be employed. The cutting tool is held against the edge of the lens on the convex (anterior) surface and with even, light pressure it is rotated up and around the lens edge in an arclike manner (Figure 8–27). Arms and hands should be braced against the edge of the modification unit or counter-top so that the cutting tool can be accurately manipulated. It is fairly difficult and takes some experience to control the cutting tool to obtain the desired contour. The edge must be inspected with a stereomicroscope after this procedure, and if further contouring is needed, the operation is repeated with the cutting tool being held at the appropriate angle to remove the necessary plastic stock in order to obtain the correct edge shape.

After an edge is shaped, it must be polished. This can be accomplished by holding a small piece of foam, saturated with polish, between the index finger and thumb. This piece of foam is then held against the area shaped with the cutting tool (Figure 8–28). A piece of hard felt, such as a felt cone, covered with a polishing compound can also be used. The piece of felt is held against the edge of the spinning lens (Figure 8–28) and rotated in an arc pattern over the edge of the lens. Other materials such as a piece of moleskin, chamois leather, or velveteen can be attached to a holder, such as a tongue depressor, and held against the edge of the lens (Figure 8–28). Again, the polishing tool is rotated around the lens edge.

Foam Cylinder Technique

Another method of edge shaping and polishing is to use a cylinder of polyester foam material with a hole down the center. The lens is mounted

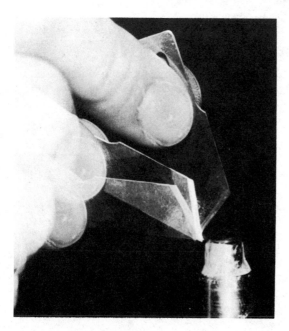

Figure 8–27. Using a razor blade or other sharp cutting tool to shape the edge. The cutting edge is held nearly parallel to the front surface and rotated up and around the edge

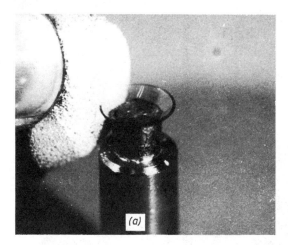

Figure 8–28. (a) Using a small piece of polyester foam; (b) felt cone; or (c) pad material on a tongue depressor to polish the edge. Polishing compound is used in each case

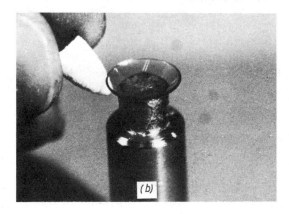

on a rod by its concave surface and then worked up and down in the foam material, which is kept moist with polishing compound (Figure 8–29)

This technique will produce a rounded, symmetrical edge but not the tapered one usually desired. The edge must be of the right thickness when this procedure is used and care must also be taken that the foam material does not polish too far in from the edge of the lens and distort the optics.

Automatic Edgers

Several companies have developed what many call automatic edgers to produce edge contours. Most of these instruments work on the principle of polishing the edge from the front and back surface for a set period of

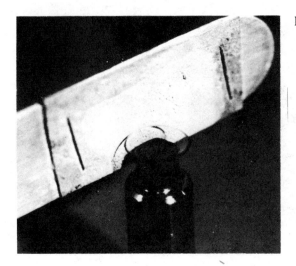

Figure 8–28. (c)

time. There are several problems that make it difficult to obtain consistently good edges with these instruments. If the edge thickness varies from one lens to the next, the final shape will be different. Lenses of varying diameters will polish differently, the amount of polish on the pad material can vary, and the pad may wear. Pressure of the lens into the pad may not be consistent, and the hardness of the plastic from one lens to the next can be different. For these reasons the amount of plastic removed in a set period of time will not be the same for all lenses and the final edge contour will be different. Good results can be obtained with most of these machines if the edge is regularly inspected after polishing, so long as it is appreciated that further shaping of the edge on the instrument may become necessary when so indicated by a poor form. It must not be assumed that a proper edge contour is automatically obtained just because the edge was polished for a set time period.

These instruments are most often used by laboratories for large-scale production of edge contours and are seldom employed in the practitioner's office because of expense and variable results.

POWER CHANGES

The power of a hard plastic contact lens can be changed by 0.50 to 0.75 diopters in the office without markedly affecting the optical quality of the lens.

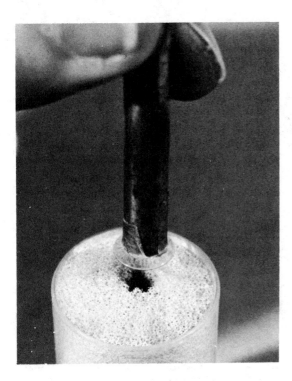

Figure 8–29. Running a lens up and down in a hole placed in the center of a rotating polyester foam cylinder to polish the edge

Adding Minus Power

To add minus power or reduce plus power a lens is first mounted on a spinner, convex surface out. The lens is held on a spinning, flat, soft polyester foam pad (as used in the edging process) and is moistened with polishing compound. The axis of the spinner is held perpendicular to the surface of the foam and near the periphery of the drum (Figure 8–30). The lens is then held against the sponge with light pressure. Greater polishing action occurs in the center of the lens, causing the front surface radius to be flattened and therefore creating a decrease in plus or an increase in minus prescription. One can rotate the lens around the periphery of the drum in the direction opposite to the rotation of the drum, which causes the power to be changed more rapidly. The lens can be allowed to spin when mounted on the spinner or the lens can be mounted on a stationary rod and slowly rotated with the fingers around the axis of the rod.

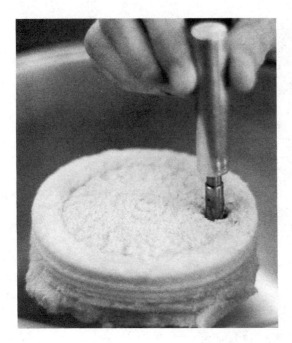

Figure 8–30. Adding minus power to a lens by holding it perpendicular to the soft pad near the periphery. The lens is allowed to rotate

Other polishing pads can be used; for example, a hollow drum with velveteen or silk stretched over it and employed in the same manner as described above.

Adding Plus Power

To increase plus power or reduce minus power the lens and pad are prepared as described above. The lens is held in the very center of the rotating pad and is prevented from rotating (Figure 8–31). In this position the center of the lens receives little or no polishing action because there is no angular rotation of the pad at this point. Going toward the periphery of the lens there is greater angular rotation. This increases polishing action. The front radius is steepened since more plastic is removed toward the periphery of the lens. The lens can be slowly rotated by hand in a direction opposite the rotation of the pad and a slight rocking action of the lens from the center of the pad will help prevent distortion of the optics.

Before changing the power on a patient's lens, one should practice on rejected lenses to learn the technique. Adding plus is more difficult than adding minus. Lens distortion may occur with changes greater than one-half diopter.

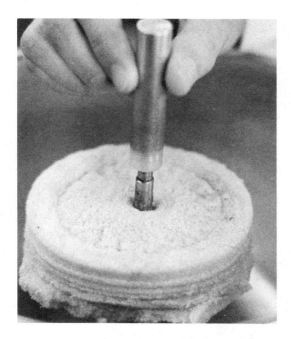

Figure 8–31. Adding plus power by holding the lens in the center of the polishing pad. The lens should be allowed to rotate only very slowly

POLISHING LENS SURFACES

After a period of wear, deposits or scratches may occur on either surface of a lens. Deposits can be removed by placing a polishing compound on the lens and rubbing it between the fingers.

To remove minor scratches from the front surface of a lens, where the majority of scratches occur, the lens can be mounted on a precision spinner with the convex surface exposed and held against a spinning, soft foam pad or soft cloth-covered drum. The spinner is held at a 45 degree angle to the surface of the drum approximately halfway between its center and the edge of the drum. The lens is then moved back and forth toward the center (Figure 8–32) and also back and forth in a path around approximately one-fourth of the pad (Figure 8–32). It should be spinning freely at all times during polishing and the foam drum must be kept moist with polishing compound at all times. It takes only several seconds to remove minor scratches. Deep scratches, of course, will not be completely removed, but their edges will be smoothed and this may make the lens wearable.

The posterior lens surface is difficult to polish, but fortunately it is not often scratched. If this surface must be polished, the lens can be mounted on a rod or spinner and placed on a soft, rotating sponge (Figure

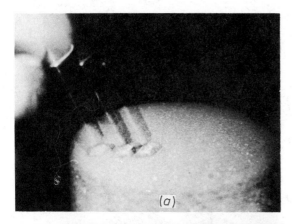

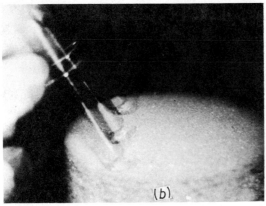

Figure 8–32. Polishing the front surface of a contact lens. (a) The spinner is held at a 45-degree angle to the pad and moved in and out toward the center and (b) back and forth on the pad

8–33) or on a radius lap covered with a soft pad. Another method is to use a wax radius lap equal to the base curve radius and polish the base curve in the same way as one would a peripheral curve.

MODIFYING LENSES WITH SPECIAL DESIGN FEATURES

Lenses with Prism Component

Methods for diameter reduction and peripheral curve fabrication are the same for prismatic as for regular spherical lenses. The method of edge treatment usually has to be changed, however. Edge thickness of a prismatic lens varies around the lens, with the apex being the thinnest portion and the base the thickest.

To contour the edge properly, unequal amounts of plastic must be

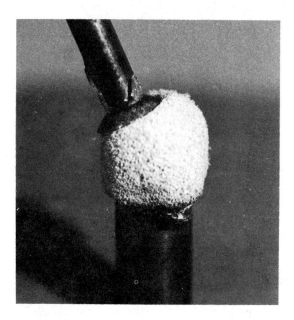

Figure 8–33. Polishing the posterior surface of a contact lens

removed from these different parts of the lens. To accomplish this, the lens should be mounted on a stationary holder, by the concave surface, and only part of the lens circumference modified at a time. It is helpful if one section of the lens, such as the base, is marked with a felt-tipped marking pen. The lens can then be held on a flat molefoam pad and approximately one-fourth of its circumference modified by a rocking action. The edge contour can be controlled at all points around the lens by varying the angle of the lens against the pad and the length of time the edge is polished at one point. If an edge is made too thin, the lens can be mounted by the opposite surface and the foam drum used. Apex thickness and shape should be the same as for a well-contoured spherical lens. The edge at the base of the prism should be either tapered from the front or relatively flat, depending on the fitting characteristic desired.

Lenses with Toroidal Surfaces

If a lens has a spherical base curve radius and peripheral curves but a toric front surface, most lens modifications, such as diameter reduction and peripheral curve fabrication, are the same as with spherical lenses. Local edge modifications may have to be carried out in the same manner as described for prismatic lenses, if there is enough toricity to cause significant variation in the edge thickness in the different meridians of the lens. Also, it is *not* possible to change the power of the lens with the normally available equipment because of the cylinder on the front surface. The surface should *not* be polished with the foam pad as this may change the cylindrical power.

If a lens has a toric base curve and a toric peripheral curve is desired, it is usually not within most practitioners' capacity to fabicate this curve. If, however, a spherical peripheral curve is desired, it can be ground or polished in the same manner as with a spherical base curve lens. It must be remembered that a spherical periphery on a toric base curve lens will result in an oval optical zone.

A lens with a toric base curve will often have a toric front curve, and thus the power of the lens cannot be changed.

Truncating a Lens

When fitting prism ballast and bifocal lenses, a truncation is often desired. Although truncation can be ordered from the laboratory, the precision and edge shape of the truncated area can be better done in the office. To do this a reference mark is placed where the lens is to be truncated and the lens is held between thumb and index finger (Figure 8–34). The lens is then truncated with a fine file, emery board, or other flat, abrasive tool. Plastic is removed until the desired diameter is obtained and the truncation shaped. Corners may be rounded off with an abrasive tool. The edge is then polished with a flat pad and foam drum as described above for a prismatic lens.

HYDROGEL LENSES

Due to the softness and flexibility of hydrogel lenses, it is not clinically feasible to make the modifications that are made with rigid lenses. In some cases, they can be properly dehydrated and modified using the general principles described above for rigid lenses. This is difficult, however, especially with the very thin and high water content lenses in use today. Therefore, these techniques will not be discussed here.

Surface Polishing

The surface of hydrogel lens can be polished. The lens is mounted on a plastic or metal holder (a radius lap will do) cut with a radius on one end (Figure 8–35) somewhat longer than that of the BCR, commonly around

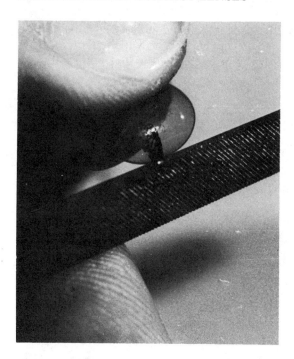

Figure 8–34. Truncating a lens using a fine hand-held file or emery board

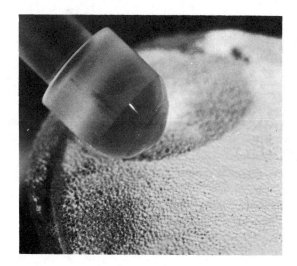

Figure 8–35. Polishing a hydrogel lens

9.0 to 11.0 mm. The lens is allowed just to begin to dehydrate to the extent that the surface becomes slightly sticky and tacky. It is then simply placed on the radius holder with the side to be polished exposed. It will be found to adhere quite well. Alternatively, double-faced tape can be placed on the lap, which is wetted on the side on which the lens rests prior to placing the lens on it. If this is not done, the lens will tend to be torn on removal.

The surface is then polished by holding the lens against a fine polyester foam or other very soft pad that has been covered with polishing compound mixed with water. XPAL can be mixed with water to make a thick polishing solution. The lens is held into the polishing pad at an angle of approximately 45 degrees and moved back and forth over it in the same manner used to polish rigid lenses.

The polishing of hydrogel lenses with this method can be helpful in removing surface deposits.

The lens should be thoroughly cleaned following polishing.

9

SOLUTIONS AND ACCESSORIES

Many solutions and accessories are utilized in the fitting, wearing, and maintenance of contact lenses. A good, in-depth understanding of these solutions is required by office personnel if they are to be used to their fullest advantage. Problems from mild discomfort to severe ocular damage can occur if the systems are not properly used. These adverse effects must be recognized and avoided through proper patient education and instruction. If problems do arise, alternatives must be understood and initiated.

Considerable experience has been gained and information is available concerning the use of solutions with polymethylmethacrylate lenses. The effect of these solutions on the eye has been extensively reported. With the advent of hydrogel lenses and other new polymers new solutions and systems had to be developed. Therefore, much research and development has occurred in recent years in this area. New products are constantly being developed and introduced into the market. These solutions must be compatible with the lens, case, eye and other solutions. To understand the clinical reports and company advertisements, as well as to be able to evaluate the effectiveness of a system with a given patient, there must be an understanding of the basic properties and terminology of contact lens pharmacology.

GENERAL PRINCIPLES OF CONTACT LENS PHARMACOLOGY

Tonicity (Osmolality)

When the cornea is bathed in a solution that has a salt concentration of about 0.9 to 1.0 percent, the cornea will maintain its normal thickness. Such a solution is called isotonic. If the salt concentration is less than this, it is called hypotonic. If the cornea is bathed in a hypotonic solution, water will flow from the solution into the cornea causing the cornea to swell. This occurs, for example, while swimmming in fresh water and with eyes open under water. There is very little salt in the water so the cornea swells. After a short period of time, a slightly cloudy or hazy vision will be noticed. To a much less extent, just excessive tearing (crying or tearing caused by an uncomfortable lens) will cause some corneal swelling. When a hydrogel contact lens is placed in distilled (water from which salts and other materials has been removed) or plain tap water, it will absorb water and swell. If this lens is then placed on the cornea, the dilute (lack of salts) water in the lens will flow into the cornea to equalize the salt concentration. This water flow creates a pressure called osmotic pressure. Thus, the lens will tightly adhere to the cornea. If this accidently occurs, forcibly trying to remove the lens may pull off some of the corneal epithelium. Waiting a few minutes until the patient's tears have time to replace the fluid in the lens will produce an isotonic condition. The lens can then be easily removed.

Should a hypertonic solution (salt concentration over 1.0 percent) be placed on the eye, water will be drawn out of the cornea to equalize the tonicity. This will cause the cornea to become slightly thinner. In some cases, such solutions are purposefully used to reduce cornea swelling caused by corneal disease.

Solutions formulated to be placed on the eye with contact lenses are usually made with a tonicity of about 0.9 percent equivalent sodium chloride (salt) solution. Other compounds, in addition to sodium chloride, also effect tonicity and may be used in solutions. The use of isotonic solutions provides greater comfort and prevents cornea thickness changes.

Hydrogen Ion Concentration (pH).

Certain substances dissociate into positively and negatively charged portions. If the positively charged portion is a hydrogen ion (H^+) the solution is acidic. If the negative ion is the hydroxyl group (OH^-) the solution is basic (also called alkaline). In case of pure water, some of its molecules (HOH) dissociate into H^+ and OH^-, the concentration of each being 1 $\times$ 10^{-7} moles per liter (at 20°C). This chemical terminology means that the solution is neutral. In order to simplify the notation for the concentration of these ions, the term pH is used.[1] The pH of pure water is then

---

[1] $pH = \log \frac{1}{(H^+)}$; the pH is the logarithm of the hydrogen ion concentration.

7.0. Values below 7.0 are acidic and above 7.0 are basic. A change of 1.0 pH unit equals a 10 times change in hydrogen ion concentration. The range of possible pH values is 0 to 14.

The pH of tears is very close to that of blood which is 7.3 to 7.4. Studies have shown considerable variation in human tears ranging from 5.2 to 8.35 with the majority at 7.0 to 7.4. If the pH of an ophthalmic solution varies considerably from neutrality, more than 1 to 2 pH units, patients may complain of discomfort. The amount of solution used, the time it is in contact with the cornea and its buffering capacity are factors which affect comfort.

The buffering capacity of a solution is its ability to maintain a given pH even when a basic or acidic solution is added. The buffering agent neutralizes the H^+ or OH^- ions. Tears have relatively good buffering capacity and thus tend to neutralize the pH of any added solution. If a solution is very acidic, basic, or itself highly buffered, the tears will not be able to neutralize this solution and thus it will cause discomfort, or in extreme conditions ocular damage.

In terms of comfort, the ophthalmic solution should ideally have a pH of about 7.4, although this is not always possible. For example, certain compounds such as polyvinyl alcohol, a wetting agent used in some contact lens solutions, are not stable at a high pH level and must be kept below 6.0 Some solutions become cloudy due to precipitate formation with high pH. They are therefore, buffered at a low pH in order to remain stable prior to use. Certain preservatives must be kept either above or below neutrality to be stable and effective. The buffering capacity of such a solution should be kept at the very minimum necessary so on contact with the eye the tears can neutralize the pH of the solution, avoiding discomfort. If a solution is stable at a pH close to 7.4, it can be highly buffered without adverse effects.

With some drugs, a high pH is required to penetrate the corneal epithelium. Such drugs are buffered at the necessary pH and ocular discomfort is an unavoidable side-effect. The buffer must be compatible with other components of the solution. Borate or phosphate are commonly used buffers. Borate buffer, however, is incompatible with the widely employed preservative benzalkonium chloride.

The pH of a solution can change with aging if exposed to the atmosphere since carbon dioxide (CO_2) may diffuse into the solution and form carbonic acid. Some CO_2 can diffuse through polyethylene containers to cause this effect. A buffered solution resists such pH changes longer than one without buffering.

It may be necessary to change the type of solution a patient uses if discomfort occurs on instilling the solution. One with a different pH level may solve the problem.

Viscosity (Thickening) Agents

Compounds which increase the viscosity are often added to ophthalmic and contact lens solutions in order to maintain it on the eye or lens for a longer time. They act as a lubricating and cushioning agent on placement of a contact lens and also help to prevent contamination through handling prior to placement. Methyl cellulose is the most commonly employed agent to increase viscosity but there are others such as hydroxyethyl or hydroxypropyl cellulose, providone, and gelatin. If an excessive amount is used, the solution will feel sticky. If spilled on the lids it may dry and leave a whitish deposit or crust. When this happens, the patient should be informed to use the solution sparingly or to lightly rinse the lens with water prior to placement.

Viscosity-increasing agents should not be confused with wetting agents which have surface active properties not enjoyed by viscosity agents. For example, polyvinyl alcohol is a very nonviscous (watery) solution but is a good wetting agent.

Preservatives

Any solution that is instilled into the eye or used with contact lenses should be sterile (no living organisms present). Sterilization may be undertaken by the manufacturer through autoclaving or some other technique and prove effective in a sealed bottle prior to being received in the office or by the patient. This is not totally sufficient, however, since any solution may become contaminated when opened and used. The solution must thus contain bactericidal ingredients, that is, chemicals capable of killing bacteria, or a bacteriostatic agent that prevents their growth. It must be compatible with the ocular tissues in the concentrations used as well as effective against organisms that can infect the eye. *Pseudomonas aeruginosa* is one type of resistant bacteria that grows rapidly and causes corneal ulcers.

Benzalkonium chloride is a compound employed as a preservative in many ophthalmic and contact lens solutions in concentrations of 0.001 to 0.01 percent. Its mode of action on organisms is not precisely known but may take place through surface active effect on the cell membranes or interference with respiration and glycolysis (metabolism) of the cells.

Benzalkonium chloride is a positively charged surface active molecule, which means it has a hydrophobic or nonpolar end and a hydrophilic or polar end. In a solution the hydrophobic ends will be attracted to any hydrophobic material such as lipids or to hydrophobic surfaces such as a contact lens. When such a surface active agent aligns itself on the lens it is held there and slowly released onto the eye. This causes irritation and prevents the tears from wetting the surface. Due to these problems, the concentration of benzalkonium chloride is kept as low as possible while maintaining its bactericidal potency.

Benzalkonium chloride can additionally be classified as a detergent. The hydrophobic portion of the molecule, also termed lipophilic, will orientate around any lipid or oily material and cause it to stay in aqueous solution since the other end of the molecule is hydrophilic (Figure 9–1). Because this molecule is generally attracted to surfaces of containers, lenses, dead as well as living cells, proteins and lipids, a large portion of the compound may not be available for activity against bacteria. It is, therefore, important that solutions containing benzalkonium chloride, such as soaking solutions, be replaced frequently. Patients must be educated to replace the solution in their cases each day.

Due to the ionic nature of the benzalkonium chloride molecule, it can be absorbed and electrostatically bound by hydrophilic materials. If a hydrogel lens is allowed to stand in a solution containing benzalkonium chloride for a period of time, it will become concentrated in the lens and slowly leach out onto the eye during wear. This causes ocular irritation and possible corneal damage.

Maximum antibacterial effect of benzalkonium chloride is at an alkaline pH, but since many contact lens solutions have an acidic pH, this compound is not operating at peak efficiency. It is also incompatible with sodium fluorescein, boric acid, silver nitrate, and argyrol. Therefore, solutions containing benzalkonium chloride should not be used to moisten

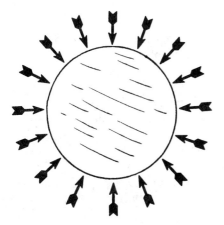

Figure 9–1. Hydrophobic ends of a compound like benzalkonium chloride or other detergent-type compound aligned around a hydrophobic material to make it soluble in an aqueous solution

fluorescein strips or in combination with other ophthalmic solutions containing boric acid.

Chlorobutanol is another preservative suitable for contact lens solutions. Its mode of action is different from that of most other bactericides in that it is thought to be taken up by the bacteria and converted to toxin, which eventually kills it. It is rather slow acting, destroyed by heat, decomposes rapidly in alkaline solution, is volatile, and loses its effect quickly with dilution. Due to these limitations, chlorobutanol is seldom used as a sole preservative. Its main function lies in combination with benzalkonium chloride which produces a synergistic effect (the effectiveness in combination is greater than the sum of the effectiveness of each compound alone), which permits a lower concentration of both compounds for the same antibacterial effect.

Chlorobutanol causes ocular irritation in some individuals even in low concentrations and it is not advisable for use with hydrogel lenses, since it is concentrated by the lens material. It also has a characteristic odor to which some patients object.

Thimerosal (sodium ethyl mercurithiosalicylate) is an organic mercury compound that is effective against bacteria, fungi, and molds. Its mode of action is by release of mercurial ions which enter the cell and inactivates respiratory enzymes. It is most active in neutral or alkaline pH and is commonly used in concentrations of 1:5000 to 1:25000. Since this compound is an organic mercurial, it does not have the adverse health and ecological effects attributed to inorganic mercury compounds.

Thimerosal is not bound to surfaces or significantly concentrated by hydrogel lenses and is, therefore, used in many of the solutions formulated for such lenses. It is compatible with sodium fluorescein but not with benzalkonium chloride because it will form a precipitate (solid particles form and the solution becomes cloudy or residue forms in the bottom of the bottle).

Phenylmercuric nitrate and acetate compounds are similar to thimerosal but not used as frequently. They are not as potent antibacterial agents as the previously mentioned preservatives. They are incompatible with chlorides, bromides, and iodides but can be kept at a slightly acidic pH level. There is also slight binding to hydrogel materials.

Chlorhexidine diacetate and chlorhexidine digluconate are very effective bactericidal agents. They are compatible with other preservatives but can be irritating to some patients, the digluconate being less so than the diacetate. Chlorhexidine has received considerable attention since it does not normally cause problems with hydrogel lenses and is thus used for chemical (sometimes called cold) sterilization. Being a surface active agent, however, it will bind to mucus and, in turn, to the lens surface, causing hydrophobic spots. Chlorhexidine also binds to proteins, apparently acting on the cell walls of the bacteria.

Ethylenediamine-tetra-acetic acid (EDTA) is not a very effective antibacterial agent itself, but is used in conjunction with other preservatives to enhance bactericidal effect. EDTA is a chelating agent, a class of materials that bind metal ions. Since bacteria need trace amounts of several metal ions to maintain normal metabolism and cell membrane integrity, a chelating agent will inhibit their growth. Bacteria can become resistant to certain antibacterial agents by incorporating metal ions into the cell membranes.

Because of these effects, EDTA is commonly added to contact lens solutions containing thimerosal, chlorobutanol, or benzalkonium chloride, enhancing the bactericidal potency of these preservatives. EDTA is most effective in alkaline pH since in acidic solutions the H^+ ions complete with the metal ions for the binding sites on the molecule. EDTA does not bind and concentrate in hydrogel lenses and has not been shown to cause ocular irritation or allergic reactions. Table 9–1 provides a summary of preservatives used in contact lens solutions.

Shelf Life

Many solution containers will have an expiration date. The reason for this is that most chemical compounds will tend to break down and change with time. The preservative may break down and not be effective against bacteria or the buffering compound might become ineffective, allowing the pH of the solution to change significantly. The breakdown products may become irritants to the eye causing the patient discomfort. Some solutions will turn color due to breakdown of some of the chemicals, commonly a yellow or brown. With many solutions, however, there is no noticeable change.

For the above reasons all solutions that are beyond the expiration date should be discarded.

SOLUTIONS FOR PMMA AND OTHER HYDROPHOBIC LENSES

Extensive knowledge has been accumulated concerning solutions to be used with PMMA plastic lenses. Many of the same solutions can be used with other relatively non-water-absorbing plastics. Before using a solution developed for PMMA on other materials, however, one should be sure that some component of the solution does not bind to or react with the material. For example, benzalkonium chloride, particularly in high concentrations, may adversely affect lenses manufactured from CAB.

Table 9–1.   Summary of preservatives used in contact lens solutions.

Preservative	Used with PMMA	Used with hydrogels	Concentrations (%)	Comments
Benzalkonium chloride	Yes	No	0.001 to 0.01	Used in many solutions.
Chlorobutanol	Yes	No	0.4–0.5	Has an odor. Slow acting.
Thimerosal	Yes	Yes	0.001–0.004	Used in majority of hydrogel solutions.
EDTA	Yes	Yes	0.01–0.2	Very slow acting. Only used with others.
Chlorhexidine	Yes	Yes	0.005	Used mostly with hydrogels.
Alkyl triethanol ammonium chloride	Could be	Yes	0.013	
Phenylmercuric cpds.	Yes	Yes		Slow Acting. Not widely used.
Hydrogen peroxide	No	Yes	3.0	Requires neutralization.

Therefore, it is best, unless further research proves differently, to avoid the use of this compound with CAB.

Contact lens solutions were developed to provide clean, safe, and comfortable lenses. In some cases, more than one type of solution is required to do this. Solutions used with rigid lenses have generally been classified into three basic groups: wetting, soaking, and cleaning.

Wetting Solutions

A wetting solution is used on a lens prior to placement to transform the surface from a hydrophobic (a surface repelling water) to a hydrophilic (a surface attracting water) state. This effect only needs to last a few seconds after placement because the mucoid layer of the tears, which is spread over the lens surface by the lids, will take over the wetting. A wetting solution helps to clean the lens, keep it clean while being placed on the eye and acts as a mechanical buffer between lens, cornea and lids.

Polyvinyl alcohol (PVA) is widely utilized as a wetting agent. It is a long chain polymer of relatively simple structure with a hydrophilic and a hydrophobic end. The hydrophobic ends of the molecules align on the hydrophobic lens surface and then an aqueous solution can wet the hydrophilic portion of the PVA, resulting in a uniform tear film. The PVA will tend to stay on the lens longer than a viscosity increasing agent alone. It is a clear liquid with low viscosity and maintains its wetting properties even in very low concentrations. It is compatible with most preservatives and has no retarding effect on corneal healing. PVA is unstable in alkaline pH. A pH of 5 to 6 is the best. Since a 5 to 6 pH is fairly acidic with respect to tears, such a solution should not be strongly buffered. This will permit the tear film to neutralize the low pH.

Most solutions, in addition to their wetting properties, contain a viscosity building agents such as methylcellulose, hydroxyethylcellulose, or hydroxypropylcellulose. Viscosity keeps the solution on the lens during placement and provides a cushioning effect. If too great, the solution will be sticky and the patient may complain of blurred vision for a few minutes after placement. Some manufacturers introduce viscosity increasing agents without a wetting agent, rationalizing that the viscosity agent remains on the lens long enough for the tear film to take over the wetting. A viscosity increasing agents does not have the hydrophobic and hydrophilic ends to the molecule.

Wetting solutions should be isotonic or slightly hypertonic to prevent discomfort or epithelial swelling on lens placement. Neutral salts such as sodium chloride or potassium chloride are added to adjust tonicity. The solution should be provided in sterile condition with a preservative incorporated. The solution should also be supplied in relatively small containers, about 25 to 50 ml (1 to 2 oz), to decrease the likelihood of contamination and inactivation of the preservative.

Soaking

There has been protracted controversy in the past over whether lenses should be stored dry or in a solution. It is now widely accepted that wet storage is the best method because lens parameters are kept stable, unlike the variation that occurs with hydration and dehydration in dry storage. Sterilization is also more effective, and although microbial growth will not occur on dry lenses, in practice few patients ever store their lenses completely dry. Some moisture or tear film remains on the lens and enhances the growth of organisms.

Soaking solutions should contain effective antibacterial agents such as benzalkonium chloride, chlorbutanol, EDTA. A combination of pre-servatives is often used to increase potency. Higher concentrations can be prescribed for soaking since this solution is not intended to contact the eye. A soaking solution may occasionally be used in place of a wetting solution as a result of misunderstanding or accident. Therefore, soaking solutions should not be capable of causing severe discomfort or ocular damage. High viscosity must be avoided as this affects lens hydration, decreases bactericidal efficiency, and slows solubility of foreign debris. A soaking solution also prevents tear proteins and mucus from becoming dried on the lens and some preparations contain solubilizing ingredients to help clean foreign matter from the lens and leach out any absorbed material.

The soaking solution in which a lens is stored should be changed regularly since the preservative may become deactivated by binding to protein and other debris introduced into the solution.

Storage Containers

Lens cases must have certain features to insure hygiene, safety, and efficiency. The case material should not react with, absorb, or deactivate the commonly used preservatives (some rubber materials may cause such actions). No substance should leach out of the case material. Sponge or porous materials should be avoided because of their tendency to accu-mulate bacteria. A lens case should be easy to clean, free of corners or crevices, and capable of withstanding boiling or autoclaving. There must be an adequate volume of solution to assure bacteriostatic effect, and the lenses should be completely submersed regardless of the case position. (The small type of case, used for mailing, is not recommended.) Lenses should be free floating and not held by clips or pressure, which could cause warpage. To decrease lens scratching, the case should be softer than the plastic of the lens. To avoid leaking, the case should seal easily and resist cracking. Each lens compartment should have a clearly marked (color coded or tactile projection) to avoid interchanging lenses. The well should be designed so it is difficult to position the lens in such a way that it can be broken when the case is closed.

Cleaning Solutions

Mucus, proteins, lipids, and other materials from the tear film and foreign debris from lens handling tend to build up on the lens surface even with regular use of wetting and soaking solutions. Specially formulated cleaners should therefore be used periodically, at least once or twice a week, to clean the lenses properly. Cleaning solutions generally contain one or more preservatives. Some manufacturers use an anionic detergent on the premise that the surface of a lens is negatively charged. Positively charged debris will thus be attracted to the surface, which in turn will be neutralized by the anionic or negatively charged detergent. A potential problem with anionic detergents is their incompatibility with cationic preservatives such as benzalkonium chloride. This stresses the importance of patients' using all solutions (wetting, soaking, and cleaning) made by the same manufacturer so that they are compatible. Some cleaning solutions have nonionic surfactants that reduce surface tension and solubilize debris.

Cleaning solutions are usually made with relatively high pH because proteins are more soluble in alkaline than in acidic solutions. Chelating agents, such as EDTA, are incorporated to remove insoluble metal ions which are frequently present.

Patients should not use dishwashing or laundry detergents, shampoos, abrasive or household cleansers on their lenses. These compounds may contain anionic detergents, which react with preservatives in other solutions forming insoluble films on the lens or may contain oils which coat it. They may also utilize ingredients that can craze (crack) the lens surface or cause ocular irritation or damage.

Cleaning solutions or gels should be formulated so that no ocular damage occurs, though most will cause discomfort. All traces should be thoroughly washed off before the lens is placed on the eye. It is best if the patient cleans the lenses after removal. They should be completely rinsed and soaked overnight. Even though patients should not use abrasive materials to clean lenses, in the office a polishing compound to clean stubborn accumulations off a lens surface may be used.

The most common method to clean lenses is to rub the surfaces between the fingers or in the palm of the hand with a cleaning solution. To prevent lens scratching, the patient's hands must be clean. Special contrivances that hold and agitate lenses in cleaning solution are available. These are especially good for patients with rough hands or jobs where they have contact with oils or abrasive materials that make it inadvisable to handle their lenses. These devices must be designed with the same safety features as for storage cases.

Combination Solutions

Preparations have been formulated and marketed to replace two or more solutions, for example, a single solution designed for wetting-soaking-cleaning. The advantage is that the patient need acquire only one or two solutions instead of three. This is sometimes less confusing to the patient. But when two solutions are combined, certain compromises have to be made. The practitioner must decide if the compromise is worth the increased convenience for the patient.

Always be aware that a combination solution, for example, may not be as good a cleaning solution as a separate cleaner. Therefore, if problems develop the patient may have to be changed to separate solutions. With any solution system (including the separate function solutions) some patients will complain of burning and discomfort on lens placement with one brand of solution and not with another. Therefore, it is necessary to have several manufacturer's solutions available in the office. Alternative solutions will then be available to use with patients.

SOLUTIONS AND STERILIZATION FOR HYDROGEL LENSES

Hydrogel lenses present special problems in relation to storage and sterilizing solutions. This is due to their ability to absorb and bind many molecules. Considerable concern and controversy has arisen over procedures to use with these lenses. Preservatives such as benzalkonium chloride and chlorbutanol are absorbed and concentrated in the lenses, causing irritation when the lenses are worn. Thus, the majority of rigid lens solutions cannot be used with hydrogel lenses. Thimerosal does not bind to or concentrate significantly in hydrogel lenses, and thus has been used extensively in solutions for these lenses. The same is true for EDTA. Chlorhexidine digluconate does bind to the lenses but does not release very rapidly; therefore, it usually does not cause problems.

Unpreserved Saline Solution

Saline solution is made up of 0.9 percent sodium chloride in distilled water. It has a tonicity that approximately matches that of the tear film when the lens is placed on the eye, which balances the osmotic pressure between lens and cornea. If the lens is equilibrated in a solution of less than 0.9 percent NaCl, hypotonic, there will be an osmotic pressure difference which causes water to move from the lens into the corneal epithelium. In addition to creating discomfort, this situation will make the lens adhere tightly to the cornea. If forcefully removed, epithelial cells may be pulled off. If a hypotonic solution is accidently used, the lens should be allowed to remain on the cornea for a few minutes until it equilibrates with the tear film. It can then be removed normally. With a hypertonic solution (greater than 1.0 percent NaCl), water will move from the cornea into the lens and also cause discomfort.

When saline solution is made with salt tablets and distilled water (Figure 9–2) it is important that the water being used does not contain minerals or other contaminates. Such impurities will affect tonicity, cause deposits on the lenses or be absorbed and bound by the lens. One should be aware of the different types of water available. Be sure that only purified, distilled water is used. Preservatives should not be present in the water from which the saline solution is made or in commercially available saline, unless it has been especially formulated for use with hydrogel lenses.

Unpreserved saline made from salt tablets must be thermally disinfected before use. The distilled water can have bacteria growing in it and the bottle in which the saline is formulated can be contaminated.

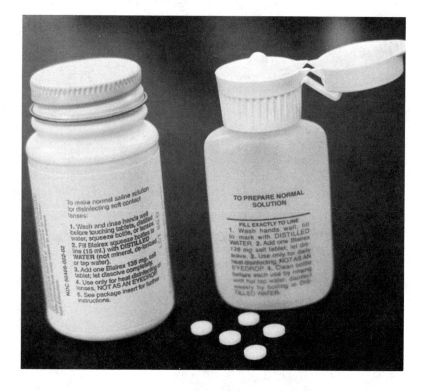

Figure 9–2. Salt tablets and bottle used to make up saline solution

The saline from the bottle can be used to rinse and clean the lens after it has been removed from the eye. The lens should then be placed in the case with fresh saline and run through the heat disinfecting cycle prior to being placed on the eye again. When preparing the lens to be placed on the eye, only the saline from the case that was disinfected should be used. The patient must be warned never to use the saline directly out of the mixing bottle on the lens prior to placement on the eye. This will negate the use of the heat cycle and again contaminate the lens. Likewise, the patient should not use the saline out of the mixing bottle as eye drops since this may result in organisms being placed directly in the eye with a greater chance of an infection. Fresh saline should be made each day to minimize the contamination. The bottle in which the saline is made should be rinsed out, cleaned, and disinfected at least once a week. This can be done by placing it in a pan of boiling water for 15 minutes.

The salt used to make up the solution should not contain iodide since it can be absorbed by the lens and leach out onto the cornea. Salt tablets made specifically for use with hydrogel lenses should be used. Other salt tablets may contain binders or other chemicals which may damage the lens.

If the above precautions are followed in the office and by the patient, then the formulation of saline from distilled water and salt tablets can be a safe and inexpensive system. Patient compliance to the system is a problem, however, making the system open to criticism. Patient education is extremely important.

One way to overcome some of the problems inherent in unpreserved saline is to use single-dose, sterile, unpreserved saline. In this case, small (unidose) packets of sterile saline are provided by the manufacturer (Figure 9–3). The patient does not have to use the salt tablets and distilled water. There is only enough saline in one packet for rinsing the lens and

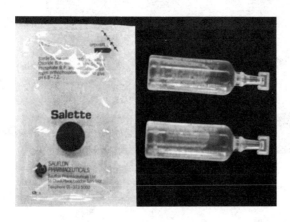

Figure 9–3. Single dose unpreserved saline (two types)

filling the case. Therefore, the solution and bottle are not kept around to become contaminated. The package is discarded after use. The disadvantage of this system over the salt tablets is the higher cost.

Preserved Saline

A third system involves the use of preserved saline. This is commercially formulated saline that has a chemical or chemicals in it to prevent the growth of organisms. The most common preservatives are thimerosal at a concentration of 0.001 to 0.005 percent and EDTA at a concentration of 0.1 percent. This prevents the growth of organisms in the bottle but is not strong enough to disinfect the lenses. Preserved saline, as may the unidose unpreserved saline, contains a buffer, such as sodium borate, to keep the pH of the solution near 7.0 to 7.4. These solutions commonly come in small bottles (1.5 oz or 45 ml) (easily carried by the patient) or larger bottles (4 ounce or 118 ml, 8 oz or 237 ml, and 12 oz or 355 ml).

The main problem with preserved saline is that a small percentage of the patients develop ocular irritation from the preservatives. These patients must be switched to unpreserved saline, either the salt tablet system or single dose packaged saline.

Chemical (Cold) Disinfection

Chemical, sometimes called cold, disinfection is a rather simple way to care for lenses. It parallels the method used with rigid lenses. One procedure uses a soaking or storage solution that contains a chemical or chemicals strong enough to kill organisms that may contaminate the lens. Several such solutions have been developed. The most common uses thimerosal (0.001 percent), chlorhexidine (0.005 percent), and EDTA (0.1 percent) as the disinfectant. If hydrogel lenses are allowed to soak in this solution for 4 to 6 hours, the organisms should be killed. The main problem with this system is that a number of patients develop ocular irritation with resultant corneal staining, injection, and discomfort. In this case, they must be switched to other solutions or to saline and thermal disinfection.

Another chemical disinfection system uses alkyl triethanol ammonium chloride and thimerosal as the disinfectant. Thus, it provides an alternative chemcial disinfection system for patients with irritation from chlorhexidine. Still another company has formulated a solution using only thimerosal and EDTA. A disadvantage of this is the long time period for disinfection. It is not as effective as the other formulations.

Thimerosal and nipastat (another disinfecting chemical) have also been used for disinfecting hydrogel lenses.

A chemical method of disinfection is the use of iodine solutions specially formulated for use with hydrogel lenses. The lens is placed in an iodide solution and then in a neutralizing agent. In about 15 minutes the disinfection is complete and the iodide is neutralized in 2 to 4 hours. The procedure and time periods vary somewhat depending upon the manufacturer.

One of the earliest systems used hydrogen peroxide as the disinfecting compound. The lens is cleaned with a surfactant cleaner and placed in a 3 percent solution of hydrogen peroxide for 10 to 15 minutes. It is then put in a neutralizing solution for 10 to 15 minutes before being placed in saline overnight. The main problem with such a system is the time the patient must attend to the disinfecting process. If it takes more than one or two steps and more than just a few minutes to complete, the patient will soon not comply.

A revised hydrogen peroxide system calls for placing the lenses in 3 percent hydrogen peroxide for 10 minutes and then transferring the lenses to a case filled with preserved saline, which has a disc containing a platinum catalyst. The catalyst breaks down any residual hydrogen peroxide so that it will not irritate the eye. A preserved saline must be used because if the saline was contaminated, the lens would end up in a contaminated solution. This system still requires two steps with a 10-minute wait, which is a disadvantage. Irritation and allergic reactions have not been reported with this system, however.

Other chemical disinfection systems have been used, one being storing the lenses in a high concentration of salt solution, the idea being that microorganisms cannot survive in it. Of course, the lens is in a very hypertonic solution and must be allowed to equilibrate in a normal tonicity sterile saline before being placed on the eye. New systems are being constantly developed. Others will certainly be on the market in the future.

Cleaning

Matter from the tear film such as proteins, lipids, and salts can coat a hydrogel lens. With time, these coatings can become dense enough to decrease visual acuity. Likewise, foreign material such as oils, handcreams, grease, and hairspray can contaminate the lens surface. This type of contamination should be avoided by properly cleaning the hands before handling the lenses and by keeping the lenses away from environments that cause coatings. This is not always possible, however, and methods of cleaning the lenses are required.

Numerous procedures and solutions have been devised to clean lenses with only partial success. Procedures include mechanical rubbing of the lens, ultrasonic, hypertonic solutions, surfactant cleaners, enzymatic cleaners, and oxidative cleaners.

Mechanical cleaning of the lens surface is an important step in preventing the build-up of materials on the lens surface. The patient should be instructed to place the lens in the palm of the hand and firmly rub both the front and back surfaces of the lens with the thumb (Figure 9–4). The use of the thumb to massage the lens helps to prevent cutting the lens with the fingernail. The index finger can be used, but the chance of lens damage is increased. The patient should be taught to rub the lens rather vigorously. Many patients rub the lens a short time and quite lightly, fearing they might tear it, and thus no cleaning action occurs. Even very thin lenses can be cleaned in this fashion. After instructing

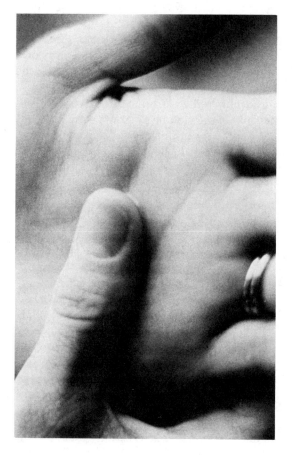

Figure 9–4. Cleaning a hydrogel lens in the palm of the hand using the thumb

the patient, have them demonstrate the procedure. Be sure they use sufficient pressure. Clean each surface at least 30 seconds and after finishing one surface, turn the lens inside out to do the other surface. Of course, the patient's hands should be clean before starting the procedure.

Although the lens can be cleaned in the above fashion using just a saline solution, special cleaners called surfactant cleaners have been formulated for this cleaning step. Surfactant cleaners can be thought of as soaps or detergents that help remove grease, oils, makeup, lipids, and some proteins from the lens surface. The surfactant cleaner dissolves these materials into solution so they can be carried away. To be useful, these cleaners normally must be used daily to remove material before it becomes baked onto the lens surface by heat disinfection or otherwise denatured ("cooked") on the surface. The lens should be cleaned in this fashion each day immediately after removal and before being disinfected. These surfactant cleaners should be thoroughly washed off the lens before being disinfected or placed back on the eye, as they will cause discomfort and may, with susceptible individuals, cause epithelial damage.

Another type, the enzymatic cleaner, has been effective in removing denatured proteins and other materials from lens surfaces and thus prolong lens life. These cleaners work by breaking chemical bonds of the contaminating material, resulting in the release of the substance from the lens surface. Both papin and pancreatic enzymes are available. In addition, some are also effervescent. These cleaners work best on coatings of tear film components that leave a fairly uniform, hazy surface coating (Figure 9–5). It does not remove crystalline deposits of calcium carbonate or calcium phosphate that form due to the use of water-containing minerals to formulate saline from salt tablets (Figure 9–6) or deposits that form on extended wear lenses.

The enzymatic cleaners are usually used once a week, although they may be used more frequently if coatings are not a particular problem. The enzyme is usually supplied in tablet form wrapped in individual foil packets. The foil wrapping is to prevent moisture from reaching the tablet, as the enzyme will become inactive in several hours if in the presence of water. Thus, if the foil wrapping is found damaged, the tablet should be discarded.

The enzyme cleaner is used by placing the enzyme tablet in the specified amount of water or preserved saline, depending on the brand, and then placing the lens in the solution for at least two hours. Commonly, the patient is instructed to leave the lens in the solution overnight, remove it the next morning, clean the lens with a surfactant cleaner (to remove the material loosened by the enzyme), and then disinfect the lens prior to placement on the eye. Leaving the lens in the enzyme solution for more than 10 to 12 hours is not effective, as the enzyme is deactivated

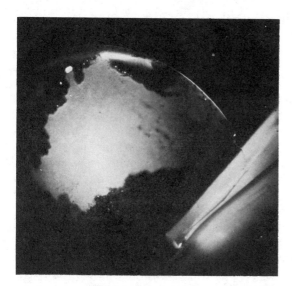

Figure 9–5. Surface coating of tear film materials on a hydrogel lens

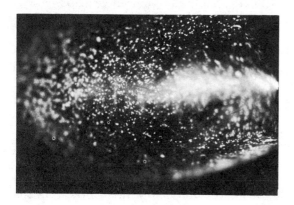

Figure 9–6. Crystalline deposits on hydrogel lenses from the use of water containing minerals

by this time. If a heavily coated lens needs additional cleaning, new enzyme should be made up and the lens run through another cycle. Be sure to clean the lens well with surfactant cleaner between enzymatic cleanings.

The enzymes used to clean hydrogel lenses appear to be safe and not cause ocular irritation. The lenses should be cleaned and disinfected, however, before being placed on the eye, as some patients could be allergic to the enzyme. It must also be remembered that enzyme cleaning does not disinfect the lenses, and thus bacterial contamination of the enzyme solution is possible, requiring the disinfection before wearing the lenses.

Another type of hydrogel lens cleaners is the oxidative cleaner.

These cleaners work by chemically breaking down materials contaminating the lens surface into small, often water-soluble, molecules. They are strong acids or bases and must be used with care since if they were accidentally placed in the eye, severe damage could occur. Therefore, most of the oxidative systems are in-office procedures. The lenses are left at the practitioner's office and cleaned by office personnel instead of at home by the patient. This decreases the chance of an error occurring, resulting in eye damage. If these harsh cleaners are used, it places a greater responsibility on the office personnel to be sure the proper procedure is followed before the lenses are returned to the patients.

The chemical composition of the oxidative cleaner and the procedure used varies with the manufacturer, but usually it consists of soaking the lens in one or two different solutions for given time periods. In some cases, the solution is heated to enhance the activity of the cleaner. Some practitioners will use a magnetic stirrer hot plate that not only heats the solution, but gives a constant stirring action. Following the one- or two-step cleaning cycle, the lenses are neutralized in another solution. The lenses must then be well rinsed.

Most of the oxidative cleaners should not be used repeatedly on a hydrogel lens, as the cleaner also tends to oxidize the lens polymer slightly. With time, it can severely damage the lens. Exceptions to this are a couple of mild oxidative cleaners that have been devised for patient use on a routine basis. Hydrogen peroxide (described earlier) is a mild oxidizing agent and can be used daily for disinfection and lens cleaning.

The advantage of harsh oxidizing agents is that they will remove some deposits that cannot be removed by other means and will also often clear discolored lenses as they are a type of bleach. As already mentioned, however, they must be used with caution as improper use can cause ocular damage, and repeated use will cause lens damage.

Other cleaning techniques such as ultrasonic cleaning and the use of hypertonic (high salt concentration) solutions to lift debris from the surface have received only limited use. The use of ultrasonic cleaning in conjunction with the enzyme cleaner reportedly increases the effectivity of the enzyme by allowing the enzyme to reach the deeper layer of the coating.

An important factor in lens cleaning, regardless of the procedure used, is educating the patient on the importance of proper, regular cleaning of the lenses.

HEAT (THERMAL) DISINFECTION

Earlier in this chapter the use of chemicals to disinfect lenses to prevent infections was discussed. One of the main problems with these chemicals is the large number of patients with irritation or allergic reactions to the chemicals. One way to avoid these reactions is to use heat to disinfect the lenses. If the lenses, case, and solutions (saline) are heated to a sufficiently high temperature for a certain time period, all the microorganisms present are killed. The higher the temperature used, the shorter the time required, and vice-versa; the lower the temperature the longer the time required. Since higher temperatures apparently accelerate the rate and type of deposits that form, most of the heat disinfecting units available today use temperatures of about 80°C (176°F) to 95°C (203°F) for 15 to 30 minutes.

Modern disinfecting units are rather compact (Figure 9–7) and have a compartment to place the lens case containing the lenses and solution. The units should be designed so that if solution leaks from the case, it will not cause damage or present an electrical hazard. It should also be easily cleaned and small enough to be carried by the patient when traveling. If the patient travels internationally, an adapter must be used if the local current is not compatible with the unit. Some have interchangeable cords or a switch to change from one current to another.

With heat disinfection, the soution used in the case is either saline prepared from salt tablets and distilled water or a preserved saline as previously described. In some cases, patients may have a reaction to the

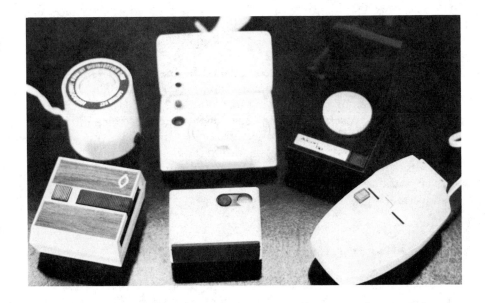

Figure 9–7.   Examples of patient heat disinfecting units

chemicals in the preserved saline and must be switched to saline formulated from salt tablets. The special precautions necessary when using unpreserved saline were pointed out earlier.

The advantages of heat are the short disinfection time and the lack of irritation or allergic reactions. The disadvantages are: deposits often develop faster with heat disinfection, difficulty carrying the unit when traveling, and using the unit where there is no electricity, such as when camping. Also, heat disinfection is not a continuous process. That is, once the heat cycle is completed, there is no further disinfection, while with chemical disinfection the chemical is always present. This means that if the patient, for example, takes the lens out of the case after heat disinfecting it, handles the lens and places the lens back in the case to soak overnight, the lens has been recontaminated and the organisms are not killed, whereas with chemical disinfection the chemicals would act against the organisms introduced. Thus, the patient should be warned not to remove the lenses from the case until they are ready to wear them. Table 9–2 gives the advantages of chemical and heat disinfection.

Sterilization differs from disinfection in that sterilization procedures kill all organisms present including spores. Disinfection, however, will not kill spores, which means that if a lens and solution are disinfected and left for several days or longer, the spores may become vegetative and could cause an infection. If the lenses are disinfected daily, this is not a problem. If lenses are allowed to sit several days without disinfection, however, they should be disinfected before being placed on the eye again. If a lens has been sterilized as done by the laboratory before being sent to the practitioner, it can stay in the sealed vial indefinitely without becoming contaminated.

Sterilization is usually accomplished by heating the lenses in solution under pressure at a minimum temperature of 121°C. This is the same principle as pressure cooking foods in the canning process.

A patient autoclave unit has been developed to use on a daily basis and provides the ultimate in safety from contamination, but seems to accelerate coatings and lens deterioration. Some practitioners use autoclave units so that lenses can be left indefinitely in their stock prior to use on patients without fear of contamination or need for repeated disinfection.

ACCESSORY SOLUTIONS

Numerous solutions, in addition to the ones described above, have been formulated for the patient and/or practitioner to use with contact lenses. These include "comfort" drops to use while wearing lenses, cleaning drops

Table 9–2. Advantages and disadvantages of disinfection procedures.

Chemical Disinfection

Advantages	*Disadvantages*
1. Continuous as long as the lens is in the solution.	1. Slow acting.
2. Easily portable for traveling.	2. Common toxic and allergic reactions.
3. Often gives longer lens life.	3. Chemicals (preservatives) may decompose with time.
4. Low initial cost.	4. May not handle large amounts of contamination.
	5. If solution not changed regularly may become ineffective.
	6. Possibly higher long-term cost.

Heat Disinfection

Advantages	*Disadvantages*
1. Few allergic or toxic reactions (especially when salt tablets are used).	1. Shorter lens life (more deposit formation).
2. Quick and complete disinfection.	2. If case is opened following heating, it can become contaminated.
3. Lower long-term cost.	3. Need for electrical source.
	4. More to carry when traveling.
	5. Higher initial cost (for unit).

to use while wearing lenses, irrigating solutions, diagnostic stains (dyes), artificial tear solutions, and decongestants.

Irrigating Solutions

These solutions are used to wash foreign material out of the eye such as sand, grit, and chemicals. They are also used to moisten fluorescein strips.

Irrigating solutions must be compatible with the eye. The salt concentration should be about 0.9 percent and the pH 7.0 to 7.5. They should be supplied in bottles that can be used to spray a constant stream of solution onto the eye.

Stains

The most common stain used in contact lens practice is sodium fluorescein. It is supplied either in solution or impregnated in dry filter paper strips. The fluorescein in the individually wrapped paper strips is most commonly used in contact lens practice since it is less likely to become contaminated and less expensive than unit dose liquid fluorescein. Liquid fluorescein is a good media for *Pseudomonas aeruginosa,* an organism that causes corneal ulcers. If liquid fluorescein is desired, unit dose packets should be used.

Fluorescein penetrates damaged epithelial cells and is used to inspect the eye prior to contact lens fitting, as well as at follow-up visits after the patient has worn lenses, to determine if there is any damage or disruption to the surface of the eye. Since fluorescein dissolves in the tear film, the stain is also used to visualize areas of tear pooling under a contact lens.

The fluorescein strip should be moistened with a compatible solution, which means an alkaline pH, and preserved with something other than benzalkonium chloride. Usually one of the common irrigating solutions is used. Be careful not to touch the tip of the bottle to the strip, as this will contaminate the whole bottle with fluorescein. Contact lens wetting solution should not be used because it is too viscous, preventing it from penetrating damaged areas, and, in the case of evaluating the fit of the lens, the viscosity causes the stain to coat the front of the lens, obscuring the pooling under the lens. To visualize the stain, ultraviolet ("blacklight") illumination is necessary. To evaluate the fit of the lens a magnifier with an ultraviolent light source can be used. In the case of evaluation of epithelial damage, the biomicroscope is used with a cobalt filter in the path of the illumination source.

Fluorescein is a relatively small, water-soluble molecule, which means it can be absorbed into a hydrogel contact lens and thus should not be placed in the eye while the patient is wearing the lens. If it accidentally gets into the gel lens, the stain will slowly leach out of most gel lenses. In this case, the lens should be purged by allowing it to soak in repeated changes of saline solution. It does not cause any problem if the patient wears a hydrogel lens with small amounts of fluorescein in it. Likewise, when fluorescein is used to inspect the eye for damage after the gel lens is removed, the eye should be irrigated prior to placing the lens back on the eye, as described in Chapter 5.

To avoid the problem of fluorescein being absorbed into hydrogel lenses, a high molecular weight fluorescein has been developed. The molecule is large enough that it will not readily penetrate the lens. One of the disadvantages of the presently available high molecular weight fluorescein is that it does not fluoresce as brightly as regular fluorescein and does not show up defects in the corneal epithelium as well. If a hydrogel lens is left in the solution too long, it will absorb some of this stain.

You should avoid getting fluorescein on the patient's clothing. Since it is water soluble, however, it will usually wash out.

Another stain occasionally used is rose bengal. It is a reddish-purple stain supplied in individual dose packets in liquid form or in paper strips. It is used to stain areas of degenerating or dying cells.

The eye is examined for areas of staining using the biomicroscope with white light. The stain must be thoroughly irrigated from the eye before a gel lens is placed on the cornea.

ARTIFICIAL TEARS—CUSHIONING AGENTS

Artificial tear solutions, also called ocular lubricants, may be used to decrease dry eye symptoms, reduce corneal staining as a result of drying, reduce irritation, lubricate lenses, and keep the surface from drying. Of course, such solutions should be nearly isotonic and have a pH and buffering capacity to be comfortable on instillation. These solutions must be supplied sterile and have a preservative to keep them from becoming contaminated.

To be useful the solution must stay on the eye for as long a time as possible. In order to accomplish this, these solutions are usually viscous. Such agents as methylcellulose, hydroxyethycellulose, gelatin, or other viscous compounds are added.

Decongestants

Decongestants are formulated to decrease conjunctival injection by constricting the blood vessels. There are several vasoconstrictors used, for example, phenylephrine hydrochloride, naphazoline hydrochloride, ephedrine, adrenaline hydrochloride, and tetrahydrozoline hydrochloride. In addition, these solutions contain preservatives, buffers, salts for proper tonicity, and often a viscosity increasing agent. Decongestants may also be made slightly hypertonic to help decrease the conjunctival swelling accompanying injection.

Decongestants, as well as artificial tears, should always be used cautiously with contact lens patients since they may only be treating the symptom and not the cause of the problem to be corrected. Many artificial tears and decongestants cannot be used with hydrogel lenses since the active ingredient may concentrate in the lens, causing irritation or exaggerating effects. Thus, be sure the solution is compatible with the type of lens material the patient is wearing.

It is also possible that the patient may be allergic to a component in the solution or develop an irritation to it. For example, if a patient has developed an allergy to thimerosal in solutions used with hydrogel lenses, do not have that patient use a decongestant preserved with thimerosal.

When any patient is prescribed a solution, be sure they are instructed as to how often to use it, how much to use, how long to use it, any possible side effects, such as allergic reactions, and how to instill it. The patient should be taught to instill drops in the same manner previously described for placing drops in the patient's eye.

Hand Cleaners

When handling contact lenses, either by the personnel in the office or by the patient, the hands must be clean to prevent contaminating the lens with microorganisms, grease, lotion, makeup, or other foreign material that can damage the eye, the lens, or affect comfort or vision. The hands should be thoroughly washed with a soap that is easily rinsed from the hands and does not contain irritants, creams, or perfumes. Examples of these are Ivory or Neutragena soap. After washing the hands, they should be thoroughly rinsed.

10

PATIENT EDUCATION

Proper education of the patient in placement, removal, and care of contact lenses, as well as educating the patient to signs, symptoms, and proper follow-up care, is extremely important for successful and safe contact lens wear. The contact lens technician in the professional office is the logical individual to carry out this function.

To teach patients proper lens usage there must be not only an understanding of the technical aspect, but also an enjoyment of working with people, along with empathy for their problems. A willingness to spend sufficient time with them to master proper lens handling and care is also required. It is helpful, but not mandatory, that the technician wear contact lenses. At the least, an ability personally to place and remove different types of lenses before teaching others is important. This ability helps to understand the patient's problems.

When working with patients, it must be remembered that some will have greater dexterity, experience, and confidence than others. Some will learn the procedures very quickly, using the first technique demonstrated. Other patients will have great difficulty, requiring several office visits before becoming sufficiently competent to take their lenses home. Different patients will require the use of different techniques due to eye and lid anatomy, the type of lenses, their dexterity, and many other factors. Thus, a technician must know and be able to teach and adapt different procedures for individual patients. It must be remembered that practically all patients can learn placement, removal, and care of their lenses if they have some desire and the paraprofessional is willing to take the time and use all the acquired skills to teach them. Many patients with the use of only one arm are able to care for and wear lenses. Likewise, patients without arms have learned placement, removal, and care utilizing their feet. Thus, always remember it is possible.

The technician's enthusiasm, encouragement, and confidence are quite important in teaching others, and are particularly necessary when working with children and the elderly, who must be made to believe they can do it.

The techniques and procedures that will be described are some of the more common and successful ones. They are by no means the only ones that can be employed. Many other methods are used successfully. In some circumstances other techniques or modifications must be made to handle a given situation.

GENERAL PRINCIPLES

Educational Aids

Many practitioners find it very helpful to use a variety of educational aids. These include written pamphlets, drawings, eye models, books, slide-tape series, movies, and videotapes. Sources for these aids are given at the end of this chapter. Such systems have the advantage in that the same basic information is given to all patients. These aids repeat the same message without forgetting specific items as people might. Thus, if a patient watches a movie or takes a pamphlet home, it is certain that the patient will have at least been exposed to certain information.

The use of educational aids supplements personal instruction. They do not replace it. When patients come into a practitioner's office, there is a certain amount of excitement and apprehension. For this and other reasons, patients do not always hear, understand, or remember everything they are told. Thus, all important points should be repeated in different forms. Likewise, to be sure the patient understands, a "test" must be given. Ask the patients to repeat instructions, and explain what should be done in different circumstances or how they are going to perform a procedure. In addition to verbal response some practitioners have patients answer written questions. In the case of procedures such as lens placement, removal, and cleaning, have the patient demonstrate how to do it, not just verbally elaborate. Never assume that if patients have been told or shown something that they will remember it.

There are many different successful ways to utilize educational aides. Some practitioners prefer to have the patient view a slide-tape series, a movie, or a videotape prior to the first examination. This educates the patient to the practice and procedures of the initial examination. The technician must constantly remember that the office and examination procedures become automatic and are second nature since they are performed each day; but for the patient, it is all new. It is the technician or assistant's duty to help put the patient at ease and to educate the patient. A movie or videotape at the first visit can also educate the patient. Knowing the pros and cons of contact lenses helps patients decide if contact lenses are desired.

Some practitioners prefer to present educational material after the fitting of lenses but prior to the visit when the patient actually receives the lenses. In some offices the patient may view a film on care of contact lenses and then have a few days to think it over before returning for the dispensing visit. More commonly, the patients are given written material, booklets or pamphlets, on lens placement, removal, and care to read over before coming in for the dispensing visit. This allows them to become somewhat familiar with the techniques at their leisure prior to being given instructions in the office.

Other practitioners prefer to present the educational material at the dispensing visit. At this time an audiovisual presentation may be shown on placement, removal, and solutions. The technician will then teach the procedures. Following the instruction another audiovisual presentation may be given on expected symptoms, what to do in emergencies, importance of follow-up care, and similar topics. In addition, patients may be given a questionnaire to determine if they understand the important points and written material on the procedures to refer to at home.

The audiovisual presentations should be shown to the patient in a quiet, relaxed atmosphere. These may be viewed by a single patient or to groups of patients at one time. The assistant must be willing to answer a patient's questions when they arise. The use of eye models and diagrams is also very helpful.

Practitioners occasionally want patients to sign forms or questionnaires indicating they have seen certain audiovisual presentations and understand lens care. In any case, a presentation given the patient should be entered on the patient's record by the technician.

Individual versus Group Instruction

Practitioners and technicians often prefer to have instruction given to patients on an individual basis. They feel this gives more individual attention, allowing better control over patient education.

Others feel that it is more efficient to have a group of patients instructed at one time. Two to six patients can be instructed by one technician. To do this an appropriate space must be available where each patient has a mirror and faces the instructor. Semicircular counter tops or desks with the instructor in the center and the patients seated around the outside work well for this.

In addition to requiring less technician time, an advantage of group education is that patients know they are not the only ones having some difficulty in the process of learning. Likewise, each can help and encourage the other. As questions are asked, the answer to one patient's questions helps all at the session.

Of course the disadvantage to this system is that each patient may not receive as much personal attention. Sufficient time must be allowed to minimize this problem. Groups should also be scheduled so that all patients will be using the same lens care procedure. Dispensing different types of lenses and care systems can be confusing.

Whether group education or individual is best depends on the size of the practice, the preference of the practitioner, along with the personality, capabilities, and preference of the technician. Either method, if handled properly, can work well.

Hygiene

The hygiene of the office, technician, and patient is important. Poor hygiene can lead to lens discomfort and increased risk of infection. This becomes increasingly important with extended wear and with patients who might be fit for pathological reasons.

The office, including sinks, counters, lens cases, vials, solution bottles, and other equipment, must be kept clean. A contaminated sink or solution bottle could spread an infection to many patients in just a few days.

The technician must set the example for the patient. A technician should be sure the hands and fingernails are clean and thoroughly wash and rinse the hands before handling a lens. No matter how hard attempts are made to try to convince the patient of the importance of good hygiene, if it is not practiced by the technician and practitioner it is not going to be followed by others.

Soaps containing perfumes or creams or those that leave residues should never be used. These were discussed in Chapter 9.

Patient Competency

As an instructor, the technician must be sure the patient can adequately place the lens on the cornea, recenter it if decentered, remove it, and properly clean and disinfect it. The patient must demonstrate a proficiency in these procedures before being allowed to leave the office with the lenses. If patients cannot properly handle the lenses, they may develop a fear or become discouraged by the problems. Sometimes they do not become satisfied lens wearers. Likewise, if the lenses are not properly cared for, they may become dirty or scratched, resulting in discomfort and poor vision. The chance of an ocular infection is also increased.

Therefore, in order to get patients started off in a positive manner, their ability must be assured even if it takes several training sessions.

Emergency Procedures

The patients should know what to do if an emergency of any kind arises. They may not be able to remove a lens, it can become lost under the lid, or a red or painful eye might be experienced. All contact lens patients should be given telephone numbers of not only the office, but also the home numbers of office personnel or someone who can help or find help for them if required. Patients should be encouraged to call if there is an emergency. Usually an explanation or verbal directions over the telephone can take care of the problem and reassure the patient.

Family members or friends should be taught how to find a lens decentered off the cornea, how to remove a lens, and what to do in an emergency. This is particularly true if a child or elderly patient is fitted. Patients should also be encouraged to have identification on them indicating they wear contact lenses. This is especially important in case of an accident, unconsciousness, or hospital incapacitation. In these situations the lenses should be removed as soon as reasonably feasible. Identification cards are often included in starter kits of solutions or are available from lens manufacturers and professional organizations. The patient should be encouraged to fill out such a card and place it in the wallet with other pieces of identification. One of the problems with such identification cards is that with time they become lost. Likewise, these may not be found by emergency personnel due to all of the other cards in a patient's wallet. This may be overcome by using a bright red or fluorescent card[1] Another method that can be used is to place a label or sticker on the patient's driver's license or other piece of identification, indicating the patient is wearing contact lenses. These may consist of just a small red sticker with "I Wear Contact Lenses" on it. Probably the best identification a patient can use is a Medic Alert Foundation ID bracelet or necklace.[2] Emergency care personnel usually look for these. In addition,

---

[1]Metroptic Services, 309 North Lake St., Mundelein, IL, 60060
[2]Medic Alert Foundation, P.O. Box 1009, Turlock, CA 95380.

other information such as drug allergies and health problems can also be indicated. A supply of Medic Alert application forms should be available to give to patients.

Often emergency personnel (emergency or ambulance personnel, firemen, policemen) or emergency room physicians do not know how to remove and care for contact lenses. Educating these people will help to correct this situation. This can be accomplished on an individual basis as they might come into the office for a vision examination. All emergency personnel should be shown how to identify a patient who wears contact lenses by pulling the lids apart and using a flashlight or penlight to see the edge of the lens. They should be shown how to remove and store different types of lenses. It is helpful to give them a small emergency contact lens kit containing a suction cup or soft rubber-type remover, a case to put the lenses in, and a small bottle of preserved saline in which any type of lens can be stored. The kit should also include a simple instruction sheet. Such kits are available from different professional organizations and some contact lens laboratories, but they can also be easily put together in the office.

To educate emergency care personnel such as police, fire departments, and emergency room personnel in a more organized fashion, you might consider short seminars. It is helpful to deliver emergency kits to the different groups on a regular basis and to educate new personnel.

RIGID LENS TECHNIQUES

Solutions

The proper use of solutions is important for hygiene, safety, initial lens comfort, wearability, and lens life. Different types of contact lens plastics may require different solutions. Additional professional judgment may be involved in chosing the appropriate solutions to be used. This depends on the patient's environment, ability to care for the lenses, and reactions to the solutions during the first few weeks. The previous chapter should be consulted for a detailed discussion and uses of solutions.

Lens Handling by the Patient

The patients should be instructed to handle the lenses gently. They should not apply undue pressure on the edge as this might warp or crack the lens. Emphasis should be placed on having absolutely clean hands. Dirt and grit will scratch the lenses and be uncomfortable on placement. Similarly, grease, nicotine, or cosmetics will coat the lenses, creating discomfort on placement. Patients must be cautioned not to use soap containing hand cream or oil. They must also be sure that all soap residue is thoroughly rinsed off before touching the lenses. Lens surfaces should not be wiped or rubbed with a towel, a tissue or other material which may contain any abrasive substance. Prior to placement on the eye, the patient should periodically hold the lens up by the edges, between thumb and index finger, toward a light background and inspect it for scratches, cracks, or chips.

A patient is best advised to perform placement and removal techniques over a table top or counter so the lenses will not be dropped on the floor and lost. Dropping a lens down a sink drain is quite common and losses could be avoided by calling attention to the hazards involved and the value of closing a sink stopper. It is easy to step on a dropped lens; therefore, patients should be told not to move around until a lost lens is found. Lenses often cling to clothing, which must be examined closely if the lens is dropped. When retrieved, a lens should be picked up by gentle contact with a wet finger tip. Always take care not to slide a lens across any surface.

A patient should not use hot water on the lenses or store them in a place where they might be exposed to high temperatures, such as near a heater, the dashboard of a car, or on a television set. In addition, the patient must be warned not to use any substance on or with the lenses except that which has been advised by the practitioner or technician.

Placing a Lens on the Eye

When instructing the placement of the lens on the cornea, it is convenient to have the patient seated at a small table with a mirror on its surface and perhaps a second mirror at a 45-degree angle in front of the patient. The assistant should be positioned so that all of the patient's movements can clearly be seen and at the same time give appropriate instructions. Lighting should be arranged so patients can see their eyes when looking down into the mirror. This can be achieved by having lights in the table top under diffusing plates beside the mirror. There should also be a sink nearby or a container of water to rinse the lenses in. All sinks in the office should have traps with holes small enough to prevent the contact lenses from going through. A supply of lint-free tissues and the required solutions should be close at hand.

The first step is to remove a lens from the storage case. Only one lens is removed at a time to avoid interchanging right and left. The patient should get into the habit of removing the same lens first each time. Soaking solution should be rinsed off under running water or in a cup. Wetting solution is then dropped on the surface of the lens and spread over both sides with the fingers. Patients should be told not to touch the tip of the bottle as this could lead to contamination of the solution. If so desired, the wetting agent may be lightly rinsed from the surface but not washed entirely off. Removing excess solution sometimes makes initial contact with the eye more comfortable. Some patients might prefer to leave excess solution on the lens or they may even add a drop to the back surface before placement. This is acceptable, although excess solution can flow out of the eye on to the lids and lashes, become dried, and leave a white residue. If this proves to be a problem, excess solution can be rinsed off by holding the lens between the thumb and forefinger under a stream of water prior to placement. Excess solution might also cause blurred vision for a few seconds after placement due to its high viscosity. Saliva to wet a lens should be avoided, even though some patients routinely use it. Good wetting action is present in saliva, but there are a large number of bacteria that could, under the right conditions, increase the risk of ocular infection.

Before attempting to apply a lens, patients should dry their hands but leave the finger on which the lens is to rest wet. They should ascertain that their lids are dry in order to obtain an adequate grip and firm hold.

There are several equally acceptable methods of placing a lens on the eye. The assistant should be familiar with all the alternatives since some patients will require different techniques than will others. Verbal instructions should be given while the patient is in the actual process of placing the lens on the cornea. This approach provides reassurance, keeps attention on the procedure, and helps to prevent natural reflex reaction— drawing away from the lens or blinking at the time it is about to touch the cornea. Specific encouragement becomes less necessary when the patient has managed to place and remove the lenses two or three times. In fact, before the patients take the lenses home they should demonstrate placement, recentering, and removal with no help or encouragement.

One of the most common methods of placement (Placement Method 1) is to grip the upper lid margin over the lashes and pull up directly above the cornea with the index or second finger of one hand. Use the left hand if the patient is right handed (Figures 10–1 and 10–2).The lid and lashes should be securely pressed against the orbital bone. The patient should not be able to close the lid forcefully if it is held correctly. An attempt should, in fact, be made to try to close the lids before placing the lens to confirm that a firm grip has been established. At first it might help to rest the hand and wrist on the forehead for stability. The lens is placed on the index finger of the other hand (right hand if right handed) and the second finger of the same hand is used to pull down the lower

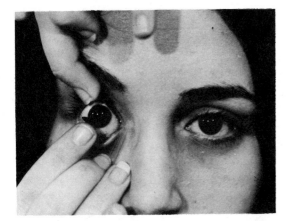

Figure 10–1. Placing lens. Notice hand resting on forehead and good grip on upper lid. Lens on index finger with good grip on lower lid and hand resting on the cheek. Opposite eye open and fixating straight ahead

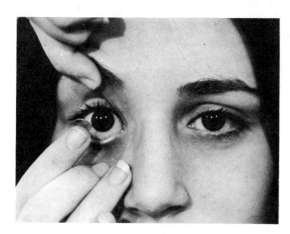

Figure 10–2. Improper grip on lids. Fingers holding lids are too far away from the lid margins

lid. Alternatively, the lens can be placed on the second finger and the index finger used to pull down the lower lid. It may be helpful to rest the thumb and hand on the cheek to steady the hand, especially when dealing with a nervous or shaky patient. The lens is then brought up and, while the patient looks "through" the lens, placed on the cornea. The instructor can help at this point by continually reminding the patient to *keep both eyes open,* to look quite steadily *straight ahead* into the mirror or at a fixation point to avoid eye movements, not to blink, and to touch the lens to the cornea. It is even helpful if the patient opens the mouth widely, as this will reflexively keep the eyes open wide. Many patients will initially be afraid to securely set the lens on the cornea. Once in place, the patient should be told to (1) look down, (2) release the lower lid, and (3) release the upper lid. Looking down will prove more comfortable for the beginner than looking up or looking to the side. The following summarizes the placement technique:

1. Wash and rinse hands
2. Close the sink trap
3. Work over counter top
4. Remove right lens from case
5. Rinse soaking solution off
6. Put wetting solution on lens
7. Lightly rinse off excess wetting solution if desired
8. Place lens on index finger of right hand
9. Dry fingers used to hold lids
10. Hold upper lid with index or second finger of left hand (rest arm on the head)
11. Hold lower lid down with second finger of right hand
12. Look straight ahead with both eyes open
13. Place lens on cornea
14. Look down
15. Release the lower lid
16. Release the upper lid
17. Blink

When using this technique for the left eye, most right-handed patients will still prefer to use the right hand to manipulate the lens and to hold the upper lid with the left hand. This is acceptable. During the learning stages the patient should be cautioned not to block the sight of the eye opposite the one on which the lens is being placed. If an eye is covered, the patient will tend to roll both eyes upward when the lens approaches, causing it to be placed on the sclera.

A second method (Placement Method 2) is to use the thumb and index finger, or the index and second finger on one hand, to hold the lids open and then place the lens on the cornea using the index finger of the other hand (Figure 10–3). Again, the patient should have a good control of the lids, not block the sight of the other eye, and follow the other general instructions previously stated.

A third method (Placement Method 3) is to place the contact lens on the second finger, and then hold the upper lid with the index finger and the lower lid with the third finger (Figure 10–4). Only one hand is thus required. This technique is the method of choice for persons with only one usable hand.

It is further possible to hold the upper lid with one hand, as explained for the first method, and put the lens on the side of the second finger of the other hand (Placement Method 4). The inside of this finger is placed

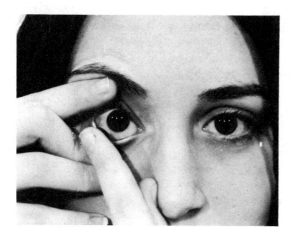

Figure 10–3. Holding the lids with the index and second finger of one hand and placing the lens with the index finger of the second hand

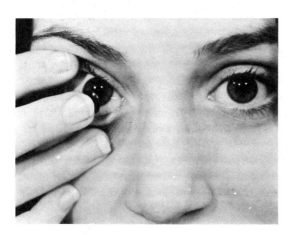

Figure 10–4. Placing the lens using only one hand

against the outside of the index finger (Figure 10–5), the inside of which is in turn positioned against the lower lid to pull it downward. By rolling the hand, the lens is placed on the cornea. This technique has advantages for the patient with long fingernails, which must be kept away from the cornea. It gives the hand a good deal of support and stability; therefore, it is recommended for those with hand tremors. Little manipulation of the fingers is required here, making it comparatively easy for patients who have trouble bending and moving the fingers.

Variations of the above techniques, where only the upper or lower lid is held or where the lens is placed on the cornea without parting the lids, can be used by the patient with experience, but such methods are not usually recommended for the beginner.

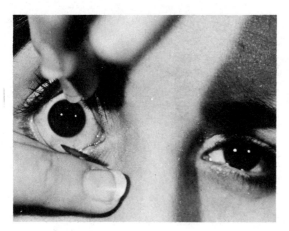

Figure 10–5. Lens placed on the side of the second finger for placement

A suction cup or similar holding device may also be used for placement. The lens is moistened and set on the holder, without suction, and brought to the cornea in the same manner as when the finger is used. The suction cup should be smaller than the lens. Dependence on such a device is normally not recommended since the patient may need on occasion to place the lens without the cup being available. A suction holder is useful, however, for those with fixation difficulties. The bottom end can be cut off, and the patient can look through the tube at a bright target or light source.

While the patient is first learning, it may be easier to use a mirror, but it is better if it can be mastered without the mirror. Occasions will arise when a mirror will not be available and sole reliance on it is therefore not wise.

Patients who have very poor acuity, without correction, may not be able to see well enough to place the first lens. To overcome this problem, a frame can be fitted with the near prescription before one eye, the lens and lower rim removed from the other side. The patient can thus see with one eye while still being able to place the lens on the other eye. A visual guideline through a tube, as already mentioned, may also prove helpful for such a situation.

Recentration

Lenses are occasionally displaced from the cornea and lodge in the conjunctival sac. This happens more frequently to the new patient on placement due to a tendency to blink or turn the eyes the moment the lens comes into contact. It is, therefore, important that the patient acquire the skills to recenter or remove the lens from the sclera before leaving the office.

To recenter the lens it must first be located. A mirror is often helpful, although the lens can usually be felt by palpating through the lids. If it is found to be above the cornea, the patient should look downward, lift the upper lid by placing the finger at the lid margin, and move it up until it is above the upper edge of the lens (Figure 10–6). By lightly pressing the lid margin against the conjunctiva above the lens, the lid can then be moved downward, hitting the edge of the lens and pushing it back on to the cornea (Figure 10–7). The procedure is sometimes more effective

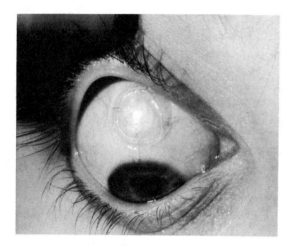

Figure 10–6. Lifting lid above decentered lens

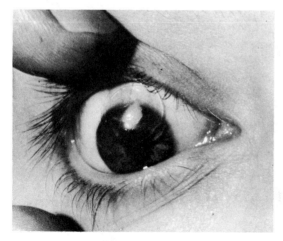

Figure 10–7. Using the upper lid to push lens back onto the cornea

if the patient is instructed to look simultaneously toward the position where the lens is lodged. If the lens is in the lower conjunctival sac, the patient looks up and uses the lower lid in a similar manner.

If the lens is located temporally or nasally from the cornea, the patient should turn the eye in the opposite direction. Then the index finger of one hand is placed on the upper lid margin and the index finger of the other hand on the lower lid margin. The lids are now pulled apart so that the margins are behind the edge of the lens. The lens is pushed back over the cornea. Alternatively, the lens can be held in place with the fingers (over the lids) and the patient instructed to turn the eye towards the lens, causing it to be pushed over the cornea (Figure 10–8 and 10–9). The lens could also be removed from the eye from its scleral position and replaced correctly.

A lens can sometimes be moved onto the cornea by manipulating it manually through the lids. The lens is held by applying light pressure through the lids and the eye turned in the direction of the lens in order to recenter it. It may be difficult for the patient to feel the lens and then move it with closed lids, especially if it is under the stiff tarsal plate of the upper lid. The lens could also be forced back against the sclera by pressure through the lids, causing a negative force under it, which in turn holds it tightly against the sclera. In such a situation, the lid margin must be positioned above the edge of the lens as described for the first centration procedure. Inward pressure must be applied against the sclera with simultaneous lateral pressure on the lens edge in order to break the negative force or suction effect. When a lens is stuck to the sclera in this manner, a patient can become quite frightened if there is not an under-

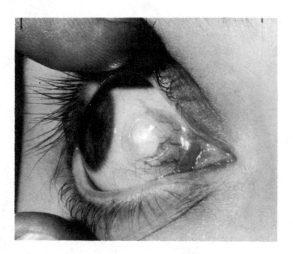

Figure 10–8. Lens displaced onto the nasal sclera

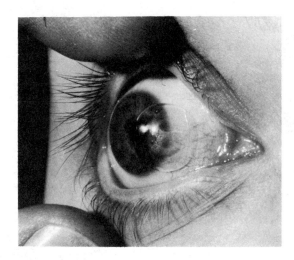

Figure 10–9. Eye turned toward lens to recenter lens

standing of what is happening. The individual must be reassured. The conjunctiva may be indented and injected for a while around the area where the lens adhered.

Lens Removal

The most common removal technique (Removal Method 1) for the patient is to tilt the head so it is parallel to the table top or mirror, looking straight ahead or slightly nasal and opening the eyelids as wide as possible. The index finger is then placed in the outer canthus and the lids pulled outward, taut against the eye. Next, the patient blinks and the lid margins should catch the edge of the lens and expel it from the eye. Comparatively light force on the lids, together with a regular blink, is all that is required to remove the lens if the technique is performed correctly. A really forceful lid action is not necessary. The other hand should be cupped below the eye to catch the lens. If the patient does not open the lids wide enough so that the lens is completely within the palpebral aperture before blinking, the lid margin cannot catch the edge of the lens. In such a situation, be sure the patient's face is parallel to the mirror so that the cornea is in the middle of the palpebral aperture before starting the removal process. Sometimes it helps to have the patient open the mouth very wide. This will cause the lids to open wider also.

If, when pulling the lids with the finger at the outer canthus, the patient pulls either upward or downward (Figures 10–10 and 10–11) instead of straight temporally, the lid margins will not catch the lens. If

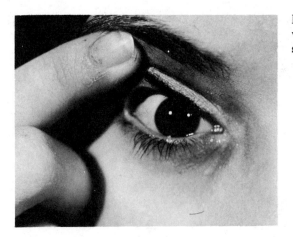

Figure 10–10. Pulling upward at outer canthus instead of straight temporally

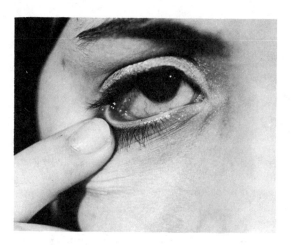

Figure 10–11. Pulling downward at outer canthus instead of straight temporally

this occurs, it may be helpful to direct the patient to hold the arm straight out to the side parallel with the palpebral aperture (Figure 10–12) until the technique is correctly mastered. A patient occasionally develops a habit of turning the head sideways so that the cornea and lens are in the temporal portion of the palpebral aperture (Figure 10–13). In this position the lids will not be tight enough against the eye and the lens will be difficult to remove. The patient should be instructed to look straight ahead or slightly nasally.

The following summarizes the steps for lens removal using this removal technique (right eye):

1.   Look straight ahead (cornea in center to slightly nasal of palpebral aperture)

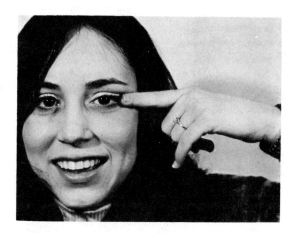

Figure 10–12. Holding arm straight out while learning lens removal to assure temporally pulling of the lids

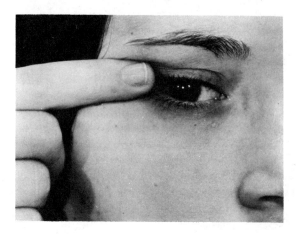

Figure 10–13. Incorrect fixation position due to head turn

2. Cup left hand under eye to catch lens
3. Open eye as wide as possible (open mouth also if this helps)
4. Place index finger of right hand in outer canthus
5. Hold right arm straight out
6. Gently pull lids (right index finger) toward right ear
7. Blink normally
8. Catch lens or lift off lashes

Another method (Removal Method 2) similar to the above is to employ the second finger of the hand opposite the eye from which the lens is being removed to pull the lids taut (Figure 10–14), or to use the thumb of the hand on the same side as the eye (Figure 10–15). The lens is caught in the same hand, providing an entirely one-handed operation. Eye position and other conditions are similar to those previously described.

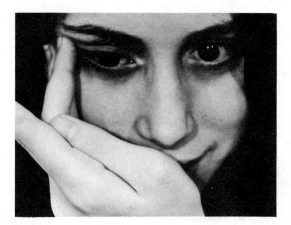

Figure 10–14. Using second finger to pull lids and same hand to catch lens

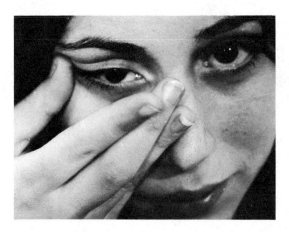

Figure 10–15. Using thumb to pull lids and same hand to catch the lens

Where the palpebral aperture is quite small or a large diameter lens is employed, the patient may have difficulty opening the lids wide enough for the margins to clear the edge of the lens. When this occurs, the patient can use the index finger of one hand on the upper lid and the index finger of the other on the lower lid (Removal Method 3). The tip of the finger is placed right at the lid margin (Figure 10–16) over the lashes and the lids spread open wide enough to clear the edges of the lens. The lid margins are then held with light pressure against the eye, brought towards each other and made to hit the edges of the lens and thus expel it. The patient should do this over a table or counter top in case the lens falls, although it will usually catch on the lower lashes or the finger on the lower lid. If the patient places the index finger a short distance away from the lid margin, the lid will roll away from the eye (Figure 10–17),

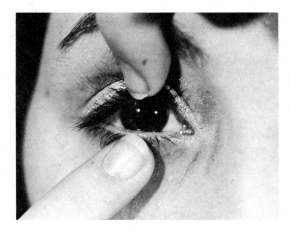

Figure 10–16. Placing index fingers at lid margins to remove lens

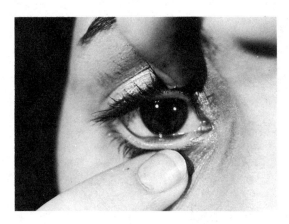

Figure 10–17. Incorrect position of the fingers on the lid margins causing the lids to be rolled away from the eye

and when they are brought together they will slide over the lens, causing it to remain on the cornea. Placing the fingers at the very lid margin is, therefore, of great importance in order to succeed with this technique.

The same general procedure can be used but the index and second finger of the same hand brought into play (Removal Method 4). One finger is placed on the upper and the other on the lower lid (Figure 10–18). The lids are separated and then brought together against the lens edge as described above. The other hand catches the lens as it falls.

The use of a rubber suction holder or soft plastic removers available from laboratories occasionally facilitates removal for those not able to master the other methods. With the head in an upright position (Figure 10–19), the patient's gaze is directed steadily forward and the lids lifted apart as already described. The holder is brought squarely onto the center

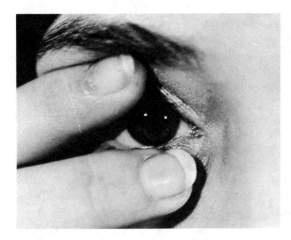

Figure 10–18. Using two fingers of one hand on the lid margins for removal

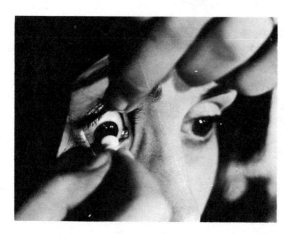

Figure 10–19. Use of a suction cup to remove the lens

of the lens, the inside of the cup having previously been moistened and pressure applied to the stem. As contact is made, pressure against the stem is released and the lens lifted off the eye as though hinged at the bottom. Caution must be exercised when using soft rubber removers which do not require pressure on the stem for suction because if accidentally placed against the cornea, they are difficult to remove. The device must be moved laterally on to the limbal area before it will release itself.

Placement, Centration, and Removal by a Third Party

When a child or a handicapped or elderly individual is fitted with contact lenses, parents or someone who will be helping the wearer must be trained to handle the lenses. They should be taught about solutions, lens care, and expected signs and symptoms just as the patient would be. They should be instructed to watch for problems such as injection and discomfort on the part of the patient as the patient may not be capable of realizing that a problem exists.

The placement, centration, and removal techniques for rigid lenses taught to a third party are the same as used by the technician or the practitioner. This is described in Chapter 6.

Lens Care

After removal the patient should be instructed to clean the lens with water or an appropriate lens cleaner to remove any lacrimal fluid. After rinsing the cleaner off with water, the lens should then be placed in a proper container filled with soaking solution when wet storage has been recommended. Emphasis should be put on placing the lens into the case very carefully, being certain that it is completely inside so that it cannot be caught by the lid when the case is closed. Lenses can easily be broken or warped in this manner. The patient should also be advised always to place the lens in the appropriate section, right or left. The solution will have to be changed according to recommended practice and the case kept thoroughly clean, washed periodically with soap and water and rinsed well before being refilled with fresh soaking solution.

Attention should further be drawn to periodic cleaning of the lenses with one of the specially formulated solutions. This should be done after removal at the end of the wearing period by placing a couple of drops on the lens and rubbing it between the fingers. The cleaning solution is then rinsed off and the lens placed into the container of soaking solution until worn the next day. PMMA lenses should normally be cleaned two or three times a week. If this is undertaken too frequently—some patients tending to do this three or four times a day—they will not wet properly when placed on the cornea. This may cause irritation, increased mucus production, and blurred vision in a short period of time. Thus, a paradoxical situation; the more a lens is cleaned, the sooner it will become cloudy with mucus. Cleaning the lens before it is stored away overnight helps to prevent irritation from residual solution left on a lens after cleaning, which will in any case be diluted in the soaking fluid. Some of the new contact lens plastics must be cleaned with the cleaning solution upon removal each day. The lenses should then be placed in the proper storage case with sufficient *new* soaking solution to keep the lens immersed.

Cosmetics

During the initial fitting and training sessions, patients should avoid wearing eye makeup. It can run and smear, get on the fingers, on the lens, and into the eye. When trapped under the lens, cosmetics can cause discomfort and corneal abrasion. In the early adaptation period the patient is advised to wear only minimal eye makeup. Being less adept at placing and removing the lenses, more tearing than usual will occur, causing a tendency to rub or touch the area around the eyes. After full adaptation and experience in handling the lenses has been achieved, eye makeup may be worn as usual with but a few precautions taken.

Only good-quality makeup should be applied after the lenses are placed. With the lens on the cornea the patient is able to see, will not spoil the makeup during placement or get the makeup under or on the lens during the procedure. The patient should be told not to change brands of cosmetics when first obtaining contact lenses. A type to which there may be an allergic reaction could be falsely attributed to the lenses or solutions. Hypo-allergenic cosmetics are best. Patients should be told not to use old cosmetics or cosmetics of others as they are often contaminated with organisms.

Certain eye shadows should be avoided. The sparkling or glittering types contain abrasive materials such as ground oyster shell that can get under the lens. Excessive amounts of eye shadow should be avoided since the surplus can easily enter the eye.

When affixing artificial eyelashes, a waterproof adhesive that has been allowed to dry to a sticky state should be used above the patient's own lashes, taking care not to get it on the lens.

A soft pencil, water-based liquid, or water-soluble, cake-type eye liner can safely be employed. If flaking occurs, a lesser amount or another type should be used. Eye liner should not be applied to the inner margin of the lid.

Creamy or water-soluble, cake-type mascara may be used, but the highly waterproof types should be avoided since a flake from this can easily become lodged under the lens or embedded in the conjunctiva. Lash build-up types of mascara that contain pieces of hair or other material should be avoided. Only light application should be administered and blotted from beneath the lashes.

Any cream or oil that is used on the hands or face can be transferred to contact lenses, causing discomfort and blurred vision. The patient should always be warned about such materials since they can remain on the skin, even overnight. Many hand soaps contain cream that persists on the hands even after rinsing.

Soaps with deodorants or antiseptics may cause irritation even if the hands are well rinsed prior to handling lenses. A mild or pure soap should be recommended, as well as thoroughly rinsing the hands before touching contact lenses.

Hair spray can cause severe problems by coating the lenses, which will then require polishing. In some cases the lens surface may be permanently damaged. Using hair spray prior to placing lenses will eliminate this problem. If it must be used after placement, however, the eyes should be tightly closed during the spraying and the patient should be advised to walk away from the spray area prior to opening the eyes.

Adaptation Sensations

The contact lens technician should explain common and expected symptoms related to adaptation. Not only will this prevent unnecessary concern, but it will alert the patient to symptoms that are not normal.

The patient should understand that lenses will move on blinking and that this is normal. Also, they may not remain in the center of the cornea at all times.

Increased tearing may be expected during the initial period, perhaps accompanied by slight nose run, but will subside after the patient becomes accustomed to the lenses. Edge reflections may be noticed at first and should decrease with adaptation. They may become noticeable at night or at the movies, whenever there is pupil dilation. If this persists after several weeks of wear, the patient should know to report it.

Minor discomfort and irritation are to be expected during the first few days because the contact lens is a foreign body to which the lids and cornea must adapt. Irritation may be more pronounced in a smoke-filled room, near an open fire, or in a dry, windy environment. If there is pain, the lens may be damaged or a foreign body trapped underneath. The lens must then be removed, examined, and cleaned before reinserting. If the pain persists, the lens should not be worn and the practitioner notified. The same applies if pain occurs after removal.

Mild burning or a warm sensation may be experienced during the first weeks of wear, especially when reading, sewing, watching television or a movie, or other concentrated visual tasks when the eyes are fixed in one position for prolonged periods. Tear exchange under the lenses is decreased in such cases, causing the discomfort. Advising the patient occasionally to look away from the work at hand and to blink normally will often alleviate the symptom. If severe or persistent, a lens design change may be indicated.

Hazy or foggy vision may occur during adaptation due to corneal swelling. The patient can be told that mild haziness may be present initially, but if it is severe or prolonged, the lenses should be removed and the practitioner notified since it might indicate a need for a modification or lens change.

The patient should be made aware of the difference between hazy or foggy and blurred vision, which may be caused by foreign matter on the lenses or uncorrected refractive error. If this occurs, the lenses should be removed, cleaned, and put back on. If the problem persists after a couple of removals and cleanings, the patient should call or come into the office.

Blurred vision with spectacles after removal of contact lenses is common and the patient must be warned. Spectacle blur should not last for a long time or be so severe that it incapacitates the patient. If this problem persists, a change in the lens fitting relationship might have to be considered.

The patient should always be encouraged to blink normally when wearing lenses since inadequate blink rate or incomplete blinking will cause stagnation of the tear reservoir with accompanying symptoms. This may result in a decentered lens position. An excessive blink rate will look unnatural and should also be avoided. Many new patients labor under a misconception that they should either not blink when wearing lenses or perhaps at a greater rate than normal and must be told to blink naturally. Some practitioners prescribe blinking exercises and have the patient practice blinking normally.

Patients sometimes develop an unnatural head tilt while wearing lenses. A backwards head tilt is common since there is less lid irritation with this position. This is undesirable and should be discouraged.

Itching of the eyes or lids may occur in the beginning and the patient should be told not to rub the eyes, but to inform the practitioner if the condition is pronounced or prolonged.

Increased sensitivity to sun and bright light is common when wearing contact lenses. A pair of plano sunglasses normally alleviates mild photophobia and even helps prevent foreign material from blowing into the eyes. If light sensitivity is not eliminated with sunglasses, the practitioner must investigate further and establish the cause.

Some patients report discomfort when lenses are placed immediately after arising in the morning. Mild corneal swelling or mucus build-up can occur during sleep, causing these problems. These problems can be avoided by waiting 15 to 30 minutes before applying the lenses.

Most lenses should not be worn during sleep as corneal swelling and abrasions may develop. It must always be pointed out that corneal lenses should not be worn while swimming as they may float or be washed out of the eye. Dusty environments are usually a limiting factor. Lenses may prove generally more difficult to wear if the patient suffers from some general illness or a head cold. Beginners' symptoms and initial reaction to lenses will differ widely, and no undue emphasis need be placed on variations experienced until the eyes have become fully adapted.

Symptoms of excessive burning or irritation causing tearing, inability to open the eyes, severe or persistent foggy, hazy vision, and haloes are all warning signals. These may be accompanied by redness of the eyes and indicate that the patient should discontinue wearing the lenses and contact the practitioner. Appropriate advice given prior to the patient leaving the office will prevent serious ocular injury and unnecessary subsequent suffering.

The patient should be encouraged to write questions down that occur between visits so they are not forgotten.

Wearing Schedules

Patients should always be given written instructions regarding wearing time. It must be strongly indicated that schedules must not be exceeded, even if the lenses are comfortable at the end of the wearing period. The rate at which adaptation is increased will depend on the practice routine and the practitioner's individual preference and judgment.

The daily wearing period for most patients should not fluctuate by more than 2 or 3 hours once full wearing time is achieved. The patient must be told that if lenses are not worn for a day or longer, or if tolerance is reduced for some reason or other, full wearing time (commonly 15 to 16 hours per day) must be reestablished gradually, starting again with 4 to 6 hours a day, or the number of hours worn on the previous day if greater than 6 hours and increasing tolerance by 1½ to 2 hours each day usually offers a safe approach. The longer a patient remains without lenses, the longer it will normally take to return to the original wearing period.

To be sure the patient understands all the procedures and wearing schedules, instruction booklets and written schedules should be given to the patient. Some practitioners also like to have the patient answer a questionnaire to be sure they understand the basic concepts. Table 10–1 is an example.

HYDROGEL LENS PROCEDURES

Solutions

Special precautions must be taken concerning the use of solutions used with hydrogel lenses. These lenses will absorb solutions. It must be pointed out to the patient in the strongest terms that only those solutions

Table 10–1.   Patient questionnaire on rigid lens care.

Yes	No	
_____	_____	1. Have you ever been instructed how to place, recenter, and remove your lenses?
_____	_____	2. Do you feel you can adequately place, recenter, and remove the lenses yourself?
_____	_____	3. Have you been instructed and do you understand the use of the wetting, soaking, and cleaning solutions?
_____	_____	4. Did you receive a case, solutions, and instruction booklet?
_____	_____	5. Did you receive a wearing schedule and understand that it must be followed?
_____	_____	6. Do you understand the importance of washing your hands prior to handling the lenses and the need not to get foreign matter such as makeup on the lenses?
_____	_____	7. Do you know what to do if the lens is uncomfortable when placed on the eye?
_____	_____	8. Have you been instructed as to what to do if pain, blurred vision, or other problems develop as you wear your lenses?
_____	_____	9. Do you know you are not to use eye drops or medications while wearing your lenses unless specifically told to by your doctor?
_____	_____	10. Do you know you are not to sleep or swim with your lenses on?
_____	_____	11. Has it been indicated to you that the lenses can be broken if not handled carefully and to close any sink drains over which you are handling lenses?
_____	_____	12. Have replacement costs and the insurance plans been discussed with you?
_____	_____	13. Have you been told what to do in case of an emergency?
_____	_____	14. Have you been scheduled for a future examination to evaluate your progress?

Date: _____   Patient's signature: _____

that they are given and recommended are to be used. Remember that the preservatives in many of the solutions formulated for rigid lenses will concentrate in the soft hydrogel lens and cause damage to the corneal and conjunctival epithelium. The same is true for many ocular medications and other chemicals that may accidentally contaminate the lens.

Patients should be instructed to call the office if they think the lens has been exposed to chemicals or solutions and before any solutions or medications are placed on the eye.

Read and understand Chapter 9, relating to solutions and lens disinfection, prior to instructing patients on the care of lenses. Likewise, read all the labels, package inserts, and literature provided by the solution and lens manufacturers prior to instructing and giving these materials to the patient.

Lens Handling by the Patient

A patient's hands should always be perfectly clean before removing a lens from its storage container. Any cream, grease, dirt, or other foreign matter on the hands may coat, scratch, or become embedded in a lens. This may result in blurred vision or lens damage.

After the hands are washed with a soap free from cream or other additives, they should be thoroughly rinsed so all residue is removed. If soap gets on the lens, when it is placed on the eye it will be irritating. If the hands are dried after washing, a clean, lint-free cloth should be used. Fine fiber adhering to the hands from other towels may get on the back surface of the lens, become trapped under it, and cause considerable discomfort.

When a soft, flexible lens is removed from its storage container, care must be taken not to tear or otherwise damage it. The ability of lenses to withstand abuse in handling varies and depends on material as well as design. A high water content lens will be more prone to tearing than one with comparably low water content. Likewise, a thin lens will tend to tear more easily than a thicker one of the same material. On the other hand, a thick lens may split sooner on flexing. The same may apply to low water content lenses. A lens should always be handled carefully to avoid damage.

When a lens is taken out of a storage container and is to be placed on the eye, solutions that are not sterile should never come into contact with the lens. If the lens is disinfected by boiling, only the saline solution in the case should be used. It has gone through the heating process and should be free of living organisms. Saline solution, which is made up by the patient from salt tablets and distilled water, cannot be assumed to be fully sterile. Microorganisms may contaminate any solution allowed to stand or obtained from a large, opened container. If additional solution is added to that in the case, it should be boiled or disinfected prior to use, unless it contains a preservative. The patient should, nevertheless, be advised to use only preserved saline solution especially formulated for the particular lens material.

If the solution in which the lenses are stored is for soaking only and not to be used for application, it must be rinsed off with saline solution. Tap water or distilled water must not be used since this would create a hypotonic situation. Water would be drawn into the cornea in order to equalize the osmotic pressure between lens and cornea. When this occurs, the lens will adhere tightly to the cornea and result in discomfort. If the lens is forcefully moved, it can take some epithelial cells with it and result in considerable pain. The patient should be told of this possiblity in case distilled water or tap water is inadvertently used. If the lens does not move with light finger pressure, do not force it but wait 5 to 10 minutes until the osmotic pressure equalizes. At this time easy lens removal will be restored.

Another important aspect of lens care involves inspection for tears or damage. The patient can do this by shaking the excess solution off the lens, placing it on the index finger, holding it up to a light and carefully looking at the lens edge and surface.

Due to its soft, flexible nature a soft lens is easily inverted (turned inside out). If placed on the cornea in this way, it will usually be uncomfortable, will not stay centered, and may be expelled from the eye on blinking. An inverted lens may be checked by holding it up on the index finger and looking at the shape of the edge. If edges tend to curl outward (Figure 10–20 left), it is inverted, whereas if it resembles the edge of a bowl, it is in its correct form (Figure 10–20 right). Similarly, when the lens is slightly folded between the thumb and index finger, it will curve inward if correct, but curl outward if inverted.

For instruction purposes a hollow rubber ball can be used. Cut it in half and allow the patient to see the change in shape when it is turned

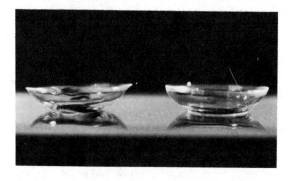

Figure 10–20. Left lens inverted, note shape of lens near the edge. Right lens is correct

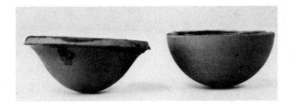

Figure 10–21. Use of a hollow rubber ball cut in half to show the appearance of an inverted lens

inside out (Figure 10–21). Once the patients see the difference on this large a scale, it will be easier for them to recognize the difference in the contact lens.

Placing a Lens on the Eye

There are several ways by which a hydrogel lens can be placed on the eye. One method is to position the lens directly on the cornea by setting it on the index finger of one hand, pulling the lower lid down with the middle finger of the same hand and holding the upper lid up and out of the way with the index or middle finger of the other hand. Lids and fingers should be dry so a secure grip can be achieved to prevent blinking as the lens approaches the cornea. Likewise, the finger on which the lens is placed should be dry to prevent the lens from folding back over the finger instead of adhering to the cornea. Also, excess solution should be shaken off the lens for the same reason. This is especially important with the thin lenses. Allowing the lens to air dry on the finger for a few seconds is also helpful. The lids must be pulled apart widely enough to allow a lens to pass. With hydrogel lenses the lid separation required is greater than for most rigid corneal lenses. The lens is then touched to the cornea (Figure 10–22). To prevent the lens from being ejected on the first blink it is helpful if the patient looks down before the lower lid is released over the lens. The upper lid can then be released. This procedure is essentially the same as that commonly employed for rigid corneal lenses, and similar instructions and precautions apply. Both eyes should remain open, with fixation straight ahead during placement. All the placement procedures described earlier in this chapter for rigid lenses can also be used for soft lenses.

One of the problems that may be experienced in placing a lens directly on the cornea is that a bubble will sometimes form under large lenses. This will usually cause the lens to be ejected on the first blink. This can be overcome by applying more pressure to the lens as it touches

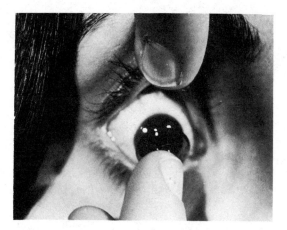

Figure 10–22. Placing the lens directly on the cornea

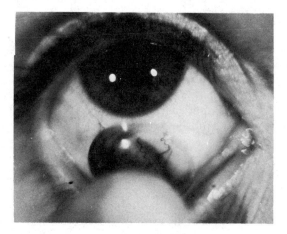

Figure 10–23. Placing the lens on the lower sclera

the cornea to force out the bubble, or a different placement procedure can be used. A common alternative, specifically with hydrogel lenses, is for the patient to look up and to place the lens on the sclera below the cornea (Figure 10–23). The lids can be held as described before, although in many cases this is not found to be necessary after the first few placements. The lens must be placed firmly against the sclera. It may actually be moved around slightly in a circular manner to ensure that all bubbles are forced out and that it is securely in place. The patient then looks straight ahead and blinks so that the lens will center over the cornea.

Patients who have difficulty handling the lenses can place them on the eye with a suction holder or on the solid holder specially designed for hydrogel materials. The lens is placed on it without applying suction (Figure 10–24). The procedure is the same as with rigid corneal lenses.

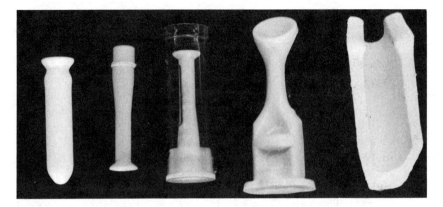

Figure 10–24. Devices used in placement and removal of lenses

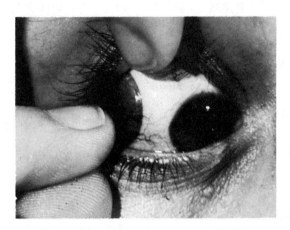

Figure 10–25. Sliding the lens onto the temporal sclera to dislodge a foreign body trapped under the lens

If there is discomfort on initial placement, it is most likely due to a foreign body such as lint or makeup trapped under the lens. One way of alleviating such a problem is for the patient to fixate nasally, place the index finger on the surface of the lens, and slide it on to the temporal sclera (Figure 10–25). The lens is then moved around in a circular manner on the sclera before being released. Then the lens is slid back on the cornea or, with absence of digital pressure, the patient is instructed to blink once or twice in order to recenter it. This will usually dislodge any foreign bodies. If discomfort persists, the lens must be taken out, rinsed in saline solution, and inspected for any damage or embedded particles. If the lens appears clean and undamaged, it can be placed on the cornea, but if the irritation is still present it should be removed and the practitioner consulted.

Lens Removal

In a few cases hydrogel lenses can be removed in the same manner as rigid corneal lenses. For example, the patient may look straight ahead or down into a mirror with the head tilted forward, voluntarily open the lids as far as possible, apply a pulling pressure at the outer canthus with the index finger and blink the lens out. Many hydrogel lens patients, however, will have difficulty with these methods because of the large overall size and softness of the lens. The palpebral aperture cannot be opened widely enough to clear the top and bottom edge. Alternative procedures must therefore be suggested.

One of these is the two-finger scissor technique as described for use with rigid lenses. The index finger of one hand is placed at the upper lid margin and that of the other hand on the lower (Figure 10–26). The lids are then opened widely enough so that the lens is within the palpebral aperture. Keeping the lid margins snug against the eye, the lids are brought together and the lens is expelled. To ensure success with this approach a few precautions must be observed. The index fingers must be held very close to the lid margin which, in turn, must be kept tight against the eye. There is a tendency to place the fingers back from the lid margins allowing them to roll away from the eye. The edge of the lens will thus not be caught and the lens not removed. In addition, the fingers on the lid margins must be directly above and below the lens, not nasal or temporal.

The easiest and most common procedure for removing flexible lenses is to have the patient look up, lift the upper lid with the index or second finger of one hand, hold the lower lid down with the second finger of the

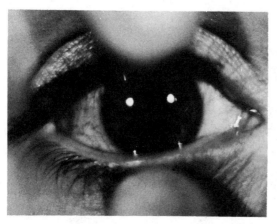

Figure 10–26. Removing a lens by placing the fingers against the upper and lower lid margins then squeezing the lens out

other hand, and then slide the lens down on to the lower sclera with the index finger of the same hand holding the lower lid (Figure 20–27). Once the lens has been moved down onto the sclera, it is pinched off using thumb and index finger (Figure 10–28). When a patient becomes proficient with this technique, it is not necessary to hold the lids. Also, a mirror does not need to be used. A criticism with this approach is that the lens can be damaged by the repeated flexure, especially in the case of rather thick or low water content lenses, which may tend to split.

This last method can be used by the technician or someone else to remove a hydrogel lens from a patient's eyes.

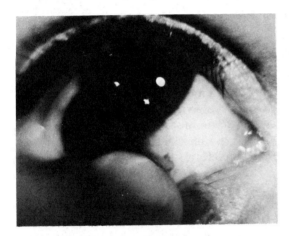

Figure 10–27. Sliding the lens down onto the lower sclera

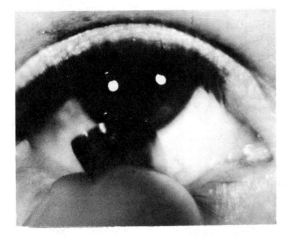

Figure 10–28. Pinching the lens off the lower sclera

Lens Care

On removal, lenses should be cleansed of all lacrimal fluid and other debris. If left on, these may develop into a heavy coating and cause permanent lens damage. A method of daily cleaning is to rub the lens in the palm of the hand with saline solution or one of the specially formulated cleaning solutions (see Chapter 9). Both surfaces should be rubbed and then thoroughly rinsed. Care must be taken not to tear or damage the lens during cleaning, although most hydrogel lenses can withstand fairly vigorous rubbing. If the thumb is used to rub the lens instead of the index finger, there is less likelihood of cutting the lens with the fingernail. Only cleaning solutions that have proved to be safe with the particular lens material should be used. New solutions and agents are constantly being developed and the instructions provided should be closely followed. Some of these, the enzymes, require that the lenses stand in the solution for a period of time.

To prevent microorganism growth, disinfection or sterilizing procedures have to be followed. One of the most effective and safe methods is to heat the lens, although it must be pointed out that if a lens is not absolutely clean, there will be an accumulation of sterile surface dirt. After cleaning, the lens is placed in a case that can withstand the heat and in which the lens remains completely immersed in saline solution at all times. The case should be designed to hold an adequate volume of solution, be easily cleaned, and permit lenses to be readily placed and removed without damage. The case containing the lenses and solution should be closed tightly to prevent loss of solution. It is then placed in the heat unit and turned on and should go through a 20- to 40-minute cycle before automatically shutting off. The patient should periodically check the unit after it has been on several minutes to be sure it is warm and functioning properly. Most units have a pilot light that is on while the unit is heating and then shuts off at the end of the cycle. If the unit does not heat up or does not shut off at the end of the cycle, the patient should be told to return it.

Normally, the patient will place the lenses in the unit and not remove them until they are ready to wear the next morning. If the lenses are needed immediately, however, the patient should be cautioned to wait 10 to 15 minutes after the unit has shut off to allow the case and lenses to cool sufficiently.

The heat technique is effective against most vegetative organisms and is usually no more time-consuming than chemical sterilization procedures. Certain problems can arise, however. If the lenses are not thoroughly cleaned prior to heating residual material from the lacrimal fluid or other foreign matter could become baked onto the lens surface. To remove this coating an enzyme or similar cleaner may have to be used or the lenses replaced if badly coated. The patient should be told not to open the case and handle the lenses until they are ready to be worn. Handling the lenses can cause recontamination. If they are placed back into the case for several hours or days without being disinfected again, a good culture of microorganisms can develop, exposing the patient to possible infection.

There are times when heating might be inconvenient or impossible. This can occur when traveling or in the absence of electricity, such as on a camping trip. The patient may even have forgotten to pack the unit prior to traveling. In such circumstances it is possible to boil the carrying case containing the lenses in a saucepan of water for 15 to 20 minutes. Care must be taken not to allow the water to boil away; otherwise the case and lenses will melt. The case should always be tightly closed to prevent water from seeping in. It should be removed before cooling takes place to avoid water being drawn into the case as it cools. The case should ideally be suspended from the side or raised from the bottom of the saucepan. This will prevent its resting on the bottom of the pan, which gets hotter than the boiling water. This will also protect the lenses from melting should the water boil away.

The disinfection of hydrogel lenses can also be achieved by use of a chemical method. This method overcomes, to a certain extent, some of the problems associated with boiling but introduces others. There are several chemical disinfection procedures and with each the instructions of the manufacturer must be followed. These solutions are described in Chapter 9. One must be sure to inform the patient of the need to clean the lenses properly prior to placing them in the disinfecting solution and to change the solution in the case daily. There is the possibility that allergic or irritation reactions with these solutions may occur during the first few days of wear or may not start for several months. The patient should be told to report any eye redness, itching, increased mucus buildup, or irritation. Keeping the lenses clean helps to minimize or prevent this problem.

Regardless of the type of disinfection used by the patient, instructions on how to clean the storage case thoroughly every few days with a mild soap followed by a good rinsing should be given. Do not use solutions beyond their expiration date or if left unstoppered for any length of time. Large bottles are best avoided as the solution may not remain sterile, the risk of contamination increasing with each use.

The patient should further be instructed on a course of action in the event of lens dehydration resulting from solution evaporation or its having been lost for sometime. Such a lens can be relatively brittle and easily broken if handled in this state. A partially dehydrated lens may firmly adhere to the surface on which it rests and be torn when the patient attempts to pick it up. In order to prevent any damage, the lens should not be disturbed, but a few drops of saline solution should be placed on it. By keeping the lens moist for five to ten minutes it will again become soft and can then be handled without danger of breakage. It should be fully hydrated and disinfected before being worn again.

If the patient must remove lenses when no case or solution is available, the patient should be told to place the lenses in a glass or bottle of tap water to keep them moist until the proper solutions can be obtained. Before wearing the lenses again they should be thoroughly rinsed with saline and placed in the proper case and solution and then disinfected.

Adaptation

Patient symptoms and length of adaptation with well-fitted hydrogel lenses are less than with rigid lenses. This is mainly due to less lid sensation from the lids hitting the lens edge. Hydrogel lenses usually are large enough that the upper lid stays over the lens. Some patients will have mild lower lid sensation from the lens edge.

At first the patient usually will have a mild awareness of the lens, but it should not be uncomfortable or painful. If it is painful, there may be a foreign body under it or the lens may be damaged. The patient may also notice some lens movement, especially with looking up or to the side.

During the first few days there may be slight injection and the eyes might feel "tired" after several hours of wear. The patient may also notice that the lenses tend to feel dry later in the day. Slight occasional blurring might also be noticed from surface drying or excessive tearing.

If there is a problem with the fit of the lenses or difficulty in adaptation, more severe symptoms may develop. Such problems are covered in Chapter 11.

Wearing Instructions

The wearing schedule given a particular patient varies depending on the type of lens fitted, individual need, and the practitioner's routine. Patients with flexible lenses can generally reach all-day wearing, 12 to 16 hours, in a substantially shorter time than with corresponding rigid lenses. The schedule may vary from a few hours on the first day with an increase of an hour or so per day to full-day wearing, to the other extreme of all-day wear immediately, provided the patient will be examined during the first few days of wear. A written as well as verbal schedule should be given to all patients with instructions not to exceed their schedules.

The patient should be forewarned of possible problems that might be encountered and what action to take if such problems arise. For example, if sudden pain or discomfort is experienced, the lens should be removed, cleaned, and inspected. If the discomfort is resolved on lens removal and there is no apparent damage, the lens can be placed on the cornea again. If discomfort persists, the lens should not be worn and the practitioner should be notified. If irritation gradually develops and remains, the lens should be removed and a rest period taken. If on reapplication or on following days the irritation recurs, the practitioner should be notified. The same advice holds if misty or cloudy vision develops with wear. If blurred or distorted sight persists following lens placement, the practitioner should be consulted as there could be an optical problem or lens damage.

It should further be explained that the wearing of lenses must be avoided in the presence of noxious fumes or risk of chemicals being splashed into the eyes. The lenses will absorb many irritants, which may slowly leach out and cause corneal damage. If any chemical splashes into the eye or on the lens while being worn, the lens should be removed immediately and the eye irrigated. The lens must not be reapplied until the practitioner has been consulted.

Hydrogel lenses should normally not be worn during swimming as contaminates from the water could easily be absorbed by them. In addition, the tonicity of water differs from that of the cornea and lens, which may cause the lens to adhere tightly to the cornea, producing discomfort and possible corneal damage if the patient tries to remove the lens immediately after emerging from the water. The chance of lens loss is very good if the lenses are worn during swimming.

If a patient removes a lens and discomfort, redness, or blurred vision does not improve, the patient should immediately call the office and seek help. The lack of improvement within a couple of hours of removal can signal a serious problem.

The use of cosmetics by the patient can cause the same problems as when used with rigid lenses and the same precautions should be followed.

As with rigid lenses, the patient should be given written schedules and instruction. The patient may be given a questionnaire to be sure the basic instructions have been understood (Table 10–2).

SOURCES OF CONTACT LENS EDUCATIONAL MATERIAL

1. A-V Scientific Aids, Inc.
    12601 Industry Street
    Garden Grove, CA 92641
2. American Optometric Association

Optometric Development or
Public Information Division
243 N. Lindberg Blvd.
St. Louis, MO 63141
3. Bernell Corporation
422 E. Monroe Street
South Bend, IN 46601
4. Better Vision Institute
230 Park Avenue
New York, NY 10017
5. Communication Centers of America
9600 Manchester Road
St. Louis, MO 63119
6. Corrective Eye Care Foundation
Suite 1717
435 N. Michigan Avenue
Chicago, IL 60611
7. Setco Audiovisual
Div. Setco Inc.
7263 Lansdowne
Webster Grove, MO 63119
8. All major contact lens and solution manufacturers

SOME SOURCES OF CONTACT LENS PLACEMENT AND REMOVAL DEVICES

1. DVM Contact Lens Company
Box 2829
Zanesville, OH 43701
2. I-Quest Inc.
P.O. Box 493
Antioch, CA 94509
3. Soft-Sert, Inc.
Cedarhurst, NY
4. Many contact lens laboratories

Table 10–2. Patient questionnaire on hydrogel lenses.

Yes	No	
————	————	1. Have you been instructed how to place and remove your lenses?
————	————	2. Do you feel you can adequately place and remove the lenses yourself?
————	————	3. Have you been instructed and do you understand the use of the solutions and accessory equipment?
————	————	4. Do you understand that cleaning the lenses does not take the place of disinfecting the contact lenses and they must be disinfected daily?
————	————	5. Do you understand that disinfecting the lenses does not clean proteins and mucous from the lenses and they must be cleaned daily?
————	————	6. Did you receive an instruction booklet?
————	————	7. Did you receive a wearing schedule and understand that you must follow it?
————	————	8. Do you understand the importance of washing your hands and the need to keep foreign matter and chemicals off the lenses?
————	————	9. Do you know what to do if the lenses are uncomfortable when you place the lens on your eyes?
————	————	10. Do you understand that you are not to use eye drops, eye medications, solutions designed for hard lenses, or any other solutions with your lenses?
————	————	11. Have you been instructed what to do if pain, blurred vision, or other problems develop during lens wear?
————	————	12. Do you know you are not to sleep with your lenses on and you are not to swim with them on?
————	————	13. Do you know how to tell if your lens is inside out?
————	————	14. Have you been told that your lenses must be handled with care to prevent tearing, splitting, or damage?
————	————	15. Have you been told what to do in case of an emergency?
————	————	16. Have replacement costs and insurance plans been discussed with you?
————	————	17. Have you been scheduled for a future examination to evaluate your progress?

Date: ———————————— Patient's signature: ————————————————

11
FOLLOW-UP
EXAMINATION

The care of the contact lens patient after the initial dispensing of the lenses is extremely important. When fitting a patient, the lens design selected must be evaluated over a long time period. Problems may develop days, weeks, or even years after the initial fit. Many factors affect lens wear, including individual physiological variation, patient health, visual needs, patient environment, and lens care.

In order to prevent serious ocular health problems and to be sure the patient is a successful lens wearer, it is imperative that the patient be seen on a regular basis. The schedule of visits will vary depending on the type of patient, as well as the fitting and wearing regime selected. For the typical, young, healthy patient fitted with a daily-wear lens for correction of refractive error, the examination schedule might be 1 week, 2 weeks, 1 month, and 3 months following dispensing. Examinations at 6-month to 1-year intervals may be recommended thereafter. In some offices, it is routine to see the patient 1 or 2 days following the dispensing. In this case, the wearing schedule can be increased more rapidly, assuming there are no apparent problems. Of course if problems develop more frequent visits will be needed. Additional visits may be required in cases dealing with pathology, extended wear, and complicated lens designs.

It is extremely important that the assistant repeatedly stress the necessity of all follow-up examinations to the patient, appropriately reschedule the patient, and be sure the patient is reminded of appointments. Since the assistant often spends the most time with the patient and has the last contact with the patient before the patient leaves the office, the assistant must take the opportunity to educate the patient of the impor-

tance of these examinations. The importance of the patients' taking responsibility for their own ocular health should be stressed. The patient
should be told to use common sense. If the eyes or lids become painful,
red or the vision becomes blurred, they should removed the lenses and
call the office.

FOLLOW-UP EXAMINATION PROCEDURES

Many tests may be performed during a follow-up examination. It is the
purpose of this text to cover only the most common procedures and problems related to contact lens wear. It takes extensive professional training,
skill, and knowledge of physiology, pathology, anatomy, and examination
procedures to diagnose and correct contact lens problems. The assistant
can help extensively in the data gathering and examination procedures.
Thus, the following is geared toward the basic understanding of these
procedures and of the common problems encountered.

HISTORY AND SYMPTOMS

The assistant usually has the first contact with the patients when they
enter the office. Much can be learned from this first few minutes about
the patient's comfort and success. It is important to observe the patient's
actions and appearance with the lenses as well as first comments. Likewise, patients will often air complaints to the assistant and not the practitioner; thus, the assistant may detect symptoms or patient unhappiness
that the practitioner would not. All such findings should be recorded in
the patient's record.

As for the formal case history taking, some practices have a written
questionnaire for the patients to fill out as soon as they enter the office
(Figure 11–1). Additional questions are then asked if problems exist. In
other practices, the assistant or practitioner verbally takes the whole case
history. Either procedure can be effective.

The patient should be asked about the average number of hours the
lenses are worn each day. If this is less than normally expected, the
patient should be asked why the lenses are not worn as long as expected.
This may be all the patient wants to wear them or it may indicate a
comfort or vision problem that needs correcting. Often wearing time can
be the best barometer of comfort and success. Patients should be questioned about the maximum number of hours that they have worn the lens
in any one day and if after wearing the lens for this time period any
problems with vision or comfort occurred. The number of hours the lenses

Figure 11–1. A sample questionnaire that the patient can be asked to fill out at the follow-up examination

Patient: _____ Date: _____

CONTACT LENS PATIENT QUESTIONNAIRE
(FOLLOW-UP EXAMINATION)

	YES	NO
I. Wearing time today (hrs)		
Average daily wearing time (hrs)		
Maximum wearing time (hrs)		
II. Comfort		
1. No sensation or awareness		
2. Slight awareness		
3. Moderate awareness		
4. Not tolerable		
5. Pain		
6. Excessive tearing		
7. Excessive movement		
8. Greater light sensitivity		
9. Burning		
10. Itching		
11. Unusual eye secretion		
12. More than normal blinking		
III. Visual Performance		
1. Better than spectacles		
2. Equal to spectacles		
3. Worse than spectacles		
4. Variable vision		
5. Distance vision blurred		
6. Near vision blurred		
7. Reading problem		

Figure 11–1. continued

		YES	NO
8.	Flare		
9.	Ghost images		
10.	Halos		
11.	Night vision problem		
12.	Require repeated cleaning		
IV.	Vision with Spectacles (after contact lens removal)		
1.	Normal		
2.	Reduced (if so, for how long?)		
V.	Handling Problems		
1.	Placement problem		
2.	Removal problem		
3.	Cleaning problem		
VI.	General Health		
1.	Have you had a recent illness?		
2.	Are you taking any medication?		

have been continuously worn at the time of the examination must be recorded. If the patient has only worn the lenses an hour or two many physiological problems such as corneal swelling may not be detectable. It is best if the patient wears the lenses at least 4 hours prior to the examination and preferably 6 or more hours. Thus, it is important that the patient be informed of this at the time the appointment is originally made and the appointment be at a time which would allow this length of wear.

Questioning the patient about the lens comfort is obviously important. The patient should be asked if there is no sensation or awareness, slight awareness, moderate awareness, or whether the lens are not tolerable. During the adaptation period, say first month of wear, there may be some sensation, especially with rigid lenses, but they should not be painful. If there is discomfort, it must be known when the discomfort occurs, if it is upon placement or not until after several hours of wear. Initial discomfort may mean a damaged lens, poor edge, decentered lens, excessive edge clearance, foreign body under the lens, or solution problems. If the discomfort is alleviated with, say, one-half hour of lens wear, this might indicate discomfort from solutions. This could be resolved by changing the brand of solution or by rinsing the lens better before placement. It could also be due to residual edema from the previous day's wear, requiring lens modification or waiting an hour or so after awakening before applying the lens. If the discomfort only occurs after several hours' wear this often indicates corneal edema from a flat or steeply fitted lens, excessive lens movement, or other lens design problems. It should also be determined if the discomfort progressively gets worse with wearing time or stays constant.

Other questions concerning comfort should also be asked. Determine if there is excessive tearing. During adaptation with rigid lenses, and to a lesser extent with soft lenses, there will be more tearing, but it should not be profuse. After the initial adaptation, the patient should not notice abnormal tearing. Again, the time course of the tearing is important. Does it occur with placement of the lenses and then subside with wear, is it constant, or does it become worse with longer lens wear? The same things that cause discomfort can cause tearing. One must also determine that the complaint is not a normal response. The patient may report excessive tearing, and upon further questioning it may be found this occurs only when going outside on a very windy, cold day. This would normally occur when lenses are not worn and may not be related to lens wear.

Patients may report excessive lens movement, which might be related to excessive tearing or to lens fit, necessitating lens modification.

Greater than normal light sensitivity (called photophobia) might also be reported. During adaptation mild light sensitivity can be reported but it should not be severe. If it is persistent or severe this is an indication of ocular irritation from a damaged, poorly finished, or improperly fitting lens that is causing corneal, lid, or conjunctival insult. Some ocular pathologies will also cause photophobia and pain.

Burning, stinging, hotness, and related symptoms can indicate a poorly fitted lens (too steep or flat), ocular insult from the lens, foreign material on the lens, or a reaction to solutions. Again, the time of occurrence, duration, and severity are important in determining the cause. Mild symptoms of this type may occur during adaptation but should be mild and decrease with time.

Excessive blinking, problems with lens comfort on eye movements, and desire to tilt the head back may be indications of improperly finished lens edges or poorly fitted lenses. Such symptoms, in the mild form, may occur during adaptation, especially to rigid lenses, but in all cases should be discouraged.

Excessive eye secretions, such as mucus strands or matter in the corner of the eye, may also be reported by some patients. Mild build-up may be normal during adaptation and particularly with extended wear, but should not persist. Irritation of the ocular tissues will cause this problem. If the conjunctiva of the underside of the lids is irritated, increased secretions develop. Likewise, allergic reactions to solutions, build-up of tear film material on the lens surface, or foreign matter will also cause excessive eye secretions.

Injection (redness) of the conjunctiva reported by the patient can indicate numerous problems. Mild redness may be normal during adaptation due to mild irritation by the lens. Marked or persistent injection can indicate a poorly fitted lens, damaged lens, mild to severe insult of the ocular tissues, allergic reaction to solutions or other substances, or mild to severe ocular disease. The time of occurrence and persistence of injection are important. If the latter occurs with lens wear and gradually gets worse with longer wear but clears in 1 to a few hours after the lens is removed, it is obviously due to the lens, lens fit, solutions, or chemicals absorbed in hydrogel lenses. If, on the other hand, it occurs immediately on placement but diminishes with lens wear, it is likely due to the solution used or foreign substances—soap or cosmetics, for example—on the lens and then washed off in the eye. If the redness continues or worsens following lens removal, this can indicate a serious problem as a conjunctivitis (infection), corneal ulcer, or other serious pathology. In any case, the patient should be seen immediately.

Questioning the patient about the visual performance of the lenses is obviously quite important. The patient should be asked if vision is better than, equal to, or worse than with spectacles. This is particularly relevant for the patient recently fitted with contact lenses and previously having a proper spectacle correction. For veteran wearers who may not customarily wear spectacles or have outdated spectacles it may be more important to determine if the vision is the same as or has gotten worse than when they first received their contact lenses. Of course, if the vision is as good as or better than with spectacles, one would not necessarily expect a problem. If the patient feels it is worse, however, the cause must be determined.

The patient may indicate that the vision is good or normal part of the time and blurred at others. Again, it must be determined when this occurs and what the patient is doing at the time. The patient may indicate no problems with normal activities but difficulty seeing small detail at both distance and near. This indicates that the acuity is not as good as the patient expects and could be due to less than fully corrected refractive error, commonly astigmatism. It might also indicate a distorted lens, poor optical quality, or a dirty, coated, or scratched lens. This can be an indication of a refractive error change or ocular pathology if it occurs when the lenses are removed and spectacles worn. The patient may complain of variable vision, at distance and/or near with things being alternately clear and blurred. This may be due to a number of conditions. The lens may be moving excessively, or, with soft lenses, the lens may be distorted with each blink. Excessive tearing, mucus accumulation, or lens surface drying may also cause variable vision. Occasionally, mild variable vision occurs during adaptation due to more than usual tearing and lens movement.

Intermittent problems during reading may occur due to decentration of the lens on downgaze, lens distortion, or surface drying due to the decreased blink rate.

Patients may complain of reflections, lines appearing to radiate from lights, and other visual disturbances around objects. This is commonly called flare. It is often due to the edge or peripheral curve portions of the lens and occurs most commonly with rigid lenses. If lenses do not center well on the cornea and the pupil enlarges, flare will occur. This may occur at night or in the movie theater. Changes in lens design may be necessary. Excessive tearing and mucus build-up on the lens may also cause this.

The complaint of ghost images may be due to a small or decentered lens, particularly in relation to a large pupil. Distorted lens optics may be a cause. Likewise, ghost images, sometimes reported as two distinct images (called diplopia), may occur due to a binocular vision problem or prism induced by the lenses.

Patients may complain of halos (often colored) around lights with lens wear. This can be due to dirty or coated lenses but more commonly is a classical sign of corneal edema. It will normally occur after several hours of wear and will remain for several minutes to hours after lens removal. This is an important symptom to be reported.

The patient should be questioned about the vision with spectacles following lens removal. If the contact lens has caused corneal edema or distortion, then the spectacle vision may be blurred. If the blurred vision lasts only a few minutes it may not be of consequence, but if it persists for an hour or more, or even weeks, it is of concern. This is often referred to as spectacle blur and is particularly a problem with PMMA lenses. This has been minimized with the use of gas-permeable rigid lenses and with soft lenses, but can be a problem even with these lenses.

Tables 11–1 and 11–2 summarize many of the patient symptoms for rigid and soft lenses. In addition, many others occur from time to time.

At each follow-up visit patients should be asked about lens handling

Table 11–1. Patient symptoms and signs, rigid lenses.

Symptom	*Cause*
1. Pain	
On placement or sudden	foreign body chipped or cracked lens improper edge shape improper placement technique chemical contamination decentered lens
Develops after a period of wear	corneal abrasion (and edema) from a flat lens limbal irritation from a flat or decentered lens edema and corneal staining from insufficient tear exchange ("tight" lens) corneal insult from sharp secondary curve junction
After removal	same as after a period of wear
2. Burning (stinging, smarting, hotness)	
On placement	improper solution or contamination foreign body
After a period of time	Corneal edema due to lack of tear exchange or flat lens foreign body
Periodic burning	dry lens surface incomplete on decreased blinking dry or windy environment foreign body smoke or environmental contamination
3. Excessive tearing	same as under pain windy or dry environment incomplete or decreased blinking
4. Itching	reaction to solutions allergy (e.g., hayfever)
5. Photophobia	same as under pain
6. Discomfort with eye movements and tilting head back	poor lens edge excessive edge stand-off lens too flat
7. Scratchy or gritty	scratch or other surface defect poor edge foreign bodies

Table 11–1.   Patient symptoms and signs, rigid lenses.

Symptom	*Cause*
8. Halos (foggy, hazy vision) usually after few hours wear and lasts during wearing	corneal edema from poor fit
9. Flare (reflections, ghost images, double vision)	decentered lens too small OZD or lens diameter
10. Blurred vision immediately on placement	wrong prescription residual astigmatism lenses switched coated lens warped or distorted lens nonwetting (dry) lens surface
Good initially, decreases with wear	edema due to poor fit build-up of debris and mucus (from irritation, allergy, etc.) drying
Fluctuating (with lens wear)	excessive lens movement decentration with reading mucus on lens or drying excessive tearing
After lens removal	spectacle blur (distorted cornea) corneal edema ocular pathology
11. Headaches	uncorrected refractive error (e.g., residual astigmatism or too much minus power) distorted or warped lens

Signs	*Cause*
1. Injection	poor edge corneal edema excessive lens movement foreign bodies placement or removal difficulties causing irritation allergic reaction to solutions allergies various ocular pathology (continues after lens removal)
2. Fluorescein staining central abrasion	result of corneal edema from poorly fitting lenses

Table 11–1. Patient symptoms and signs, rigid lenses.

Signs	Cause
Peripheral (3 and 9 o'clock)	incomplete blinking thick lens edge
Scattered line abrasions	foreign body
Arc	from edge of decentered lens sharp junction at secondary curve
Lines or rub area near limbus	poor placement or removal
Fine stippling over cornea	dirty lens reaction to solution or chemical contamination edema dry, nonwetting lens
3. Decreased VA	same as for blurred vision above
4. Lid swelling or redness	poor edge excessive lens movement allergy (systemic or to solutions)
5. "Squinting" or "Screwing" up the eyes	any problem that decreases vision uncomfortable edge poor lens centration

Note: Some patient symptoms (subjective complaints) and signs (problems visible to the examiner) with rigid contact lens wear. This is not meant to be an exhaustive list or the only cause of certain problems but only as a guide to some of the most common problems.

and care. Are they able to place and remove the lenses without difficulty? If they report problems you will need to spend additional time instructing them. The patient has some experience at this point and just a little help or a few pointers can make the difference between a successful or unsuccessful patient. Have the patients describe to you the way they care for the lenses. It will be surprising how many patients tend to change the procedures and solutions with time. This results in many comfort and vision problems and may create potentially dangerous circumstances that could result in infections and vision loss. Do not hesitate to have patients show you how they handle and clean their lenses if there is any question.

In taking the case history, be sure to LISTEN. It is easy to get into the habit of asking questions and expecting certain answers and not really listening to what the patient is saying. Give the patient adequate time

Table 11–2. Patient symptoms and signs, soft lenses.

Symptom	Cause
1. Pain	
On placement or sudden	foreign body
	chipped or cracked lens
	decentered lens
	improper placement technique
	dehydrated on placement
	chemical contamination
	lens inside out
Develops after a period of wear	limbal and conjunction irritation from a flat lens
	edema from a tight lens
After removal	edema from tight lens
2. Burning (stinging, smarting, hotness)	
On placement	improper solution
	allergy or sensitivity to solution
	contaminated lens
	foreign body
After a period of wear	edema from a tight lens
	allergy or sensitivity to solution
	foreign body
Periodic	lens surface drying (wind, incomplete blink), smoke or other environmental contaminate
3. Excessive tearing	same as under pain and burning
4. Itching	reaction to solutions
	reaction to lens
	surface coating (associated with conjunctival changes)
5. Photophobia (sensitivity to bright light)	same as under pain and burning
6. Discomfort with eye movements and blinking	flat lens which moves excessively
	edge stand-off with edge hitting lower lid
7. Scratchy or gritty feeling	loose and/or decentered lens
	poor edge
	contaminated lens
8. Halos (foggy, hazy vision)	edema
	contaminated lens
9. Flare (reflections, ghost images, double vision)	decentered lens
	too small optic zone

Table 11–2.   Patient symptoms and signs, soft lenses.

Symptom	Cause
10. Blurred vision	
Immediately on placement	wrong prescription
	residual astigmatism
	lenses switched
	lens inside out
	coated lens
	a flat or steep lens
Good initially, decreases with time	edema
	surface build-up
Fluctuating	lens distortion on blink due to steep or flat lens
	excessive lens movement
	excessive tearing
After removal	spectacle blur (distorted cornea) rare
	ocular pathology
11. Headaches	wrong prescription
	residual astigmatism
	lens distortion (steep or flat lens)
12. Excessive lens movement	lens inside out
	poor fit
	surface coating

Signs	Cause
1. Injection	poor edge
	wrong solution
	reaction to solutions
	contaminated lens
	foreign bodies
	lens inside out
	excessive lens movement
	edema
	ocular pathology (continues after lens removal)
2. Fluorescein staining	foreign body
	edema
	reaction to solutions or wrong solutions
	decentered lens
	dirty lens
	poor placement or removal
	infection

Table 11–2. Patient symptoms and signs, soft lenses.

Signs	Cause
3. Decreased VA	same as blurred vision above
4. Lid swelling or redness	reaction to solution or lens contamination allergy poor edge excessive lens movement
5. "Squinting"	any problem that decreases vision or causes discomfort

to think about the question and to answer it fully without you interrupting. Do not be in a hurry or give patients the impression you are rushing them. Also listen to what patients are implying by the answer to a question. Often they will not come right out and say what is really bothering them. Pay attention as to how they answer. Do they seem hesitant or assured of the answer? If they do not seem sure or convinced of the answer, question them in more detail about it. You sometimes have to be a detective and ask the right questions. Likewise, do not use terms that are not understood by the patients. Do not be afraid to repeat a question using different wording. Under no circumstances do you want to make patients feel that their comment or question is a poor or "stupid" one. Encourage the patient to communicate openly. Also be sure to clearly record all the patient's symptoms, problems, and complaints.

During the case history, patients may have many questions about the lenses and their progress. You may want to answer the questions that have obvious answers and that you are sure of, but do not try to answer all their questions. Many of them cannot be answered until all the tests of the examination are completed and analyzed. By trying to answer them at this point, you might be absolutely wrong and find it difficult (or the practitioner will find it difficult) to explain the results at the end of the examination. It may cause the patients to lose confidence in you and make it difficult to get them to follow the correct recommendations. Thus, if not sure, the best thing is not to give the patient the answer at this time in the examination.

Visual Acuity

The order of testing during the examination will vary somewhat, depending on the practitioner's preference and the individual patient's needs and requirements. Normally, if a patient reports for the examination wearing lenses, all the tests performed with the lenses on are done before the lenses are removed. The first test is the visual acuity with the lenses on. The acuity with each eye and binocularly is measured as described in Chapter 5. The near visual acuity should also be determined, particularly if the case history indicates reading or near vision difficulties.

If the contact lenses are found in a later part of the examination to be coated or scratched, the visual acuity will be repeated after the lenses are cleaned and/or polished.

Overrefraction

With the patient still wearing the lenses the practitioner will usually want to perform an overrefraction to determine if the contact lenses fully correct the patient's refractive error or if an additional prescription is required. This will often be performed even if the patient has good visual acuity with the contact lenses because a young person, for example, could require considerably more correction for farsightedness or be wearing too strong a minus lens and still see quite well.

The retinoscope may be used during the refractive procedure to help determine the overprescription but also to evaluate the optical quality of the lens on the eye.

The refractive finding, as well as the visual acuity with these lenses, should be recorded.

Evaluation of Lens Fit

Prior to removing the lenses, the way in which they fit should be determined and recorded. The procedure is the same as discussed in Chapter 6 on fitting. With a rigid lens, fluorescein is instilled and the lens centration, movement, and lens-cornea relationship is determined. A lens may change shape—for example, the base curve radius might flatten—or the patient's corneal shape, lid tension, or other factors may change. It is important to make these determinations to be sure the lenses are fitting as desired.

With hydrogel lenses the usual procedure is to examine the lens performance using the biomicroscope. The lens movement, centration, and lag, for example, are determined and recorded. Again with tear chemistry changes, lens aging, contamination, or damage, the lens may not be fitting as it did on original fitting or the previous visit.

Biomicroscopy

While evaluating the lens fitting relationship the biomicroscope may also be used to look at certain health aspects of the eye. As soon as the lens is removed the eye is examined in detail for insult and pathology.

This is one of the more important examination procedures and gives the practitioner much information on the lens performance, eye health, and necessary lens changes. Only some of the more common findings will be explained here.

Corneal staining is a common abnormality detected with biomicroscopy. If the epithelial cells of the cornea are disrupted and damaged, the fluorescein will go into them and be seen as bright green areas. It often helps to visualize these by using a blue (often called ultraviolet or "black") light. With most biomicroscopes this is accomplished by placing a blue (cobalt) filter in the light beam of the instrument. This, with the magnification of the instrument, will allow minor epithelial defects to be detected.

A rather common finding is foreign body staining or tracking. This is where foreign matter such as sand, eye makeup, or the like gets under the lens. With blinking, the eye is scratched and the epithelium is damaged (abraded). With the rigid lenses, one may see many tracks where the lens has moved the particle over the eye (Figure 11–2). With soft lenses, they will normally not move as much, leaving a small, but possibly deeper abrasion.

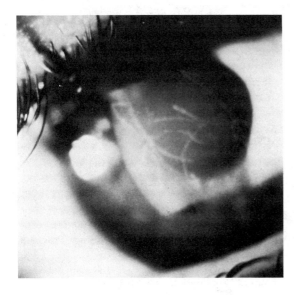

Figure 11–2. Abrasion of the cornea from a foreign body being trapped under a lens

More discrete, spotty type staining may result from a variety of corneal insults. Common causes are dirty, heavily coated lenses, lenses contaminated with chemicals, or corneal edema. This type of staining is called stippling (Figure 11–3). If the stippling coalesces and forms larger patches of staining, it is called punctate staining.

A type of corneal staining that was particularly a problem with PMMA lenses, but can occur with any lens type, is an area of rather deep staining near the center of the cornea (Figure 11–4). This has been called

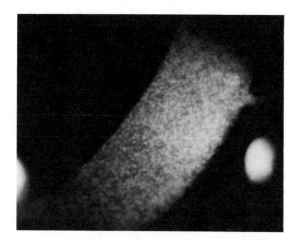

Figure 11–3. Corneal stippling

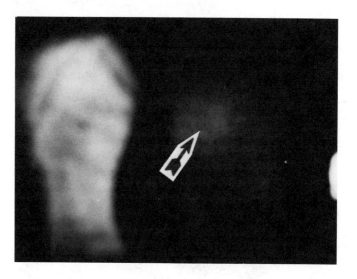

Figure 11–4. Central corneal staining typical of an overwear abrasion

the "overwear syndrome". It is the result of significant corneal edema, which softens the corneal tissue allowing the mechanical rubbing of the lens to abrade the cornea. The patient usually wears the lenses longer than normally but does not notice any significant discomfort until the lens has been removed for an hour or longer. Commonly, the patient will have worn the lens all day, gone out for the evening, come in late, and have gone to bed to be awakened in a couple of hours in great pain. This common time sequence has resulted in practitioners naming it the "3:00 A.M. syndrome" as this is the time the patient usually calls. Due to the pain and often extreme photophobia, the patient can be very frightened. If one is certain this is the problem, as can usually be determined by questioning the patient about wearing time, activities, and time course, the patient is reassured it will improve, told to stay in a darkened room, preferably going back to bed. If it helps, they can use cool compresses and take aspirin. The patient should be examined the first thing the next morning to be sure of the diagnosis, to see that no infection is present, and, if severe enough, to recommend antibiotics to prevent a secondary infection. The patient will not be able to wear lenses for at least several days. The lens and lens fit must be reevaluated prior to reassuming wear. Severe or repeated episodes can lead to corneal scarring (corneal opacities) with the loss of vision.

Another type of corneal staining is called peripheral corneal staining or three and nine o'clock staining (Figure 11–5). This is most common

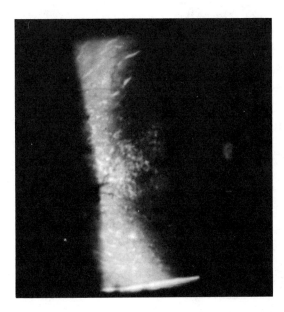

Figure 11–5. Peripheral corneal staining

with rigid lenses and is a breakdown of the epithelium in the peripheral portion of the cornea near the limbus in between the lid margins. It is due to a drying of the corneal surface in this area from incomplete blinking or a thick lens edge, which prevents the eyelid from wetting this region of the cornea. In severe cases, this can lead to ulcerated areas and corneal scarring.

Arc areas of corneal staining (Figure 11–6) may also be seen when a rigid lens is decentered or where the junction between the posterior curves are quite demarcated.

Corneal edema is another problem often detected with the biomicroscope. With rigid lenses, this may take the form of a central patch of swelling called central corneal clouding (CCC). It is a hazy or cloudy region (Figure 11–7) but does not absorb stain unless quite severe and mechanically abraded by the lens. With soft lenses the edema is more generalized and difficult to detect. High magnification with special illumination techniques may make it visible as a bubbly or roughened appearance to the epithelium. With edema there may also be folds in the deep layers of the cornea called striae. These usually appear as fine white lines, somewhat similar to the normally visible corneal nerves. The striae are usually near the center of the cornea and do not extend to the limbus.

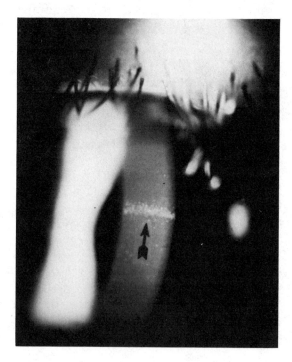

Figure 11–6. Arc staining of the cornea

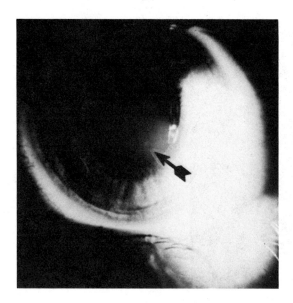

Figure 11–7. Central corneal clouding (central edema)

They are a good clinical indicator of corneal edema but occasionally are present without contact lens wear.

The biomicroscope is valuable in viewing the blood vessels of the conjunctiva and limbal area. This is important because irritation and corneal edema can cause these vessels to dilate and even invade the normally clear cornea. This must be avoided as vision loss can occur. If severe, contact lens wear must be discontinued. With mild cases, lens design and/or material must be changed to alleviate the problems. These patients must be followed very closely.

With some allergic reactions and infections, corneal infiltrates can develop. These are whitish areas of corneal clouding, often rather discrete in nature (Figure 11–8). These may occur with an allergic reaction to solutions. Lens wear commonly must be discontinued. The causative agent must be removed before lens wear is resumed.

Allergic and toxic reactions to solutions, reactions to lens surface coatings and irritation of the conjunctiva of the underside of the eyelid can cause the development of raised areas called papillae (Figure 11–9). These may be rather small or can become 1 mm or larger in size. With large papillae formation this condition is called giant papillary conjunctivitis (GPC). The upper lid should be everted to see them. Small ones are made more visible with the use of fluorescein (Figure 11–10). The conjunctiva can be graded as I for a smooth normal appearance, II for uniformly spread small papillae, III for nonuniformly spread small papillae, and IV for giant papillae. If the papillae are not uniformly distributed,

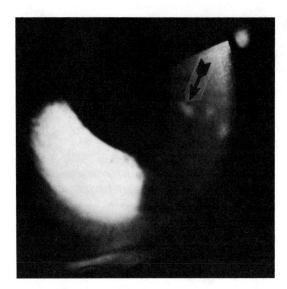

Figure 11–8. Corneal infiltrates

they may be classified into zones by numbering the zone at the fold of the lid one, the middle area two, and that near the lid margin three. If they only occur at the inner and outer canthi areas, these can be regions four and five (see Figure 11–11).

Keratometry

One may want to perform keratometry on the surface of the contact lens while on the patient's eye to discern the optical quality. This is most helpful with soft lenses since a poorly fitted lens may result in lens distortion and resultant blurred vision. Coated surfaces will also cause distortion. In this case, the quality of the mires—that is, clear and sharp or distorted—is the determination to be made. If they are distorted an assessment as to mild, moderate, or severe distortion should be made and recorded. The actual dioptric value is usually not of concern. Over keratometry with rigid lenses may be used to determine if the lens is flexing on a toric eye. In this case, the difference in power of the major meridians (toricity) is of concern.

Following lens removal, keratometry is important in determining the effect of the contact lens on the shape of the cornea. With the average patient wearing contact lenses for cosmetic reasons no change in corneal shape is desired. Thus, the K-readings are taken in the usual fashion and will be compared to the prefitting K-readings. In addition to the actual

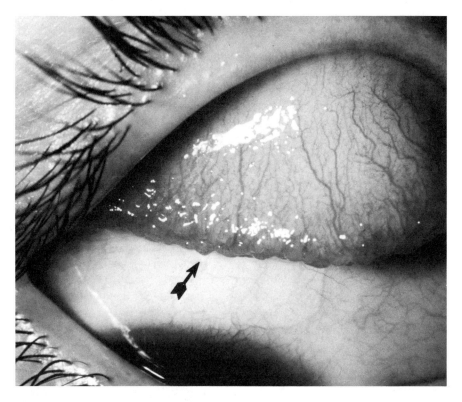

Figure 11–9. Conjunctival papillae seen on an everted upper lid

dioptric values, the clarity of the image (mires) must also be assessed. Ideally, they should be as sharp, clear, and uniform after lens removal as they were prior to contact lens fitting. Changes of 0.50 D or more in K-readings and/or distortion of the mires may indicate corneal edema and insult. If found, a change in lens design or material may be required. As always, proper recording of the values and mire quality is necessary at each visit.

Spectacle Refraction

The spectacle correction following contact lens removal should be determined for comparison to the spectacle correction prior to fitting. In most cases, one does not want the contact lenses to change the spectacle refractive finding as a change indicates corneal edema and/or mechanical

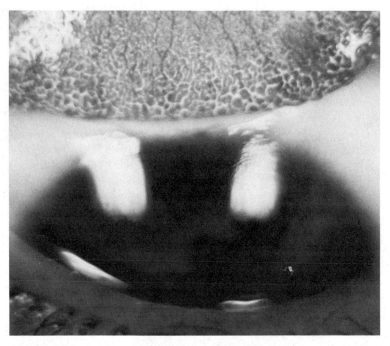

Figure 11–10.   Conjunctival papillae as seen with fluorescein and blacklight

insult to the cornea. Likewise, the patient should be able to switch back and forth between contact lenses and spectacles without vision problems. If the prescription changes, the patient may have difficulty seeing with spectacles. Therefore, they may tend to overwear the contact lenses and wear them even with ocular irritation.

In addition to the spectacle lens power, the visual acuity with this best prescription must be determined and recorded. If the best acuity finding is reduced with spectacles, this may indicate that the cornea has been distorted by the contact lens. This is an undesirable finding requiring reevaluation of the fitting.

Lens Inspection

The contact lenses should be inspected at each visit. Surface scratches, edge nicks, cracks, tears, surface coatings, and other lens damage can easily occur with lens handling and wear. Chapter 7 can be consulted for

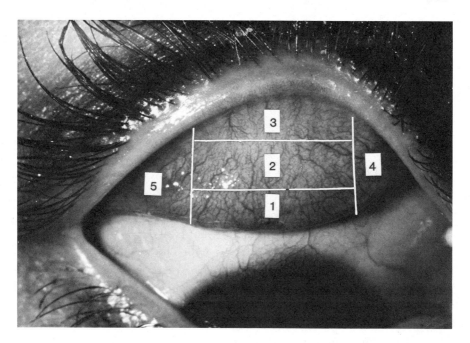

Figure 11-11. Areas of the palpebral conjunctiva for recording purposes

the inspection techniques. If the lenses are permanently damaged, they must be replaced. If, however, a rigid lens is scratched, it may be polished and still be usable. Likewise, some coated hydrogel lenses may be cleaned and worn.

The base curve radius should be routinely checked when rigid lenses are worn. Instability of some materials, inappropriate handling by the patient, or exposure to heat may cause base curve changes resulting in a change in the lens fit. Likewise, the base curve radius of soft lenses should be checked as lens environment, coatings, and degeneration of the material might change the lens dimensions.

Other lens parameters such as power, diameters, and center thickness may be checked to ascertain if lens reversal (right lens in the left eye) has occurred. It is also possible that a patient might have been examined by another practitioner since the last visit to your office and had a lens replacement or modification. Thus, the patient could be wearing quite different lenses than your records indicate. Patients might forget or be embarrassed to indicate they had been to another office. Of course, if a contact lens patient is in the office for the first time, the lenses must be completely inspected and all dimensions recorded.

Special Test Procedures

The above-discussed examination procedures are just the more common, routine tests performed. Others including pachometry (corneal thickness measurement), corneal sensitivity, photography, and tear film smears may be performed. These techniques are described in Chapter 5. The results found at a follow-up visit are compared to the prefitting baseline.

Lens polishing and modifications may be required at a follow-up visit to improve lens fit and comfort. Chapter 8 covers these procedures.

General ocular examination must be completed on any patient not examined in the preceding few months or where the history or other findings indicate the need. These may include binocular vision testing, fundus examinations, neurological examination, visual fields, and other procedures. It must be remembered that contact lens patients can develop the same problems as non–contact lens wearing patients, in addition to the lens-related problems.

Emergency Appointments

The majority of follow-up examinations will be for routine preventive care or to solve minor wearing problems such as gradual loss of tolerance, discomfort while wearing the lenses, or a decrease in corrected acuity. There are cases, however, where immediate emergency care is required.

Often the assistant takes the call from a patient and must decide if the patient needs immediate attention or if the problem wait, with the patient scheduled in the usual fashion. If the patient complains of pain even after the contact lens is removed, has a red or injected eye that does not improve after the lens is removed, has a loss of vision that is present with contact lenses and spectacles, has double vision, or has a loss of part of their field of vision, these are signs indicating the need for immediate examination. Likewise, if the patient reports trauma to the eye, a lens lost or damaged in the eye, or a chemical splashed in the eye, immediate examination is appropriate. Problems usually of less urgent nature are mild lid irritations where the patient should be seen within a couple of days. Problems that only occur when the lens is being worn, such as pain, irritation, redness, and blurred vision, but cease and clear up on lens removal, are not emergencies if the patient can discontinue contact lens wear and go to spectacles. Exceptions are patients who must wear lenses, such as pathological cases and keratoconus patients.

To many patients minor irritation during lens wear or a lost or broken lens is a dire emergency, but as far as their health is concerned it is not. These patients should be taken care of as soon as possible, but the whole office routine should not be upset over each lost contact lens. Some of these problems can be overcome by encouraging each patient to have an up-to-date spectacle correction, an extra pair of contact lenses, and a good recall system to get the patient in for routine examinations to correct problems before they become emergencies.

One must remember that when a patient calls with a problem that might be an emergency, if there is any question, the practitioner should be consulted or the patient seen. It is always better to be conservative and examine the patient.

If it is an ocular emergency of traumatic nature, the patient should be informed not to rub, apply pressure, or disturb the eye and to come into the office or emergency room as soon as possible. If a chemical accident has occurred, the lens should be immediately removed and the eye profusely irrigated with water or irrigating solution for 30 minutes to 1 hour and the patient report for treatment. If the eye is painful, irritated, red, and/or vision is reduced, the lens should not be worn, the eye should not be rubbed or irritated, nothing should be put into the eye, and the patient should come in immediately.

12

SPECIAL CASES

The majority of patients wear contact lenses on a daily basis for appearance, sports, convenience, or related reasons. There are special circumstances and conditions, however, where contact lenses give considerably better vision than spectacles, protect the eye, or prevent visual loss. These special cases can present unique problems for the patient and professional staff managing the patient. To be effective in helping and advising such patients, assistants and technicians must have an understanding of these conditions and know the procedures for handling them. Some of these areas are whole fields of study in themselves, so only limited, clinical information on each will be given here. One must also realize that the principles previously explained in this text generally apply in these special cases.

EXTENDED WEAR

With the development of new lenses, materials, and designs, the wearing of contact lenses 24 hours a day has become a possibility for at least some patients. It is a very attractive proposition for patients as it eliminates the necessity of daily lens removal, cleaning, disinfection, and placements and gives good vision on awakening. Such a wearing schedule is particularly an advantage to those individuals who are not able to easily remove lenses due to age, disability, ocular disease, or occupations requiring good vision where lens placement, removal, and care are not possible—for example, military personnel on maneuvers.

    The term permanent wear was originally used to describe this type of wearing schedule but should not be used as these lenses are not permanent but must be removed and replaced at least occasionally.

Numerous physiological requirements of the cornea and eye must be met if such lenses are to be tolerated. This can be particularly difficult since the eye does not have any period during the day or night to recover from any insult that might occur. In addition, at night with the eye closed over the lens, special circumstances and problems exist. For example, with the open eye the anterior surface of the contact lens is exposed to air containing 21 percent oxygen and is available to diffuse through the lens and be pumped under the lens via the tears and blinking. During sleep with the lids closed only oxygen diffusing from the blood vessels of the conjunctiva is available at the surface of the lens. This is equivalent to about 6 to 8 percent oxygen environment. Thus a lens that can transmit sufficient oxygen with the open eye may be totally inadequate with the closed eye. In fact, most present hydrogel extended wear lenses only give marginally adequate oxygen supply at best. Thus, corneal swelling with the resultant problems of cloudy vision, injection, possible new blood vessel growth into the cornea, and other detrimental effects can occur. If this swelling is significant during sleep it may not adequately resolve during the day.

High water content and/or very thin hydrogel lenses have been used most extensively for extended wear due to their higher oxygen permeability. Silicone lenses with very high oxygen permeabilities have also been used and offer promise. Rigid gas permeable lenses have likewise been studied for extended wear.

If the contact lens does not move adequately to flush waste products, mucus, and other debris from under the lens, the patient can experience pain, blurred vision, and a very injected eye. This is usually first noticed on awakening and requires lens removal for the eye to recover. The patient must also be examined by a professional to assess the insult and course of therapy. This may occur with patients who have successfully worn lenses for weeks or months. Usually they can resume lens wear but the episode may sporadically occur again. Extended wear patients should be warned of the possibility of such an occurrance and to remove their lenses and seek professional care when it happens.

Extended wear patients can have other clinical problems. They may complain of blurred vision on awakening, especially during the first few weeks of wear. This can be due to the edema created during sleep and/or mucus build-up on and under the lens. It should clear in 10 to 20 minutes. Some patients find it helpful to put a couple of drops of a cushioning agent or saline in the eye on awakening to clear the vision and to increase lens movement and comfort. These problems usually diminish the longer the patient wears the lens. The lens may also feel "dry" or "sticky" on awakening.

Lenses are commonly lost during sleep, again more frequently during the first weeks of extended wear. If the eye is not closed completely during sleep the lens can dehydrate and then be rolled out of the eye with rubbing or with eye movements. Patients should be warned to check to see that the lenses are on when they get up. This can be done by alternately covering the eyes to determine if they can see with each eye. Some practitioners even have patients wear a mask or patch during sleep the first few weeks in order to catch any lens ejected from the eye.

The accurate fitting and follow-up care of the extended wear patient is most important. On initial fitting, where possible, some practitioners prefer to have the patient wear the lenses on a daily basis for 2 to 4 weeks to determine if daily wear is possible since if patients cannot wear lenses on a daily schedule, they certainly will not be able to wear them on an extended basis. In addition, the normal adaptative process can occur before the patient sleeps with the lenses. Of course in many cases the patient may have to be started initially on extended wear. In either case it is best to see the patient the morning following the first night's wear. The patient should be seen frequently during the first 3 months of wear and then at 3-month intervals.

Hygiene in caring for the lenses in the office is of utmost importance since when the lens is placed on the eye it may be left there for several days or weeks. If the lens is contaminated or a foreign body is under the lens severe ocular damage could occur. Likewise, patients must be educated about the importance of good hygiene when they do remove, clean, and replace the lens.

Patient education is the most important and critical factor in extended wear. The patient, or someone who cares for them, if they cannot themselves, must know how to remove the lens. They must also know to remove the lens if discomfort, pain, injection, or blurred vision occurs. A patient can be examined and doing wonderfully one day and have a serious infection, abrasion, or insult the next. The longer the lens is worn on an unhealthy eye, the greater chance for permanent damage. Thus the patient must know to remove the lens immediately when symptoms or signs develop and to seek care and not wait and see if it gets better. A matter of hours can be important in some cases of corneal infection.

Lens coatings and deposits can also develop on extended wear lenses, causing discomfort and decreased vision if severe enough. Once significant deposits develop on hydrogel extended wear lenses, they usually have to be replaced.

HIGH MYOPIA

Patients with high degrees of myopia, particularly over 8 to 10 diopters, can often obtain better vision with contact lenses than with spectacles. High minus spectacles minify objects as compared to contact lenses so these patients will often remark that things appear larger and brighter with their contact lenses. Also the peripheral vision is better.

The fitting and lens care procedures are similar to those of the low myopes. Lenticular lens designs are required to achieve thin edges.

HIGH AMOUNTS OF ASTIGMATISM AND RESIDUAL ASTIGMATISM

If there is a large difference in the radius of curvature of the two principal corneal meridians (the cornea is shaped like the side of a football rather than a basketball) a rigid, spherical contact lens may not give an acceptable physical fit to the cornea. This can be a problem with corneal toricities above 2 or 3 diopters. A soft lens will flex and conform to the shape of the cornea, and if it only has spherical power the astigmatism will not be corrected.

In order to fit a highly toric cornea with a rigid contact lens, the lens may have to be made with a toric back surface. In this case, the lens fits on the eye like a saddle on a horse. If the toricity is sufficient the lens will not rotate significantly. This is important because if the lens rotates the correction will not be proper and will cause blurred vision. With a toric base curve lens the front surface usually must also be toric, giving what is commonly referred to as a bitoric lens. On verification, in addition to the toric base curve, the lens will have a cylindrical power. The shortest and longest base curve radii and the power in the two meridians are specified.

In order to have a round optical zone the peripheral curve or curves of a toric base curve lens must have a toricity equal to the base curve toricity. For example, if the base curve radii are 7.5 mm/8.0 mm, the secondary curve radii could be 8.4 mm/8.9 mm, that is, 0.5 mm difference in the two meridians.

To correct a patient as above or any patient with enough astigmatism to require correction even without significant corneal cylinder with soft contact lenses requires a toric soft lens. Since the soft lens will conform to the cornea only one lens surface needs to be made toric. This is not for fitting purposes but to correct the astigmatism. Some are made with the front surface toric, others with the back surface. To maintain the axis of the cylinder in the proper orientation the lens cannot rotate. One method of preventing the lens from rotating is to add prism. Since a prism is thin at one edge and thicker at the opposite edge (wedge shaped in cross-section) the thick portion (base) is heavier and positions near the lower lid. This weight difference, plus the lid forces against the thin portion (apex), usually keeps the lens in one position. The lens can be placed on the cornea in any position and after a few blinks will rotate to the correct position. In addition to the prism, the lens can be truncated, one edge cut off flat. This also helps keep the lens in the proper position. Another method of preventing rotation is not to use prism, but to thin both the top and bottom portion of the lens, leaving the center horizontal portion of the lens thick. The lid forces against this thicker portion keep the lenses from rotating.

Lenses of the above type do not always perform as well as hoped. Due to lid forces and lid movement with blinking the lenses may rotate excessively, causing blurred vision. In some cases the vision may be clear, then blur as the lens rotates due to eye movements and blinking, and then clear again.

In addition to vision problems with these prism lenses, there can be significant corneal edema since the lenses are relatively thick.

Many toric soft lenses are marked to indicate the base (thickest portion) and/or the normal horizontal position of the lens. These may be just engraved dots (Figure 12–1), lines (Figure 12–2), or just the truncation that is normally placed at the base perpendicular to the base-apex line. These markings can be used to determine the stability of the lens on the eye and to measure the position of the apex to position the cylinder axis properly.

In cases where there are less than 2 diopters of corneal toricity and a spherical rigid lens results in significant uncorrected astigmatism, if a rigid lens is desired, a front surface cylinder, prism ballast lens is used. In design and use it is similar to the prism ballast soft lens described above. It is smaller in diameter than soft lenses but can be round or truncated. It may also be marked by a black dot at the base, or a fluorescent dot at the base or at the base and apex. The fluorescent dots are only visible under the ultraviolet light and are used to measure the lens orientation. Due to the thickness, weight, and rotation such lenses do not have the same success rate as simpler, spherical lenses.

The possible problems with toric lenses should be discussed with the patient prior to fitting. Also, due to the complicated design of such lenses, the cost is greater.

APHAKIA

Following cataract surgery, where the crystalline lens is removed from the eye, a high plus prescription is required. If this is provided in spectacles there are some major difficulties. For one, the spectacles are quite heavy and are not cosmetically appealing. The high magnification and distortion produced by the lenses make activities such as walking, pouring a cup of coffee, and other general activities difficult. Likewise, there is

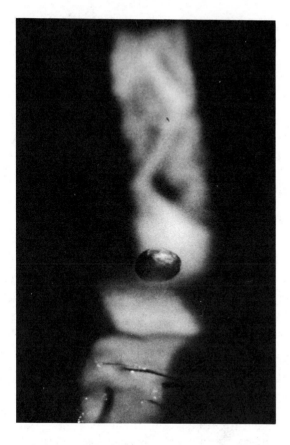

Figure 12–1. An engraved dot on a hydrogel lens to identify the base of the prism

a small field of view, making objects to the side of the patient difficult to see or putting them in a blind area. In addition, the large magnification effect makes binocular vision (simultaneous use of both eyes) impossible for the patient who has had cataract surgery on only one eye.

Contact lenses have the advantage over spectacles of markedly decreasing the weight and cosmetic problems, distortions, blind areas, and magnification. Contact lenses allow the patient to function normally. The major problem with contact lenses for these patients is the fear of the contacts and the difficulty handling the lenses because of decreased vision and dexterity. It must be remembered that the majority of these patients are elderly, have more physical problems, and lack desire. Many, however, do quite well with proper instruction and the younger or young at heart have no difficulties as the great advantage of contacts over spectacles is soon realized. For the patients who have difficulty handling lenses, extended wear lenses are recommended.

Many different types of lenses can be used to correct aphakia. These

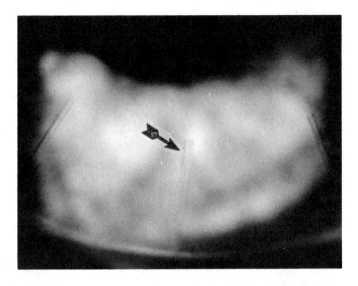

Figure 12-2.   Lines engraved on a hydrogel lens to determine orientation

include scleral (haptic), rigid corneal, and soft lenses. The major fitting problems with most aphakic contact lens corrections are the thickness required, the weight, and plus lens shape (thin edge, thick center) of the lenses. To overcome many of these problems lenticular designs (see Chapter 2) are used with rigid as well as soft lenses. This decreases the weight and thickness. Likewise, the peripheral portion of the lens can be designed to utilize lid forces to hold the lens up in position.

The thickness of the lenses can create edema problems. With hydrogel and rigid gas-permeable lenses not enough oxygen may be able to diffuse through the thick lens adequately to supply the cornea. One helpful factor in this respect is that corneas of many aphakic eyes do not require as much oxygen as normal corneas. Lens decentration, lack of movement, and pumping action compound this problem.

The type of lens used for a particular patient depends on the patient's need. A hydrogel lens often centers and stays centered on the eye better than a rigid lens. It may be more difficult to handle and may also tend to tear, however. A soft lens will not mask cornea distortion as a rigid lens might. Numerous other factors go into the lens choice.

Aphakic patients do not have any ability to accommodate for near and must have a reading correction. This usually is provided in a pair of spectacles as bifocal contact lenses are difficult with aphakia although new developments in this field may change this. Bifocal or trifocal spectacles are normally best, as they give the patient good distance as well as near vision. If there is residual refractive error, as astigmatism, it can be corrected in the distance portion as well. The aphakia patient is usually older, already accustomed to wearing bifocals, and not concerned about the appearance of spectacles. The improvement in optical performance is the concern.

One of the assistant's most important jobs with aphakic patients is to encourage them. As mentioned, they are often very apprehensive about putting a lens on their eye and about caring for the lens. A positive attitude by the office personnel can do much to overcome this.

Considerable time may be required to teach the patient to place, remove, and care for the lenses. Patience is required and usually rewarded by success and patient appreciation. The patient should remove the lens from the case and prepare it for placement while wearing an aphakic spectacle correction, then remove the spectacles and place the lens on the cornea. If this proves too difficult for the binocular aphakic patient, a spectacle correction with a lens before one eye only with the eyewire cut away from the other side (Figure 12–3) can be used as a last resort. The use of special placement and removal devices (see Chapter 10) may also be necessary. In addition to teaching the patient the procedures, signs, and symptoms, other individuals who are around the patient should also be taught these things. This is especially true if the patient is senile or disabled.

When working with these aphakes, remember to be patient, understanding; take your time and go over and over the procedures. The end result can be very gratifying.

KERATOCONUS

Keratoconus is a degenerative process where the cornea becomes thinner than normal and protrudes centrally in the general form of a cone. This typically begins to develop during the adolescent years but may begin in much older patients. Astigmatic changes often occur early and the best vision with spectacles decreases. Next corneal distortion, thinning, and biomicroscopy changes can be detected on close examination. In most cases it develops in one eye first, but in practically all cases both eyes will be involved, although one may always be worse than the other. Vision with spectacles can deteriorate to the point of legal blindness. It is impossible to predict the extent of progression or the time course. Some patients will have fairly rapid deterioration for a few months to a couple of years, then stabilizing for the rest of their lives. Others will have periods of stabilization following by periods of progression. The condition will not improve.

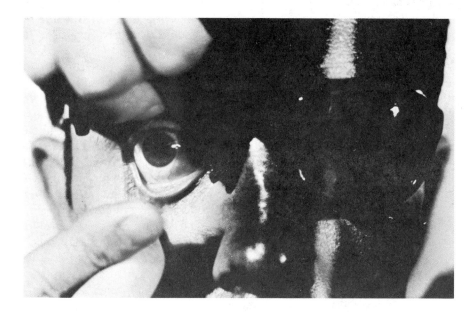

Figure 12–3.   Lens and rim removed from one side of a spectacle frame so that a lens can be placed while being able to see with the opposite eye

The cause of keratoconus is not known. Due to the common incidence at puberty it has been theorized that endocrine changes initiate it. Other possibilities as allergies, eye rubbing, and heredity have been suggested and each appears to be involved in some cases but not all. There may be multiple factors.

Since the vision of the keratoconus patient is decreased due to distortion of the cornea, contact lenses are the only correction that can give these patients good vision. In most cases the difference is remarkable. The best vision with a spectacle correction may be 20/60 to 20/400 and on placement of a contact lens be improved to 20/20. The tear layer under the contact lens neutralizes most of the distortion and the front of the contact becomes the major refracting surface of the eye. Rigid lenses are usually used to obtain this effect. This remarkable improvement with contact lenses is a blessing for the patient but can also create difficulties. These patients are totally dependent on their contact lenses for daily functioning. They cannot go to work, read, drive, or do other visual functions without them. Therefore, they will wear the lenses all waking hours regardless of comfort or other problems. Thus, ocular problems related to lens wear are common. These patients must be warned of this danger and seen on a routine basis. Likewise, they should certainly have a second pair of lenses in case of lens loss or damage.

Since a soft and flexible lens will conform to the cornea, the corneal distortion will be transmitted through the lens and will not substantially improve vision. For this reason the majority of keratoconus patients are fitted with some type of rigid lens. This may be a scleral, PMMA corneal, or a gas-permeable rigid lens. The type of lens material and design used depends on the corneal condition and practitioner's preference. The fitting of these conical corneas, especially in advanced cases, can be quite challenging. Due to the necessity of contact lenses for these patients and the difficulties, considerable effort has been put forth and numerous publications are available on the topic. The introduction of gas-permeable rigid lenses has greatly aided the fitting. In some cases a rigid lens (to provide good optics) has been fitted over a soft lens (to provide comfort).

A poorly fitted lens, and in some cases even the best available fit, on a keratoconus patient can cause corneal damage. In cases where a patient cannot tolerate a contact lens or where visual acuity is not acceptable, a corneal transplant is often performed. This is, however, usually done only as a last resort. It is also possible, but very rare, for the cornea to thin enough to rupture. Usually scarring will occur and strengthen the cornea, preventing this.

As previously mentioned, patient education and continued care of the keratoconus patient are a necessity. Many of these patients must be continually reassured as they have great concerns about their vision.

PRESBYOPIC PATIENTS

With increasing age, the ability of the crystalline lens to change decreases. At about the age of 40 to 45 one can no longer accurately focus at the normal reading distance. This ability to change focus is lost by everyone. The most common method of correcting this problem is the use of reading glasses, bifocals, or trifocals.

For those patients who start wearing contact lenses prior to reaching this age and who then need correction (referred to as an add) or a patient who needs an add when fitted, there are several possibilities. One of the simplest is to have a pair of reading glasses or half-eye spectacles (ones the patient looks over the top of for distance vision) to use with the contact lenses for reading. For some patients this is an acceptable solution to the problem. Others do not want to wear spectacles at any time.

A mode of correction that is relatively simple for the practitioner is to use what has been termed the monovision technique. With this procedure, one eye is fitted with a contact lens to correct the distance vision and the other fitted and corrected for near vision. The patient must learn to use the eye with the clear vision for the object being viewed. For some patients this is relatively easy and a satisfactory correction. Other patients, however, cannot adapt. Still others do adapt, but with some difficulties. One of the problems, in addition to the blurred vision in one eye, is the decrease or loss in stereopsis (good depth perception). For those patients requiring good stereopsis this type of correction cannot be used or they must be given a third contact lens, so there will be a pair for distance. The patient can then change to the distance pair for long periods of driving, tennis, or other activities requiring good distance vision and/ or depth perception. A pair of half-eyes, reading glasses, or bifocals can even be prescribed to be occasionally used over the distance pair when needed. With monovision, any type of lens—hydrogel, silicone, rigid corneal, or haptic—can be used.

Another method of correcting the patient is to use a simultaneous vision lens. This means that the contact lens has at least two zones that are within the area of the patient's pupil. This gives two focuses at once, one for distance and a second for near. If an object is at near, light rays from it going through the near portion are in-focus on the retina while the rays going through the distance portion are out-of-focus (very blurred). Only this in-focus image from the object the patient is viewing is noticed. For distance objects the same principle holds. Of course some patients cannot learn to ignore the blurred images.

Simultaneous vision contact lenses may consist of two concentric zones. Usually a very small central zone (like the optical zone on regular single vision lenses) is surrounded by a wide near zone (like a wide secondary curve on regular single vision lens). Another popular simultaneous vision lens design is the aspheric lens. Here there is a gradual change in radius from the center to edge of the lens. This creates a corresponding, continuous power change with more plus power toward the edge. This can allow for good vision at all distances since it acts as a multifocal lens. The aspheric surface or combination of spherical and aspheric can either be on the front or back surface of the lens. This principle can be used on any type of lens, rigid or soft.

An advantage of simultaneous designs is that one can obtain good near vision with upgaze, for example when reading a label on a shelf above the head, as well as down in the normal reading position.

Segment bifocals can also be used. In this case, the contact lens looks like a miniature bifocal spectacle lens. It can be fused from two different plastics or have two different front surface radii. This lens must be fitted to prevent rotation to keep the add or segment in the inferior position. This is usually achieved by incorporating prism in the lens. When the patient looks down to read, the thicker base of the lens hits the lower lid and is pushed up so the segment is over the pupil, allowing the patient to see at near. Sometimes these lenses are also truncated to help prevent rotation and to give adequate vertical movement on down gaze.

There are several potential problems with the segment bifocals. First, they must be made to very exacting standards due to the small dimensions. The anatomy of the lids and eye is important in order to obtain the proper lens position at the right time. In addition, the lens thickness and weight affect the fit, so that corneal edema and associated problems are common. With the proper patient, however, when they perform correctly the patient will have clear, sharp vision at distance and near.

The segment bifocals, as described above, and concentric designs that depend on translation of the lens with near gaze are called alternating bifocals.

ORTHOKERATOLOGY

Orthokeratology is a procedure where contact lenses are used to change the shape of the cornea to reduce or eliminate the refractive error. The idea is to give the patient good vision without wearing any correction. The common procedure is to fit a rigid lens to a myopic patient somewhat flatter than the cornea in order to flatten the cornea slightly. When a flattening occurs so that the lens now nearly matches the cornea another, still flatter lens is prescribed and worn. This process is accomplished over a period of several months until on lens removal there is no refractive error or no further reduction in refractive error can be induced. Of course during this process the patient must be followed closely to ascertain that no adverse effects develop.

Normally a 2 to 3 diopter reduction is the maximum change that can be achieved. It is usually a temporary change—that is, if the wearing of the contact lenses is discontinued the refractive error will gradually return to the original value. Therefore, lenses must continue to be worn on a periodic basis from a minimum of several hours every few days to 8 hours or more each day. These lenses are called retainer lenses.

Orthokeratology has been somewhat controversial due to the potential of corneal distortion and high cost in dollars and time as well as the fact it is not a permanent change. Some patients, however, can benefit from the procedure.

FITTING INFANTS AND CHILDREN

Certain pathological and developmental anomalies require contact lens correction at a very young age to allow the child to see and for the visual system to develop. Such problems as high myopia, distorted corneas, congenital cataracts, albinism, aniridia (no iris), and nystagmus (constant eye movements) are examples. Some of these problems, such as myopia, can be corrected with standard contact lenses. Soft lenses are usually more comfortable and with some infants and children using extended wear lenses can be the best mode of correction. Others require special lenses such as cosmetic lenses with artificial pupils or rigid lenses to cover a distorted eye.

The method in which the child is handled depends on the child's age and maturity. Many children 4 to 5 years old or older can be handled similarly to other patients by taking extra time, patience, and care. Of course the parents must be taught to place, remove, and care for the lenses.

For younger children and infants, other methods may be required. In some cases, it may be necessary to do the initial examination and fitting or taking of an eye impression with the child under anesthesia in the operating room. In other cases, a sedative may be sufficient to calm the child enough to carry out the procedures. The child may have to be restrained by a parent or the office assistant. It may be helpful to wrap a towel or blanket around the child for restraint. Once children have learned that the procedures are not painful, they will gradually become easier to handle. Care and gentleness are important. The end result makes the whole process worthwhile.

THERAPEUTIC APPLICATIONS

There are certain pathological conditions that require the use of contact lenses. One of the more notable cases is bullous keratopathy, where the patient is in great pain due to corneal edema and a breakdown of the corneal epithelium. An extended wear hydrogel lens will alleviate the pain so that the patient can continue, although it does not cure the condition. In some cases of recurrent erosions, that is, where an area of

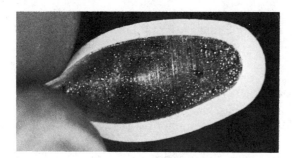

Figure 12–4. A small polymer device that slowly releases a drug when placed in the cul-de-sac

epithelium is repeatedly pulled off, causing pain and prevention of healing, an extended wear lens will protect the cornea, allowing the epithelium to heal. Severe dry eyes is another case where a lens can protect the eye by retarding evaporation. In all these and similar cases, care of the lenses and patient education are important. Some of these eyes are more prone to infections and trauma, so the use of sterilized lenses and proper handling must be followed.

Hydrogel lenses have also been used to maintain medications on the eye for longer periods of time than would occur with no lens. Although not a contact lens, a similar device has been developed to slowly release drugs into the eyes (Figure 12–4). This has been used to treat glaucoma patients. It is placed in the cul-de-sac, where it does not affect vision.

HAPTIC (SCLERAL) LENSES)

Haptic lenses are commonly 20 to 25 mm in diameter and thus are much larger than other types. This is an advantage for keeping the lens in the eye and for covering the whole front of the eye if cosmesis is indicated. These lenses are fitted so that the lens is totally supported on the sclera, with no corneal or limbal touch. This can also be an advantage.

The first useful contact lenses were haptic lenses but have been generally superseded by corneal and hydrogel lenses. There are still occasions, however, where this type of lens is the best correction and is used by those practitioners with the skills to fit them.

These lenses can either be fitted using diagnostic lenses (called preformed lenses) or by taking an impression of the eye from which the lens is made (called molded lenses). The molding is relatively simple and comfortable and results in an exact copy of the front of the eye and usually gives a better fit to unusual, distorted, or disfigured eyes.

Teaching the patient to place, remove, and care for the lenses is somewhat different from procedures with other types. The lenses are made of rigid plastic and therefore solutions that can be used with rigid corneal lenses can be used with haptic lenses. The lens can be moistened with a wetting solution. The wetting solution should then be rinsed off with water and a few drops of saline solution (as used with hydrogel lenses), or irrigating solution can be placed in the lens if desired.

The lens is placed on the eye by holding it between the thumb and second finger. The other hand is used to hold the upper lid up. The patient looks down and the lens is slid up under the upper lid, keeping the edge of the lens parallel to the sclera (Figure 12–5). Next, the upper lid is pulled down over the lens and held there by the finger. The patient next looks up slowly and the lower lid is gently pulled out from under the lens. The whole procedure takes just a couple of seconds and is quite comfortable. In fact, due to the large size of the lenses, they should be comfortable immediately because of no lid irritation. This technique for placement is used both by you placing the lens on the patient as well as the patient placing the lens themselves.

To remove the lens, the patient looks down as far as possible. The index finger is placed on the upper lid margin on the nasal portion of the lid. The lid is kept taut against the eye by the finger and the same finger is then moved along the lid margin toward the temporal side. The lid must be above the upper edge of the lens, and as the finger is brought around the lid, the lid should hit the lens edge and go under it (Figure 12–6). Move the finger all the way along the lid to the temporal extreme; do not stop with the finger directly above the lens. When the procedure is properly performed, the lens will just roll out of the eye as the finger reaches the temporal side of the eye (Figure 12–7). It may be helpful to pull the lower lid lightly away from the lens with the other hand and use this hand to catch the lens. If the lens does not naturally roll out when

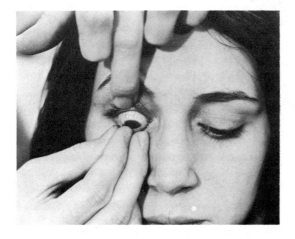

Figure 12–5. A scleral lens being placed under the upper lid as the patient looks down

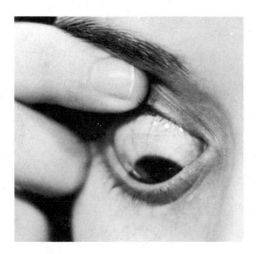

Figure 12–6. Removing a scleral lens using the upper lid starting at the nasal side moving the finger toward the temporal side

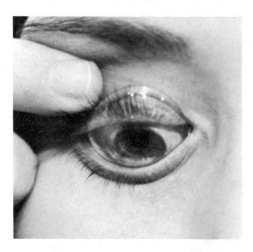

Figure 12–7. The lens coming out of the eye as the upper lid goes under it and the patient slowly looks up

the finger reaches the temporal side and the lid is under the top portion of the lens, then have the patient look up and the lens will come right out.

An alternative method of removing the lens is to use a suction cup or soft rubber remover.

After the lens is removed, it should be cleaned with a good contact lens cleaner. The lens can then be placed in a case with soaking solution or dried well with a clean, soft tissue and stored dry.

COSMETIC LENSES OR SHELLS

Cosmetic lenses may be fitted to patients who desire to change their eye color or want special effects for plays, movies, or the like. Most cosmetic lenses, however, are fitted to patients who have disfigured eyes from trauma, surgery, birth defects, or ocular disease. These problems may include patients with disfigured irises, those born with no iris (aniridia), and those with scarred corneas that appear white. In some cases, the eyes are blind and a lens with no optics, sometimes called a cosmetic shell, is used. Where there is vision, optics must be incorporated into the lens as well as the coloring. These lenses or shells are painted to match the good eye as closely as possible, if only one eye is fitted.

Several different types of lenses can be used. Rigid corneal lenses can be painted for cosmetic effect, but the thickness required to sandwich the colored portion inside the plastic adds excessive thickness and weight. Furthermore, these lenses must be made about the size of the cornea to be cosmetically appealing. The added thickness, weight, and size, as well as lens movement, make it difficult to obtain wearable lens with good appearance.

Hydrogel lenses can also be painted to give a good cosmetic match to the fellow eye. Due to the larger diameter, it centers and does not move as noticeably as the rigid corneal lens. Also, due to the lens size the iris can be painted large enough to match the other eye. Again, the painted portion is within the lens. A disadvantage of the cosmetic hydrogel lens is the thickness to allow for the painted portion, which decreases the oxygen transmission. If it is for a scarred cornea that has been invaded by blood vessels this may not be a problem, but if it is for a normal cornea, edema may occur. Many cosmetic hydrogel lenses should not be heat disinfected as this may eventually fade the colors. Otherwise, the care and handling of these lenses are the same as standard hydrogel lenses.

In some cases, the lens does not have to be painted to match the other eye, but just a darkly tinted portion corresponding to the cornea will suffice. This works best on patients with dark irises.

A problem with both rigid corneal and hydrogel lenses is that many blind eyes are strabismic, that is, not pointed straight ahead, and with these lenses their eyes still do not look straight. The only way to overcome this problem is to use a haptic shell. It is large enough so that the painted iris can be positioned at a different position from the real iris so the eye appears to be looking straight ahead. Likewise, the scleral portion can be painted and vessels included to cover the displaced true iris and to cover any scleral disfigurement. Such shells give a most realistic appearance.

The scleral shell is fitted, placed, removed, and taken care of in the same fashion as described for other scleral lenses.

Scleral cosmetic lenses can also be used for seeing eyes as optics can be incorporated.

PROSTHETIC EYES

In some unfortunate circumstances due to pathology or injury an eye must be removed. In this situation, a prosthetic (artificial) eye is fitted. In most cases when an eye is removed an implant is placed in the orbit. The implant is an approximately round piece of inert material to which the muscles are sutured to or around. This is then completely covered with conjunctiva such that the implant is not visible when one looks into the orbit (Figure 12–8). The implant can often be seen to move when the other eye moves and can be felt if palpated. In some cases all the contents of the orbit must be removed including the muscles, and thus there is no movement.

The prosthetic eye is similar to the haptic shell, but considerably thicker (Figure 12–9). The additional thickness gives a more realistic appearance than the shell as there is a thick layer of clear plastic over the iris. The eye fits over the implant, and if the implant moves the eye will usually have some movement.

Early prosthetic eyes were made of blown glass. These were hollow, quite thin, and fragile, with breakage being a problem. Today's prosthetic eyes are made of solid PMMA and are very durable. It is difficult to break one.

During the fitting procedure different diagnostic eyes are used to

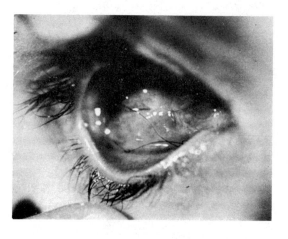

Figure 12–8. The appearance of the orbit without the prosthetic eye in place

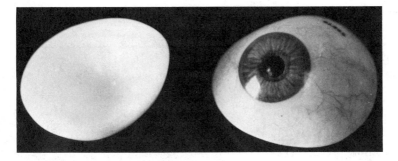

Figure 12-9. Prosthetic eyes. The back surface of the eye is on the left and the front surface is on the right

determine the correct size and shape. The eye may also be modified by grinding plastic off or adding stock by building up wax that is later replaced with plastic by the laboratory. The position, size, and color of the iris are determined. It is best to match the color of the good eye to that of diagnostic eyes using natural daylight. In addition to the iris color, the iris detail, scleral coloring, vessels, and detail are specified. The scleral color is not white as normally assumed but does have some pigment, giving it a yellowish appearance. The scleral coloring varies with age, bluer in children and yellowing with age, and with the pigmentation of the patient.

The prosthetic eye can be placed in the orbit in the same fashion as haptic lenses. It is more comfortable if the eye is wetted with a standard contact lens wetting solution.

The eye can be removed by holding the upper lid up with the index finger of one hand and then placing the index finger of the other hand on the nasal side of the lower lid. The lower lid is pulled down and gently pushed in and the finger is slid along the lower lid so that the lid slides under the eye. As the finger goes toward the temporal side the eye will come out over the lower lid.

An alternative removal technique is to use a suction cup or soft lens remover as used with contact lenses. The suction cup is placed on the eye, the lower lid pulled down, and the eye lifted out from the lower lid first.

The prosthetic eye can, and should, be worn day and night. The eye must be removed occasionally for cleaning. The frequency of removal and cleaning will depend on the patient. Some patients feel the need to remove it daily to clean off mucus that accumulates. This is especially true if the patient has a slow blink rate, the lids do not close completely on each blink, or if there is irritation. An increase in mucus and need for cleaning may indicate an infection. Other patients can go several days or longer without the need for removal. It is good practice to remove it at least once every week or two for cleaning.

The eye can be cleaned with a rigid lens cleaner or a mild soap. It should then be rinsed well with water. If it is to be left out of the socket for some time, it should be dried with a soft tissue. When it is placed back into the orbit, it should be wetted with wetting solution.

Prosthetic eyes need occasional polishing. Dried ocular secretions can build up that are not removed by normal cleaning. Likewise, scratches from handling may occur. Those problems cause the eye to become dull-looking and uncomfortable. The eye can be polished using a sponge or soft tool on the modification unit, the same one as used with contact lenses, and a contact lens polish. The eye will not be damaged due to the layer of clear plastic over the coloring and veining. The eye can just be held by the fingers and placed against the rotating sponge, turning the eye to polish the whole surface (Figure 12–10).

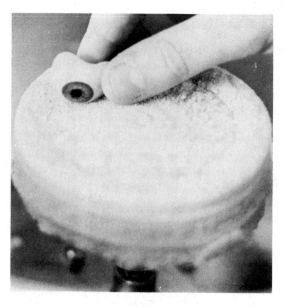

Figure 12–10. Polishing a prosthetic eye by holding it against a rotating soft pad

13

OFFICE PROCEDURES

There are many business aspects, organizational details, and housekeeping duties that must be properly handled if a practice is to be efficient and grow. There are numerous books and journals dealing with practice administration and related topics. It is not within the scope of this text to give a comprehensive coverage of the topic. Only a few aspects relating to contact lens practice will be discussed.

SCHEDULING

Usually the first contact a patient makes with an office is by the telephone to make an appointment. The impression that is made at this time is of great importance. If the greeting the patient receives is friendly, polite, helpful, and enthusiastic, the patient will likely enter the office on the first visit with a positive attitude. On the other hand, if the receptionist is not friendly, seems too busy to help, or is rude, the patient will come into the office for the first visit on the defensive and with a negative attitude. When on the phone to the patient, be pleasant and willing to answer all the patient's questions that can reasonably be answered. The same principles hold when the patient first comes into the office. That first impression of the office can determine the patient's attitude for the duration of the patient's care.

In order to be effective when a patient calls for an appointment, the appointment book must be well organized. A binder that opens flat and has ample room for writing in appointments is best. One should be able to tell at a glance which time slots are open. A messy appointment book can lead to mistakes, confusion, and disorganization. The appointment schedule should be made well in advance so that holidays, vacations, and meeting times can be crossed out to prevent the necessity of calling patients to reschedule appointments. All personnel in the office should understand the time period required for each type of patient. Different time periods are necessary depending on whether it is a new fitting, a dispensing, or follow-up examination.

When patients call, their needs must be determined. Are they presently wearing contact lenses, are they interested in being fitted, are they having particular problems, or are they just calling for information? If an appointment is to be made and the patient has not requested a specific time, it is usually helpful to give two or three open appointment times, even though there may be many openings. This makes the process much easier for the patient and saves time. For example, you could say, "Mrs. Jones, we have openings at two o'clock on Tuesday or ten o'clock Wednesday morning." If they choose one of the times, then the appointment can be made. On the other hand, if there is a problem with the times you suggest, patients will be more specific as to the days and times they are able to come in, and then you can suggest a time or two within their time block. Also remember that patients wearing contact lenses should normally be seen after they have worn their lenses at least 4 to 6 hours, usually necessitating afternoon scheduling. New fittings and dispensings can, of course, be scheduled in the mornings.

A certain minimal amount of information should be recorded in the appointment book. Included should be the patient's name, phone number (both home and business phone), address, and whether the patient is a "new" or "previous" patient (not an "old" patient). Other information, relating to present or previous lens wear or specific problems the patient is having, should be determined. A list of these questions can be kept near the phone to insure that all the necessary information is obtained.

After making the appointment, be sure to repeat the day and time of the appointment so that you are sure the patient understands. If the patients are new to the practice, be sure they know how to find your office, where to park, and so forth. If they are wearing contact lens, tell them whether they are to wear them in for the appointment, bring previous prescriptions if not former patients, and bring their lenses if not wearing them.

If the appointment is made several days or more in advance, the patients should be called the day before the appointment to remind them or a card should be sent a few days ahead of the appointment. Patients should be told at the time the appointment is made that they will be reminded. Remember that when patients do not show up for an appointment it is costly. The office expenses continue.

A daily schedule should be posted at convenient spots around the office, such as the laboratory and examination rooms. Everyone should know which patients are in the office, who is expected in next, and the service each patient is to receive. This helps everyone to keep on schedule and to be able to greet each patient by name.

PATIENT HANDLING

To do the best possible job of providing vision care to patients, one must enjoy working with people and convey this to the patient. The patients must be cared for as individuals. There are good office assistants who are very outgoing and talkative while others are more quiet and reserved. Both can do an equally good job if they are sincere and willing to put forth the effort. One must do this even on those days when not feeling the best.

As previously mentioned, the patient's first impression when coming into the office is important. If the office is disorganized, dirty, and messy and personnel are unfriendly, the patient is not going to be eager to return or recommend the office to friends. It is important to keep the office in good order by seeing that things are kept in their place and clean. Personal cleanliness, neatness, and proper dress are a must. One should not smoke, chew gum, or drink coffee around patients in the office. Likewise, the positive, friendly greeting of the patient is very important. Common courtesy is a big factor. If the schedule is running slightly behind, be sure to inform patients of this; apologize to them and indicate that they will be taken care of as soon as possible.

Know exactly what is to be done with each patient and be sure the office is ready for all of them. For example, be certain the previous patient is out of a room before bringing the new patient in. Be sure equipment is there. For example, one looks disorganized if one starts to do visual acuities and does not have a cover paddle or takes a lens off the patient's eye and does not have a case to put it in or solutions to use. Each day a general instrument and supply check should be made. When necessary, items should be reordered or replaced. A checklist including such items as solutions, fluorescein strips, cases, tissues, and the like should be used.

In addition to the general organization of the office, movement of patients through the office, and specific duties assigned each employee, everyone should be involved in patient education. Some office personnel will be more directly involved than others, but there is constant opportunity to inform patients about their vision and professional vision care. The more patients understand their vision, their correction, and their need for care, the more likely they are to seek and accept care. Likewise, they will spread the word to others. Patient education can involve just answering the patient's questions. In order to do this, learn as much about vision care and office procedures and policies as possible. Do not, however, try to answer something you do not understand or know the answer to. If an incorrect answer is given, your credibility with the patient will be lost. It is far better to say you do not know and ask someone else than to make something up.

Other methods of patient education should also be used. One is to give the patient printed material. There are numerous sources of such material including professional organizations, laboratories, and literature generated especially for your practice. The patient should not be just loaded down with printed material but be given selective readings. If patients have a certain problem or question, give them material pertaining to that question or problem.

Slides, slide-tape series, and films can also be used. To be effective, they must be on a topic of interest to the patient and should be short and easily understood. Some practitioners find it helpful to have each patient watch a film or slide-tape series at the first visit on the examination process and vision care.

Patient education concerning lens care and the problem of handling emergency patients have been covered in Chapter 10.

Handling the patient with complaints takes certain skills and patience. Everyone hopes that all the patients in his or her practice will be perfectly satisfied and happy. Everything is done to achieve this, but there will still be a few patients who will have misunderstandings or be dissatisfied. If an irate patient either calls or comes into the office, first of all stay calm yourself; keep your dignity and assurance. The worst thing that can be done is to lose your temper and become upset. Do not try to defend your position or your doctor or argue the point. If the patient comes into the reception room, take the patient to a room away from other patients, or if it is on the phone, take the call or transfer it to a phone where a private conversation can be held. Show sympathy toward such patients and try to see their point. Above all, listen to the patients and let them get it off their chest. Being a good, interested listener will usually do more to calm the patient and solve the problem than anything else. Try to find out what the patient's real complaint or problem is. Sometimes there is an underlying problem that they are not giving. For example, they may complain that the lenses are uncomfortable or do not give good vision when the real problem is difficulty putting the lenses on, a misunderstanding over fees, a negative comment by a friend, or another problem that the patient does not want to divulge or feels embarrassed about. Remember never to ridicule or belittle a patient. Many will have some major misunderstanding about their eyes, vision, or correction and it may seem humorous, but it is not to the patients. Do not embarrass them by acting as if it is a ridiculous or funny question. Encourage their questions. Just remember that there are many things outside your realm of knowledge that you are just as ignorant of and which the patient may understand better. Likewise, do not use terms that the patient does not understand. Giving the patients a long line of specialized ophthalmic terms that they do not understand may make you feel intelligent and important, but just further frustrates and belittles the patient. A sign of an intelligent person is one who can simplify difficult concepts for others. Remember that their complaint or misunderstanding may be due to your inadequate job of patient education or communication in the first place.

Practically all irate patients and patient complaints can be solved to the satisfaction of all concerned if these principles are followed. Do not hesitate to do further testing, checking, or rescheduling of the patient to solve the problem.

If a call from an unhappy patient is taken by a receptionist or technician who, after listening to the patient, cannot solve the patient's problem or if the patient wants to talk to the doctor, then the doctor should talk with the patient. It is often best, however, if the receptionist will tell the patient that the doctor is either busy with another patient or is out of the office and that the doctor will call back. Set a specific time with the patient, for example, in 15 to 30 minutes, when you know the doctor will be free to call. This gives such patients a little time to calm down after they have had a chance to talk to an understanding and sympathetic receptionist. Often the patients have had to build up the anger and nerve to call the office over a long time, and once they have vented their frustrations, they will calm down and can be reasoned with. When a time is set for the doctor to call back, be sure the doctor or someone gets back to the patient at the prescribed time. Never ignore or put the patient off hoping the problem will go away. This just makes it worse. No one wants unhappy patients campaigning against the practice or bringing a malpractice suit even if it is unfounded.

In today's climate, malpractice suits are of concern. These can normally be avoided by proper patient handling, facing the unhappy patient as described, showing concern for the patient, and being available and willing to help the patient when help is needed. Patient education and a good recall system are also important. This prevents most serious problems from developing.

There a few legal aspects that should also be considered. For example, if a report is to be sent to the patient's physician, dentist, teacher, employer, insurance company, or other person, the patient must sign a consent form allowing the release of the information. Do not give information out over the phone or if it is not authorized. Also, do not talk about patients outside the office or to other patients. What patients say is to be held in confidence.

FEES

In order to equip an office properly, pay laboratory bills, buy supplies, pay the rent, utilities, and taxes, hire proper help, attend educational meetings, learn new techniques, and cover all the many other costs of providing vision care, fees must be charged. One need not be apologetic for doing so, nor should one be afraid to discuss fees with a patient questioning them. There should be no problem justifying them.

An office should have a well laid out policy concerning fees and should have a written fee schedule. If this is available, all the office personnel will tell and charge all the patients the same. In addition, if a fee schedule is available, the patient will feel more assured that a fair and well thought out fee is being charged. If the fee appears to the patients to have been pulled out of the air, then they are more likely to question it and be unhappy.

Fees should be discussed with the patient prior to the rendering of extensive services such as contact lens fitting. The patients should be fully aware of what a fee includes and does not include. For example, does it include follow-up visits, solutions, supplies, or lens loss? What happens if they cannot wear the lenses? The upkeep cost must be discussed with the patient prior to fitting: the cost of solutions, replacement lenses, how often must they be replaced, how often the patient must be examined, and the cost of each examination. If the patient fully understands the costs and procedures, there will be no surprise later to cause unhappiness. Being honest and straightforward with the patient from the outset will build patient confidence in the practice.

It is best that the total cost to the patient be divided into a fee for professional services and material costs. From advertising and other sources, many patients know the approximate laboratory cost of lenses. Thus, if you tell them contact lenses cost $350 and they know that the actual lens cost is $40 to $100, they will feel that the fee is exorbitant. If, however, the patient is charged $100 for materials and the remainder for professional service, you are telling the patient how the fee is really derived. The patient is paying for the professional care and all the costs of providing it. This is easy to justify, and people are accustomed to paying for service since they do it constantly for other professionals, repairmen, and service personnel.

Some practitioners extend credit to patients while others require full payment early in the fitting process either by cash, check, or credit card. If credit is extended, the likelihood of collecting the fee later is increased by the way the initial fee is presented. If patients understand what they are paying for, they will readily pay on time.

WARRANTIES, SERVICE CONTRACTS, AND INSURANCE

Some contact lens companies have warranty policies on their lenses that allow a lens replacement at no charge or at a reduced charge for a specific time, commonly 6 months. Often the laboratory cost is slightly higher if the lenses are covered by warranty and only includes replacements for damaged lenses or incorrect parameters, but not lost lenses. The policies vary with the company.

Some practitioners provide a self-warranty on lenses for a short time after fitting during which lost or damaged lenses are replaced at a reduced rate.

Service contracts are offered by other practitioners following the initial fitting and adaptation period. A patient pays a certain amount for the service contract for a period of time, such as 1 year, which may cover or partially cover the cost of one or two routine examinations and allow lens replacements at a reduced rate. The advantage of such a system is that the patients prepay at least part of the fee if they come in for the visits or not. Therefore, patients are more likely to seek proper aftercare. It is also a financial advantage to the practice and helps keep patients with the practice. There are many different ways to arrange the service contract and different coverages can be arranged. One must be careful that it does not violate the state insurance laws.

Many companies offer insurance policies to cover contact lenses. These function similar to other types of insurance where the patient pays a premium for a year's coverage. With the insurance the lens (material charge) is usually paid for by the insurance company. In some cases, the insurance company will charge the patient a deductible fee each time a lens is lost. The insurance company normally does not pay for the professional fee of the practitioner for ordering, verifying, and dispensing the lens. Thus, the cost of replacing a lens even with insurance can be relatively expensive. Often there is no advantage to having the insurance unless several lenses are replaced. Before patients purchase the insurance they should be aware of all the costs involved and how it operates. To obtain insurance coverage, application forms may be given to the patient to send in. In other cases the office may collect the premium and send it to the insurance company. In a few instances, patients can insure lenses under their homeowner's policy.

RECALL SYSTEMS

The importance of periodic examinations, often every 6 months to a year for daily wear lenses and more often for extended wear, has been stressed. In order to get most patients to come in for these visits they must be reminded. A factor that is very important in determining if a patient will come in when reminded is, once again, patient education. If patients understand the need for these examinations even if they do not perceive a problem, then they are more likely to heed a recall notice. Patients should be told when they should return and that they will be receiving the recall notice.

A recall system can be a card or letter sent to the patient indicating the need for an examination and to call for an appointment. Some offices have patients address the card or envelope to themselves. It is then filed by month and year to be sent out and then mailed at that time. Patients receive it in their own handwriting. Other practices just use a card-filing system by year and month and make up the notice and address it when it is time to be sent.

Others use a telephone recall system, which has been shown to be more effective in terms of number of patients making appointments. The patient is called and an attempt is made to schedule an appointment. Some practitioners feel this takes too much of the office assistant's time or is too aggressive.

Another system involves scheduling an appointment 6 months to a year ahead of time. At each visit, the next appointment is made. The advantage of this is that patients know of the appointment and the need. They are then reminded of the appointment a few days in advance. Problems with this system are that patients do not know what day and time they will be able to keep an appointment that far in advance and the practitioner may not know of a meeting or vacation schedule.

Regardless of the type of recall system used, it is important to have one to give good, continuing care and to detect problems before they become severe.

ORDERING AND LABORATORY CONTROL

An important duty of an assistant or technician is to deal with the laboratories. When lenses are ordered for a patient, it is important that the order form be properly and completely filled out and that the lenses be correctly ordered. Most offices will call the order to the laboratory as this saves time. The sooner a lens can be received, the happier the patient will be.

Proper records of lens orders must be kept. This includes a copy of the order in the patient's record as well as on a control sheet (Figure 13–1). Each order, including the patient's name, lens ordered, and date ordered, should be recorded. There can be a separate sheet for each company used. This sheet can be used to determine, at a glance, if a lens or lenses have not been received in the expected time period. In this case, the company can be called to determine the problem. Likewise, the control sheet can be used to record whether the lens has been verified and to note if it had to be rejected. By inspecting these sheets an usually high rejection rate can be quickly determined.

For lenses with control or lot numbers, these numbers should be recorded on the patient's record and the laboratory control sheet. This information would be useful if it were found that a batch of lenses had to be recalled and replaced by the company due to a manufacturing problem. Likewise, serial numbers of other supplies, particularly heat disinfection units, should be similarly recorded.

INVENTORY MAINTENANCE

Keeping the necessary supplies in the office is mandatory. With respect to the contact lens aspect of a practice this includes keeping diagnostic or stock lens sets up to date, supplies such as solutions, starter kits, cases,

---

Figure 13–1. Laboratory control sheet to keep track of lenses on order and those waiting to be dispensed

LABORATORY CONTROL SHEET

Patient	Company	Date ordered	Date rec'd	Lot #	Accepted/ rejected	Patient notified	Dispensed

disinfection units, identification cards, fluorescein, tissues and the multitude of other necessary supplies. A list containing each item, the minimum number that should be maintained, and order information should be developed. Then the inventory must be checked on a periodic basis, for example, once a week or once a month, and replacement supplies ordered.

The diagnostic or stock lenses kept in the practice must be maintained clean and disinfected. Each time a lens is used on a patient it must be properly cleaned before being placed back into the set. The procedure depends on the type of lens and practitioner's preference. Hydrogel lenses should be cleaned with a surfactant cleaner, rinsed well, and then either heat disinfected or placed in the proper chemical disinfection system. If the same few lenses are repeatedly used as diagnostic lenses, they should also be cleaned periodically with an enzyme cleaner. Any damaged or coated lenses should be replaced.

The storage of rigid lenses depends on the type of lens and frequency of use. For example, PMMA lenses that may not be used frequently should probably be cleaned and dried well before being stored. If they are kept in solution, the solution should be replaced every couple of weeks so it does not evaporate and leave a residue on the lenses. Lenses of some of the newer polymers should be kept in solutions even if they are not used frequently. For example, CAB lenses change shape considerably on hydration. The surfaces of others may lose some of their wettability if kept dry. In these cases, do not forget to check all the lenses periodically and keep sufficient solution in the cases.

EQUIPMENT MAINTENANCE

Equipment must be kept clean and in good working order. Precision optical instruments must be handled with extreme care. They should be protected from dust and dirt and kept covered when not in use. Lenses and other precision parts should not be touched, handled roughly, or exposed to moisture.

The phoropter, used to determine the patient's refractive error, has a large number of lenses. One should never place a finger into the apertures the patient looks through as this will smear the lenses or possibly damage them. Do not allow patients to do this; children are especially curious and likely to do so. If a lens does get smeared, it may be gently cleaned using a cotton-tipped swab and an alcohol solution. Do not use excess solution. Cans of compressed air can be obtained to dry the lenses. They can also be used to blow dust off the lenses. Also, never force any of the controls on the instrument if they do not move easily.

The shields on the back of the instrument, which touch the patient's face, should be replaced frequently if they are the paper type or removed and washed if plastic (Figure 13–2). Alcohol swabs can be used to clean and sterilize them between patients. Likewise, the forehead rest should be cleaned.

When not in use, the instrument should be rotated back out of the way and the arm locked so it cannot be accidentally hit.

The keratometer is another instrument that must be cared for. The calibration and use of this instrument is described in Chapter 5. In addition, the headrest and chinrest must be kept clean. Another occasional problem is that the bulb will burn out and require replacement. Before doing this, be sure the instrument is unplugged. With the Bausch and Lomb or similar keratometer, hold the lamp housing with one hand and loosen the two screws which hold it. Remove the lamp housing, which now exposes the bulb (Figure 13–3). Unscrew the bulb, being careful not to touch the surrounding mirror. Replace it with an identical 15-watt bulb.

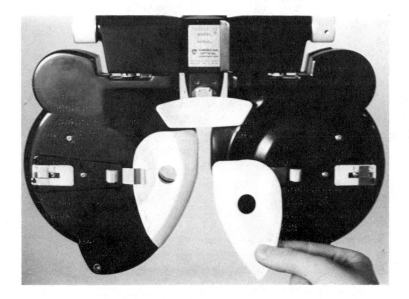

Figure 13–2. Back of phoropter showing the face and forehead shields

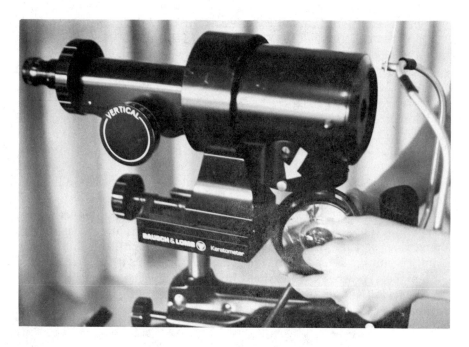

Figure 13–3. Removing the bulb from the keratometer. Arrow indicates one of the screws that must be loosened to remove the housing

To replace the bulb in the American Optical CLC Ophthalmometer, the bulb housing is removed after loosening a single screw under the main body of the instrument just in front of where the patient would be (Figure 13–4). The bulb is then removed by pressing down on it and turning it slightly counterclockwise.

The biomicroscope is another instrument receiving a lot of use in the contact lens practice. Again, it should be kept clean with the headrest cleaned with alcohol swabs and new chinrest tissues kept in place on the instruments requiring them. Again, bulbs must be occasionally replaced. The procedure varies with the type of instrument (Figures 13–5, 13–6, and 13–7). Always be careful to replace the bulb with the one specified by the company. Many of these instruments use bulbs that must be pressed down slightly and turned a partial rotation to remove or put in place. Be careful when doing this as the bulb could break, resulting in a badly cut hand. It is best to place a handkerchief, piece of foam rubber, or other protection over the bulb before trying to remove and replace it. Do not forget to be sure the bulb is cool before trying to remove it as it can become very hot. With most instruments, the position of the bulb can

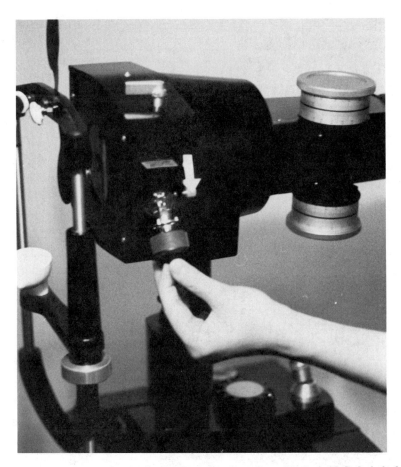

Figure 13–4. Removing the bulb from the American Optical CLC Ophthalmometer. The arrow indicates the screw that must be loosened to remove the bulb housing

be adjusted so that it is in the proper alignment to give maximum illumination. This may be accomplished by adjusting two or three screws near the base of the bulb or by twisting the bulb housing. Each time a bulb is replaced this adjustment should be checked. This is done by positioning the slit image, which would normally be on the patient's eye, on a distant wall. With the aperture (slit) fully open, the image of the light filament should be in focus and in the middle of the field. If not, use the adjustment screws to obtain proper focus and centration. If this adjustment is not done, the field illumination on the patient's eye will appear uneven and not as bright as it should be.

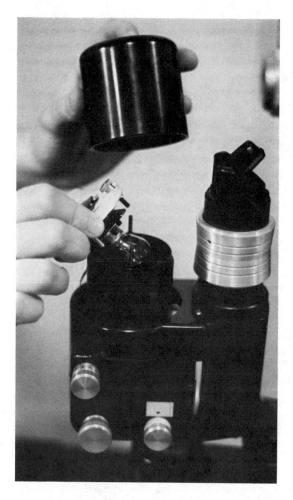

Figure 13–5. Removing the bulb from an American Optical slit-lamp

The projector used to project the distance acuity chart must also be maintained. The calibration was explained in Chapter 5. It should, of course, be kept dust free and the lenses occasionally cleaned. Again, bulbs must be changed. The method will depend on the make. With the projector unplugged, the cover over the bulb region of the lens must first be removed (Figure 13–8). With some projectors there is a second bulb covering that contains a mirror. This must be carefully removed to get to the bulb. The bulb is removed by a slight downward pressure and a partial counter-clockwise rotation. Be careful not to break the bulb during removal or replacement and protect the hand with a cloth or other type of covering. Remember to replace the bulb with an identical one as recommended by the manufacturer.

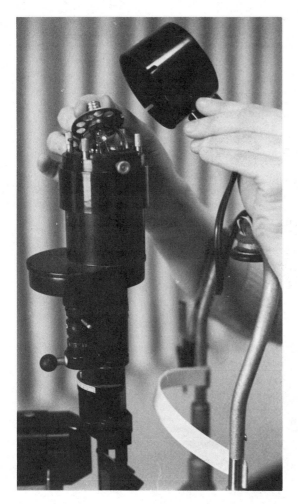

Figure 13–6.   Removing the bulb from an Haag-Striet slit-lamp

In the laboratory the radiuscope must be maintained. Again, bulb replacement is common. The procedure will vary with the make. On the most common make the bulb is in the housing on the back of the instrument (Figure 13–9). A screw holds the bulb housing. Loosen it and remove the bulb with its socket. Remove the bulb by applying slight pressure and a partial counterclockwise rotation. After the bulb is replaced, be sure to check the alignment of the bulb. This is done by placing a lens in the instrument as taking a reading. Focus the instrument so that the image of the filament is in view (see Chapter 7 for use of the radiuscope). If the filament is not centered in the field, adjust the three screws on the lamp

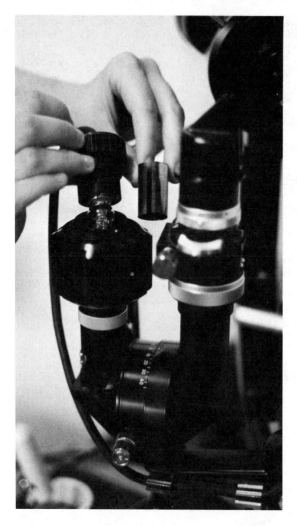

Figure 13-7. Removing the bulb from a Nikon slit-lamp

housing while looking into the instrument until the filament is centered. This will give maximum illumination with the instrument.

Another maintenance job that must occasionally be done with the radiuscope is to relubricate the stage. The stage plate is held in place only by a thin layer of grease. After a time this lubricant is lost and the plate will not slide or move smoothly. The plate should be lifted up, being careful not to hit the objective (Figure 13–10). A thin layer of lubricant provided with the instrument or any lubricant for fine instruments can be spread lightly over the bottom of the plate and the plate on which it rested (Figure 13–11). It can then just be pressed back into place.

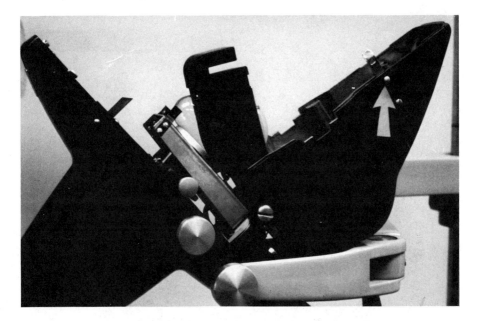

Figure 13-8. Removing the bulb from an acuity projector. The arrow indicates the release button to allow the projector to be opened as shown. The black bulb cover in the center of the projector is partially removed, exposing the top of the bulb. It must be completely removed to take the bulb out

The bulb in the lensometer (vertexometer) must be occasionally replaced. Again, the method depends on the type and make. One common make just requires loosening a screw on the back of the instrument and pulling the cover back, unscrewing the bulb and replacing it (Figure 13-12). The projection lensometers must be laid down, as the bulb is under the instrument. A screw on a small door is loosened, the door is opened, and the bulb is removed by pressing down on it and turning counterclockwise (Figure 13-13).

The bulb on some projection magnifiers is changed in the same fashion as the projection lensometers.

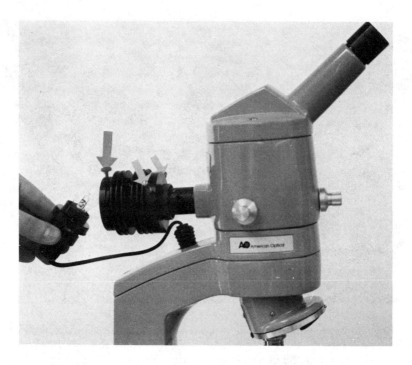

Figure 13–9. Removing the bulb from the radiuscope. The arrow to the left indicates the screw to loosen the bulb housing. The two other arrows indicate two of the three adjustment screws to align the bulb properly (see text)

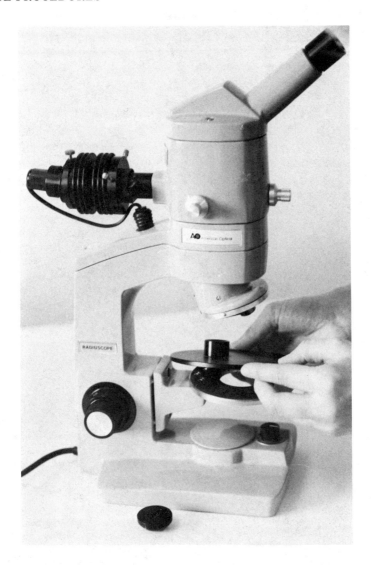

Figure 13–10.   Removing the stage plate of the radiuscope

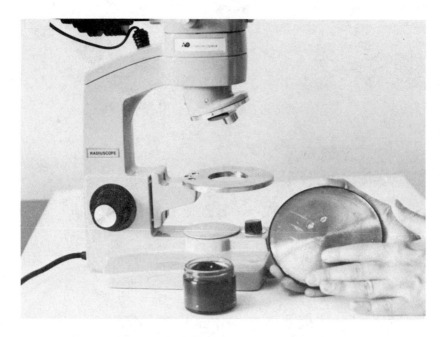

Figure 13–11. Lubricating the bottom of the stage plate of the radiuscope

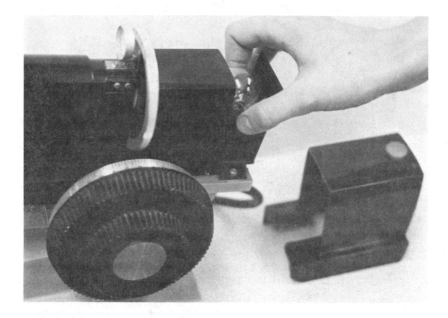

Figure 13–12. Removing the covering and replacing the bulb in the lensometer

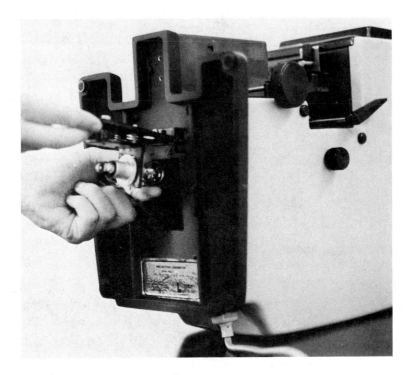

Figure 13–13. Removing the bulb in a projection lensometer

Appendix I

CONVERSION OF RADIUS TO SURFACE POWER

Conversion of radius (mm) to surface power (D) for the situations and refractive index differences indicated.

Radius (mm)	CLC opthometer (1.336–1.00)	B&L keratometer (1.3375–1.00)	Common hydrogels (1.43–1.00)	PMMA lenses (1.49–1.00)
5.00	67.20	67.50	86.00	98.00
5.05	66.53	66.83	85.15	97.03
5.10	65.88	66.18	84.31	96.08
5.15	65.24	65.53	83.50	95.15
5.20	64.62	64.90	82.69	94.23
5.25	64.00	64.29	81.90	93.33
5.30	63.40	63.68	81.13	92.45
5.35	62.80	63.08	80.37	91.59
5.40	62.22	62.50	79.63	90.74
5.45	61.65	61.93	78.90	89.91
5.50	61.09	61.36	78.18	89.09
5.55	60.54	60.81	77.48	88.29
5.60	60.00	60.27	76.79	87.50
5.65	59.47	59.73	76.11	86.73
5.70	58.95	59.21	75.44	85.97

Radius (mm)	CLC opthometer (1.336–1.00)	B&L keratometer (1.3375–1.00)	Common hydrogels (1.43–1.00)	PMMA lenses (1.49–1.00)
5.75	58.43	58.70	74.78	85.22
5.80	57.93	58.19	74.14	84.48
5.85	57.44	57.69	73.50	83.76
5.90	56.95	57.20	72.88	83.05
5.95	56.47	56.72	72.27	82.35
6.00	56.00	56.25	71.67	81.67
6.05	55.54	55.79	71.07	80.99
6.10	55.08	55.33	70.49	80.33
6.15	54.63	54.88	69.92	79.68
6.20	54.19	54.44	69.36	79.03
6.25	53.76	54.00	68.80	78.40
6.30	53.33	53.57	68.25	77.78
6.35	52.91	53.15	67.72	77.17
6.40	52.50	52.73	67.19	76.56
6.45	52.09	52.33	66.67	75.97
6.50	51.69	51.92	65.65	75.38
6.55	51.30	51.53	65.55	74.81
6.60	50.91	51.14	65.15	74.24
6.65	50.53	50.75	64.66	73.68
6.70	50.15	50.37	64.18	73.13
6.75	49.78	50.00	63.70	72.59
6.80	49.41	49.63	63.24	72.06
6.85	49.05	49.27	62.77	71.53
6.90	48.70	48.91	62.32	71.01
6.95	48.35	48.56	61.87	70.50
7.00	48.00	48.21	61.43	70.00
7.05	47.66	47.87	60.99	69.50
7.10	47.32	47.54	60.56	69.01
7.15	46.99	47.20	60.14	68.53
7.20	46.67	46.88	59.72	68.06
7.25	46.35	46.55	59.31	67.59
7.30	46.03	46.23	58.90	67.12
7.35	45.71	45.92	58.50	66.67
7.40	45.41	45.61	58.11	66.22
7.45	45.10	45.30	57.72	65.77
7.50	44.80	45.00	57.33	65.33
7.55	44.50	44.70	56.95	64.90
7.60	44.21	44.41	56.58	64.47
7.65	43.92	44.12	56.21	64.05
7.70	43.64	43.83	55.84	63.64
7.75	43.36	43.55	55.48	63.23
7.80	43.08	43.27	55.13	62.82

Radius (mm)	CLC opthometer (1.336–1.00)	B&L keratometer (1.3375–1.00)	Common hydrogels (1.43–1.00)	PMMA lenses (1.49–1.00)
7.85	42.80	42.99	54.78	62.42
7.90	42.53	42.72	54.43	62.03
7.95	42.26	42.45	54.09	61.64
8.00	42.00	42.19	53.75	61.25
8.05	41.74	41.93	53.42	60.87
8.10	41.48	41.67	53.09	60.49
8.15	41.23	41.41	52.76	60.12
8.20	40.98	41.16	52.44	59.76
8.25	40.73	40.91	52.12	59.39
8.30	40.48	40.66	51.81	59.04
8.35	40.24	40.42	51.50	58.68
8.40	40.00	40.18	51.19	58.33
8.45	39.76	39.94	50.89	57.99
8.50	39.53	39.71	50.59	57.65
8.55	39.30	39.47	50.29	57.31
8.60	39.07	39.24	50.00	56.98
8.65	38.84	39.02	49.71	56.65
8.70	38.62	38.79	49.43	56.32
8.75	38.40	38.57	49.14	56.00
8.80	38.18	38.35	48.86	55.68
8.85	37.97	38.14	48.59	55.37
8.90	37.75	37.92	48.31	55.06
8.95	37.54	37.71	48.05	54.75
9.00	37.33	37.50	47.78	54.44
9.05	37.13	37.29	47.51	54.14
9.10	36.92	37.09	47.25	53.85
9.15	36.72	36.89	46.99	53.55
9.20	36.52	36.69	46.74	53.26
9.25	36.32	36.49	46.49	52.97
9.30	36.13	36.29	46.24	52.69
9.35	35.94	36.10	45.99	52.41
9.40	35.74	35.90	45.74	52.13
9.45	35.56	35.71	45.50	51.85
9.50	35.37	35.53	45.26	51.58
9.55	35.18	35.34	45.03	51.31
9.60	35.00	35.16	44.79	51.04
9.65	34.82	34.97	44.56	50.78
9.70	34.64	34.79	44.33	50.52
9.75	34.46	34.62	44.10	50.26
9.80	34.29	34.44	43.88	50.00
9.85	34.11	34.26	43.66	49.75
9.90	33.94	34.09	43.43	49.50

Radius (mm)	CLC opthometer (1.336–1.00)	B&L keratometer (1.3375–1.00)	Common hydrogels (1.43–1.00)	PMMA lenses (1.49–1.00)
9.95	33.77	33.92	43.22	49.25
10.00	33.60	33.75	43.00	49.00
10.05	33.43	33.58	42.79	48.76
10.10	33.27	33.42	42.57	48.52
10.15	33.10	33.25	42.36	48.28
10.20	32.94	33.09	42.16	48.04
10.25	32.78	32.93	41.95	47.81
10.30	32.62	32.77	41.75	47.57
10.35	32.46	32.61	41.55	47.34
10.40	32.31	32.45	41.35	47.12

Appendix II
CORRECTION FOR VERTEX DISTANCE

Ocular refraction for indicated spectacle refraction (in diopters) is given for various vertex distances.

Spectacle refraction	Ocular refraction				
	8 mm	10 mm	12 mm	14 mm	16 mm
+2.00	+2.03	+2.04	+2.05	+2.06	+2.07
+2.25	+2.29	+2.30	+2.31	+2.32	+2.33
+2.50	+2.55	+2.56	+2.58	+2.59	+2.60
+2.75	+2.81	+2.83	+2.84	+2.86	+2.88
+3.00	+3.07	+3.09	+3.11	+3.13	+3.15
+3.25	+3.34	+3.36	+3.38	+3.40	+3.43
+3.50	+3.60	+3.63	+3.65	+3.68	+3.71
+3.75	+3.87	+3.90	+3.93	+3.96	+3.99
+4.00	+4.13	+4.17	+4.20	+4.24	+4.27
+4.25	+4.40	+4.44	+4.48	+4.52	+4.56
+4.50	+4.67	+4.71	+4.76	+4.80	+4.85
+4.75	+4.94	+4.99	+5.04	+5.09	+5.14
+5.00	+5.21	+5.26	+5.32	+5.38	+5.43
+5.25	+5.48	+5.54	+5.60	+5.67	+5.73
+5.50	+5.75	+5.82	+5.89	+5.96	+6.03
+5.75	+6.03	+6.10	+6.18	+6.25	+6.33
+6.00	+6.30	+6.38	+6.47	+6.55	+6.64
+6.25	+6.58	+6.67	+6.76	+6.85	+6.94
+6.50	+6.86	+6.95	+7.05	+7.15	+7.25

Spectacle refraction	Ocular refraction				
	8 mm	10 mm	12 mm	14 mm	16 mm
+6.75	+7.14	+7.24	+7.34	+7.45	+7.57
+7.00	+7.42	+7.53	+7.64	+7.76	+7.88
+7.25	+7.70	+7.82	+7.94	+8.07	+8.20
+7.50	+7.98	+8.11	+8.24	+8.38	+8.52
+7.75	+8.26	+8.40	+8.54	+8.69	+8.85
+8.00	+8.55	+8.70	+8.85	+9.01	+9.17
+8.25	+8.83	+8.99	+9.16	+9.33	+9.50
+8.50	+9.12	+9.29	+9.47	+9.65	+9.84
+8.75	+9.41	+9.59	+9.78	+9.97	+10.17
+9.00	+9.70	+9.89	+10.09	+10.30	+10.51
+9.25	+9.99	+10.19	+10.40	+10.63	+10.86
+9.50	+10.28	+10.50	+10.72	+10.96	+11.20
+9.75	+10.57	+10.80	+11.04	+11.29	+11.55
+10.00	+10.87	+11.11	+11.36	+11.63	+11.90
+10.25	+11.17	+11.42	+11.69	+11.97	+12.26
+10.50	+11.46	+11.73	+12.01	+12.31	+12.62
+10.75	+11.76	+12.04	+12.34	+12.65	+12.98
+11.00	+12.06	+12.36	+12.67	+13.00	+13.35
+11.25	+12.36	+12.68	+13.01	+13.35	+13.72
+11.50	+12.67	+12.99	+13.34	+13.71	+14.09
+11.75	+12.97	+13.31	+13.68	+14.06	+14.47
+12.00	+13.27	+13.64	+14.02	+14.42	+14.85
+12.25	+13.58	+13.96	+14.36	+14.79	+15.24
+12.50	+13.89	+14.29	+14.71	+15.15	+15.62
+12.75	+14.20	+14.61	+15.05	+15.52	+16.02
+13.00	+14.51	+14.94	+15.40	+15.89	+16.41
+13.25	+14.82	+15.27	+15.76	+16.27	+16.81
+13.50	+15.13	+15.61	+16.11	+16.65	+17.22
+13.75	+15.45	+15.94	+16.47	+17.03	+17.63
+14.00	+15.77	+16.28	+16.83	+17.41	+18.04
+14.25	+16.08	+16.62	+17.19	+17.80	+18.46
+14.50	+16.40	+16.96	+17.55	+18.19	+18.88
+14.75	+16.72	+17.30	+17.92	+18.59	+19.31
+15.00	+17.05	+17.65	+18.29	+18.99	+19.74
+15.25	+17.37	+17.99	+18.67	+19.39	+20.17
+15.50	+17.69	+18.34	+19.04	+19.80	+20.61
+15.75	+18.02	+18.69	+19.42	+20.21	+21.06
+16.00	+18.35	+19.05	+19.80	+20.62	+21.51
+16.25	+18.68	+19.40	+20.19	+21.04	+21.96
+16.50	+19.01	+19.76	+20.57	+21.46	+22.42
+16.75	+19.34	+20.12	+20.96	+21.88	+22.88
+17.00	+19.68	+20.48	+21.36	+22.31	+23.35
+17.25	+20.01	+20.85	+21.75	+22.74	+23.83
+17.50	+20.35	+21.21	+22.15	+23.18	+24.31

Spectacle refraction	Ocular refraction				
	8 mm	10 mm	12 mm	14 mm	16 mm
+17.75	+20.69	+21.58	+22.55	+23.62	+24.79
+18.00	+21.03	+21.95	+22.96	+24.06	+25.28
+18.25	+21.37	+22.32	+23.37	+24.51	+25.78
+18.50	+21.71	+22.70	+23.78	+24.97	+26.28
+18.75	+22.06	+23.08	+24.19	+25.42	+26.79
+19.00	+22.41	+23.46	+24.61	+25.89	+27.30
+19.25	+22.75	+23.84	+25.03	+26.35	+27.82
+19.50	+23.10	+24.22	+25.46	+26.82	+28.34
+19.75	+23.46	+24.61	+25.88	+27.30	+28.87
+20.00	+23.81	+25.00	+26.32	+27.78	+29.41
+20.25	+24.16	+25.39	+26.75	+28.26	+29.96
+20.50	+24.52	+25.79	+27.19	+28.75	+30.51
+20.75	+24.88	+26.18	+27.63	+29.25	+31.06
+21.00	+25.24	+26.58	+28.07	+29.75	+31.63
+21.25	+25.60	+26.98	+28.52	+30.25	+32.20
+21.50	+25.97	+27.39	+28.98	+30.76	+32.77
+21.75	+26.33	+27.80	+29.43	+31.27	+33.36
+22.00	+26.70	+28.21	+29.89	+31.79	+33.95
+22.25	+27.07	+28.62	+30.35	+32.32	+34.55
+22.50	+27.44	+29.03	+30.82	+32.85	+35.16
+22.75	+27.81	+29.45	+31.29	+33.38	+35.77
+23.00	+28.19	+29.87	+31.77	+33.92	+36.39
+23.25	+28.56	+30.29	+32.25	+34.47	+37.02
+23.50	+28.94	+30.72	+32.73	+35.02	+37.66
+23.75	+29.32	+31.15	+33.22	+35.58	+38.31
+24.00	+29.70	+31.58	+33.71	+36.14	+38.96
+24.25	+30.09	+32.01	+34.20	+36.71	+39.62
+24.50	+30.47	+32.45	+34.70	+37.29	+40.30
+24.75	+30.86	+32.89	+35.21	+37.87	+40.98
+25.00	+31.25	+33.33	+35.71	+38.46	+41.67
+25.25	+31.64	+33.78	+36.23	+39.06	+42.37
+25.50	+32.04	+34.23	+36.74	+39.66	+43.07
+25.75	+32.43	+34.68	+37.26	+40.27	+43.79
+26.00	+32.83	+35.14	+37.79	+40.88	+44.52
+26.25	+33.23	+35.59	+38.32	+41.50	+45.26
+26.50	+33.63	+36.05	+38.86	+42.13	+46.01
+26.75	+34.03	+36.52	+39.40	+42.77	+46.77
+27.00	+34.44	+36.99	+39.94	+43.41	+47.54
+27.25	+34.85	+37.46	+40.49	+44.06	+48.32
+27.50	+35.26	+37.93	+41.04	+44.72	+49.11
+27.75	+35.67	+38.41	+41.60	+45.38	+49.91
+28.00	+36.08	+38.89	+42.17	+46.05	+50.72
+28.25	+36.50	+39.37	+42.74	+46.73	+51.55
+28.50	+36.92	+39.86	+43.31	+47.42	+52.39

Spectacle refraction	Ocular refraction				
	8 mm	10 mm	12 mm	14 mm	16 mm
+28.75	+37.34	+40.35	+43.89	+48.12	+53.24
+29.00	+37.76	+40.85	+44.48	+48.82	+54.10
+29.25	+38.19	+41.34	+45.07	+49.53	+54.98
+29.50	+38.61	+41.84	+45.67	+50.26	+55.87
+29.75	+39.04	+42.35	+46.27	+50.99	+56.77
+30.00	+39.47	+42.86	+46.87	+51.72	+57.69
−2.00	−1.97	−1.96	−1.95	−1.95	−1.94
−2.25	−2.21	−2.20	−2.19	−2.18	−2.17
−2.50	−2.45	−2.44	−2.43	−2.42	−2.40
−2.75	−2.69	−2.68	−2.66	−2.65	−2.63
−3.00	−2.93	−2.91	−2.90	−2.88	−2.86
−3.25	−3.17	−3.15	−3.13	−3.11	−3.09
−3.50	−3.40	−3.38	−3.36	−3.34	−3.31
−3.75	−3.64	−3.61	−3.59	−3.56	−3.54
−4.00	−3.88	−3.85	−3.82	−3.79	−3.76
−4.25	−4.11	−4.08	−4.04	−4.01	−3.98
−4.50	−4.34	−4.31	−4.27	−4.23	−4.20
−4.75	−4.58	−4.53	−4.49	−4.45	−4.41
−5.00	−4.81	−4.76	−4.72	−4.67	−4.63
−5.25	−5.04	−4.99	−4.94	−4.89	−4.84
−5.50	−5.27	−5.21	−5.16	−5.11	−5.06
−5.75	−5.50	−5.44	−5.38	−5.32	−5.27
−6.00	−5.73	−5.66	−5.60	−5.54	−5.47
−6.25	−5.95	−5.88	−5.81	−5.75	−5.68
−6.50	−6.18	−6.10	−6.03	−5.96	−5.89
−6.75	−6.40	−6.32	−6.24	−6.17	−6.09
−7.00	−6.63	−6.54	−6.46	−6.38	−6.29
−7.25	−6.85	−6.76	−6.67	−6.58	−6.50
−7.50	−7.08	−6.98	−6.88	−6.79	−6.70
−7.75	−7.30	−7.19	−7.09	−6.99	−6.90
−8.00	−7.52	−7.41	−7.30	−7.19	−7.09
−8.25	−7.74	−7.62	−7.51	−7.40	−7.29
−8.50	−7.96	−7.83	−7.71	−7.60	−7.48
−8.75	−8.18	−8.05	−7.92	−7.80	−7.68
−9.00	−8.40	−8.26	−8.12	−7.99	−7.87
−9.25	−8.61	−8.47	−8.33	−8.19	−8.06
−9.50	−8.83	−8.68	−8.53	−8.38	−8.25
−9.75	−9.04	−8.88	−8.73	−8.58	−8.43
−10.00	−9.26	−9.09	−8.93	−8.77	−8.62
−10.25	−9.47	−9.30	−9.13	−8.96	−8.81
−10.50	−9.69	−9.50	−9.33	−9.15	−8.99
−10.75	−9.90	−9.71	−9.52	−9.34	−9.17
−11.00	−10.11	−9.91	−9.72	−9.53	−9.35
−11.25	−10.32	−10.11	−9.91	−9.72	−9.53

Spectacle refraction	Ocular refraction				
	8 mm	10 mm	12 mm	14 mm	16 mm
−11.50	−10.53	−10.31	−10.11	−9.91	−9.71
−11.75	−10.74	−10.51	−10.30	−10.09	−9.89
−12.00	−10.95	−10.71	−10.49	−10.27	−10.07
−12.25	−11.16	−10.91	−10.68	−10.46	−10.24
−12.50	−11.36	−11.11	−10.87	−10.64	−10.42
−12.75	−11.57	−11.31	−11.06	−10.82	−10.59
−13.00	−11.78	−11.50	−11.25	−11.00	−10.76
−13.25	−11.98	−11.70	−11.43	−11.18	−10.93
−13.50	−12.18	−11.89	−11.62	−11.35	−11.10
−13.75	−12.39	−12.09	−11.80	−11.53	−11.27
−14.00	−12.59	−12.28	−11.99	−11.71	−11.44
−14.25	−12.79	−12.47	−12.17	−11.88	−11.60
−14.50	−12.99	−12.66	−12.35	−12.05	−11.77
−14.75	−13.19	−12.85	−12.53	−12.23	−11.93
−15.00	−13.39	−13.04	−12.71	−12.40	−12.10
−15.25	−13.59	−13.23	−12.89	−12.57	−12.26
−15.50	−13.79	−13.42	−13.07	−12.74	−12.42
−15.75	−13.99	−13.61	−13.25	−12.90	−12.58
−16.00	−14.18	−13.79	−13.42	−13.07	−12.74
−16.25	−14.38	−13.98	−13.60	−13.24	−12.90
−16.50	−14.58	−14.16	−13.77	−13.40	−13.05
−16.75	−14.77	−14.35	−13.95	−13.57	−13.21
−17.00	−14.96	−14.53	−14.12	−13.73	−13.36
−17.25	−15.16	−14.71	−14.29	−13.89	−13.52
−17.50	−15.35	−14.89	−14.46	−14.06	−13.67
−17.75	−15.54	−15.07	−14.63	−14.22	−13.82
−18.00	−15.73	−15.25	−14.80	−14.38	−13.98
−18.25	−15.92	−15.43	−14.97	−14.54	−14.13
−18.50	−16.11	−15.61	−15.14	−14.69	−14.27
−18.75	−16.30	−15.79	−15.31	−14.85	−14.42
−19.00	−16.49	−15.97	−15.47	−15.01	−14.57
−19.25	−16.68	−16.14	−15.64	−15.16	−14.72
−19.50	−16.87	−16.32	−15.80	−15.32	−14.86
−19.75	−17.06	−16.49	−15.97	−15.47	−15.01
−20.00	−17.24	−16.67	−16.13	−15.63	−15.15
−20.25	−17.43	−16.84	−16.29	−15.78	−15.29
−20.50	−17.61	−17.01	−16.45	−15.93	−15.44
−20.75	−17.80	−17.18	−16.61	−16.08	−15.58
−21.00	−17.98	−17.36	−16.77	−16.23	−15.72
−21.25	−18.16	−17.53	−16.93	−16.38	−15.86
−21.50	−18.34	−17.70	−17.09	−16.53	−16.00
−21.75	−18.53	−17.86	−17.25	−16.67	−16.14
−22.00	−18.71	−18.03	−17.41	−16.82	−16.27
−22.25	−18.89	−18.20	−17.56	−16.97	−16.41

Spectacle refraction	Ocular refraction				
	8 mm	10 mm	12 mm	14 mm	16 mm
−22.50	−19.07	−18.37	−17.72	−17.11	−16.54
−22.75	−19.25	−18.53	−17.87	−17.25	−16.68
−23.00	−19.43	−18.70	−18.03	−17.40	−16.81
−23.25	−19.60	−18.86	−18.18	−17.54	−16.95
−23.50	−19.78	−19.03	−18.33	−17.68	−17.08
−23.75	−19.96	−19.19	−18.48	−17.82	−17.21
−24.00	−20.13	−19.35	−18.63	−17.96	−17.34
−24.25	−20.31	−19.52	−18.78	−18.10	−17.47
−24.50	−20.48	−19.68	−18.93	−18.24	−17.60
−24.75	−20.66	−19.84	−19.08	−18.38	−17.73
−25.00	−20.83	−20.00	−19.23	−18.52	−17.86
−25.25	−21.01	−20.16	−19.38	−18.66	−17.98
−25.50	−21.18	−20.32	−19.53	−18.79	−18.11
−25.75	−21.35	−20.48	−19.67	−18.93	−18.24
−26.00	−21.52	−20.63	−19.82	−19.06	−18.36
−26.25	−21.69	−20.79	−19.96	−19.20	−18.49
−26.50	−21.86	−20.95	−20.11	−19.33	−18.61
−26.75	−22.03	−21.10	−20.25	−19.46	−18.73
−27.00	−22.20	−21.26	−20.39	−19.59	−18.85
−27.25	−22.37	−21.41	−20.54	−19.72	−18.98
−27.50	−22.54	−21.57	−20.68	−19.86	−19.10
−27.75	−22.71	−21.72	−20.82	−19.99	−19.22
−28.00	−22.88	−21.88	−20.96	−20.11	−19.34
−28.25	−23.04	−22.03	−21.10	−20.24	−19.46
−28.50	−23.21	−22.18	−21.24	−20.37	−19.57
−28.75	−23.37	−22.33	−21.38	−20.50	−19.69
−29.00	−23.54	−22.48	−21.51	−20.63	−19.81
−29.25	−23.70	−22.63	−21.65	−20.75	−19.93
−29.50	−23.87	−22.78	−21.79	−20.88	−20.04
−29.75	−24.03	−22.93	−21.92	−21.00	−20.16
−30.00	−24.19	−23.08	−22.06	−21.13	−20.27

Appendix III
EXTENDING THE RANGE
OF THE KERATOMETER

Diopter and radius values when a $+1.25\,D$ spectacle trial lens is placed over the objective.

Drum reading	Corneal power in diopters	Radius in mm	
		Convex	Concave
43.000	50.134	6.732	6.759
43.125	50.279	6.712	6.739
43.250	50.425	6.693	6.720
43.375	50.571	6.674	6.701
43.500	50.717	6.655	6.681
43.625	50.862	6.636	6.662
43.750	51.008	6.617	6.643
43.875	51.154	6.598	6.624
44.000	51.299	6.579	6.605
44.125	51.445	6.560	6.587
44.250	51.591	6.542	6.568
44.375	51.737	6.523	6.550
44.500	51.882	6.505	6.531
44.625	52.028	6.487	6.513
44.750	52.174	6.469	6.495
44.875	52.320	6.451	6.477
45.000	52.465	6.433	6.459
45.125	52.611	6.415	6.441
45.250	52.757	6.397	6.423
45.375	52.903	6.380	6.405

Drum reading	Corneal power in diopters	Radius in mm	
		Convex	Concave
45.500	53.048	6.362	6.388
45.625	53.194	6.345	6.370
45.750	53.340	6.327	6.353
45.875	53.486	6.310	6.335
46.000	53.631	6.293	6.318
46.125	53.777	6.276	6.301
46.250	53.923	6.259	6.284
46.375	54.069	6.242	6.267
46.500	54.214	6.225	6.250
46.625	54.360	6.209	6.233
46.750	54.506	6.192	6.217
46.875	54.651	6.175	6.200
47.000	54.797	6.159	6.184
47.125	54.943	6.143	6.167
47.250	55.089	6.126	6.151
47.375	55.234	6.110	6.135
47.500	55.380	6.094	6.119
47.625	55.526	6.078	6.103
47.750	55.672	6.062	6.087
47.875	55.817	6.046	6.071
48.000	55.963	6.031	6.055
48.125	56.109	6.015	6.039
48.250	56.255	5.999	6.024
48.375	56.400	5.984	6.008
48.500	56.546	5.969	5.993
48.625	56.692	5.953	5.977
48.750	56.838	5.938	5.962
48.875	56.983	5.923	5.947
49.000	57.129	5.908	5.931
49.125	57.275	5.893	5.916
49.250	57.421	5.878	5.901
49.375	57.566	5.863	5.886
49.500	57.712	5.848	5.871
49.625	57.858	5.833	5.857
49.750	58.003	5.819	5.842
49.875	58.149	5.804	5.827
50.000	58.295	5.789	5.813
50.125	58.441	5.775	5.798
50.250	58.586	5.761	5.784
50.375	58.732	5.746	5.769
50.500	58.878	5.732	5.755
50.625	59.024	5.718	5.741

| Drum reading | Corneal power in diopters | Radius in mm | |
		Convex	Concave
50.750	59.169	5.704	5.727
50.875	59.315	5.690	5.713
51.000	59.461	5.676	5.699
51.125	59.607	5.662	5.685
51.250	59.752	5.648	5.671
51.375	59.898	5.635	5.657
51.500	60.044	5.621	5.643
51.625	60.190	5.607	5.630
51.750	60.335	5.594	5.616
51.875	60.481	5.580	5.603
52.000	60.627	5.567	5.589

Diopter and radius values when a $-1.00\,D$ spectacle trial lens is placed over the objective

| Drum reading | Corneal power in diopters | Radius in mm | |
		Convex	Concave
36.000	30.874	10.931	10.964
36.125	30.981	10.893	10.926
36.250	31.089	10.856	10.889
36.375	31.196	10.819	10.851
36.500	31.303	10.782	10.814
36.625	31.410	10.745	10.777
36.750	31.518	10.708	10.740
36.875	31.625	10.672	10.704
37.000	31.732	10.636	10.668
37.125	31.839	10.600	10.632
37.250	31.946	10.564	10.596
37.375	32.054	10.529	10.561
37.500	32.161	10.494	10.526
37.625	32.268	10.459	10.491
37.750	32.375	10.425	10.456
37.875	32.482	10.390	10.421
38.000	32.590	10.356	10.387
38.125	32.697	10.322	10.353
38.250	32.804	10.288	10.319
38.375	32.911	10.255	10.286
38.500	33.018	10.221	10.252
38.625	33.126	10.188	10.219
38.750	33.233	10.155	10.186
38.875	33.340	10.123	10.153

Drum reading	Corneal power in diopters	Radius in mm	
		Convex	Concave
39.000	33.447	10.090	10.121
39.125	33.554	10.058	10.088
39.250	33.662	10.026	10.056
39.375	33.769	9.994	10.024
39.500	33.876	9.963	9.993
39.625	33.983	9.931	9.961
39.750	34.090	9.900	9.930
39.875	34.198	9.869	9.899
40.000	34.305	9.838	9.868
40.125	34.412	9.807	9.837
40.250	34.519	9.777	9.806
40.375	34.626	9.747	9.776
40.500	34.734	9.717	9.746
40.625	34.841	9.687	9.716
40.750	34.948	9.657	9.686
40.875	35.055	9.628	9.656
41.000	35.162	9.598	9.627
41.125	35.270	9.569	9.598
41.250	35.377	9.540	9.569
41.375	35.484	9.511	9.540
41.500	35.591	9.483	9.511
41.625	35.698	9.454	9.483
41.750	35.806	9.426	9.454
41.875	35.913	9.398	9.426
42.000	36.020	9.370	9.398

Appendix IV
CONVERSION OF KERATOMETER READINGS TO CONVEX AND CONCAVE RADII

Keratometer power reading	Convex radius	Concave radius
36.00	9.38	9.42
36.25	9.31	9.35
36.50	9.25	9.29
36.75	9.18	9.22
37.00	9.12	9.16
37.25	9.06	9.10
37.50	9.00	9.04
37.75	8.94	8.98
38.00	8.88	8.92
38.25	8.82	8.86
38.50	8.77	8.80
38.75	8.71	8.75
39.00	8.65	8.69
39.25	8.60	8.63
39.50	8.54	8.58
39.75	8.49	8.52
40.00	8.44	8.47
40.25	8.33	8.37
40.50	8.39	8.42
40.75	8.28	8.31

Keratometer power reading	Convex radius	Concave radius
41.00	8.23	8.26
41.25	8.18	8.21
41.50	8.13	8.16
41.75	8.08	8.11
42.00	8.04	8.07
42.25	7.99	8.02
42.50	7.94	7.97
42.75	7.89	7.92
43.00	7.85	7.88
43.25	7.80	7.83
43.50	7.76	7.79
43.75	7.71	7.74
44.00	7.67	7.70
44.25	7.63	7.65
44.50	7.58	7.61
44.75	7.54	7.57
45.00	7.50	7.53
45.25	7.46	7.49
45.50	7.42	7.44
45.75	7.38	7.40
46.00	7.34	7.36
46.25	7.30	7.32
46.50	7.26	7.28
46.75	7.22	7.24
47.00	7.18	7.21
47.25	7.14	7.17
47.50	7.11	7.13
47.75	7.07	7.09
48.00	7.03	7.05
48.25	6.99	7.02
48.50	6.96	6.98
48.75	6.92	6.95
49.00	6.89	6.91
49.25	6.85	6.88
49.50	6.82	6.84
49.75	6.78	6.81
50.00	6.75	6.77
50.25	6.72	6.74
50.50	6.68	6.70
50.75	6.65	6.67
51.00	6.62	6.64
51.25	6.59	6.61
51.50	6.55	6.57

Keratometer power reading	Convex radius	Concave radius
51.75	6.52	6.54
52.00	6.49	6.51

Index

thickness measurement of, 117–118
Cornea, toric, and keratometry, 90
Corneal lens. *See also* Hydrogel lenses;
   Rigid lenses
   anterior surface, 21–23
   displaced, 135, 136
   fenestrations of, 26–27
   manufacture of, 4–5
   overall size of, 19
   peripheral curve widths, 20–21
   posterior central curve, 15–16
   posterior optical zone diameter, 20
   posterior peripheral curve radii, 16–17
   refractive power of, 24–26
   terminology for, 13
   thickness of, 23–24
   tints for, 26–27
Cosmetic lenses, 27, 123, 359–360
Cosmetics
   and hydrogel lenses, 313
   and lens handling, 297–299
Crystalline lens, 73
Cushioning agents, 275–276
Cutting tools size reduction with, 218–221
Cylindrical powers, fabrication of, 25–26

Dallos, J., 4
Danker Laboratories, 8
da Vinci, Leonardo, 1
DeCarle, John, 7
Decongestants, 275
Descartes, René, 1
Descemet's membrane, anatomy of, 64, 67
Diabetes, as contraindication to contact
   lens wear, 124
Dies, size reduction with, 223
Diopter, defined, 24
Disinfecting units, 271
Disinfection
   chemical (cold), 265, 273
   heat (thermal), 270–272, 273
DK value, 31
Double eversion, 105
Dow Corning, Inc. (USA), 8
Dreifus, M., 5

Edema, corneal
   cause of, 4
   metabolism of, 68–69
   and PMMA, 32

Edge contour
   evaluated by projection magnifier,
      188–190
   of hydrogel lens, 208–211
   measurement of, 185–190
Edge contouring
   automatic edgers for, 241–242
   cutting tool for, 239–240
   foam cylinder technique, 240–241, 242
   shaping edge with flat pad and foam
      took, 236–239
   thinning thick edge, 235–236
EDTA (ethylenediamine-tetra-acetic acid),
   257, 258, 261, 265
Education. *See* Patient education
Elderly, lens placement for, 350, 351
Electronic Digital Pachometer, 118
Emergencies
   appointments for, 340–341
   and patient education, 281–282
Emery board, size reduction with, 220
Emmetropia
   defined, 11
Endocrine disorders, as contraindication
   to contact lens wear, 124
Endothelium, 67
Enzymatic cleaners, 268–269
Eosinophils, on ocular smear, 111
Epithelium, corneal, 64–66
Equipment, maintenance of, 372–384
Equivalent oxygen percent (EOP), 31, 68
Ethylenediamine-tetra-acetic acid
   (EDTA), 257, 258, 261, 265
Examination
   external
      lid eversion, 103–105, 106
      slit-lamp biomicroscopy, 97–100
      use of stains, 100–103
   eye
      and contraindications for contact lens
         wear, 123–125
      and indications for contact lens wear,
         122–123
      photography in, 118–122
   follow-up (*see* Follow-up)
   of lids, 113–114
   tear film
      break-up time, 106–108
      ocular smears, 109–112
      Schirmer test, 108–109
   vision, 77
      case history in, 78–80, 81–82